RENAL DISEASE IN CANCER PATIENTS

RENAL DISEASE IN CANCER PATIENTS

Edited by

KEVIN W. FINKEL

UTHealth Science Center- Medical School, Houston, TX, USA
and University of Texas MD Anderson Cancer Center, Houston, TX, USA

SCOTT C. HOWARD

St. Jude Children's Research Hospital, Memphis, TN, USA

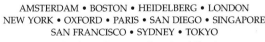
AMSTERDAM • BOSTON • HEIDELBERG • LONDON
NEW YORK • OXFORD • PARIS • SAN DIEGO • SINGAPORE
SAN FRANCISCO • SYDNEY • TOKYO
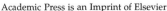
Academic Press is an Imprint of Elsevier

Academic Press is an imprint of Elsevier
32 Jamestown Road, London NW1 7BY, UK
225 Wyman Street, Waltham, MA 02451, USA
525 B Street, Suite 1800, San Diego, CA 92101-4495, USA

Medicine is an ever-changing field. Standard safety precautions must be followed, but as new research and clinical experience broaden our knowledge, changes in treatment and drug therapy may become necessary or appropriate. Readers are advised to check the most current product information provided by the manufacturer of each drug to be administered to verify the recommended dose, the method and duration of administrations, and contraindications. It is the responsibility of the treating physician, relying on experience and knowledge of the patient, to determine dosages and the best treatment for each individual patient. Neither the publisher nor the authors assume any liability for any injury and/or damage to persons or property arising from this publication.

Permissions may be sought directly from Elsevier's Science & Technology Rights Department in Oxford, UK: phone (+44) (0) 1865 843830; fax (+44) (0) 1865 853333; email: permissions@elsevier.com. Alternatively, visit the Science and Technology Books website at www.elsevierdirect.com/rights for further information

Notice

No responsibility is assumed by the publisher for any injury and/or damage to persons or property as a matter of products liability, negligence or otherwise, or from any use or operation of any methods, products, instructions or ideas contained in the material herein. Because of rapid advances in the medical sciences, in particular, independent verification of diagnoses and drug dosages should be made.

British Library Cataloguing-in-Publication Data
A catalogue record for this book is available from the British Library

Library of Congress Cataloging-in-Publication Data
A catalog record for this book is available from the Library of Congress

ISBN : 978-0-12-415948-8

For information on all Academic Press publications visit our website at www.store.elsevier.com

Typeset by TNQ Books and Journals

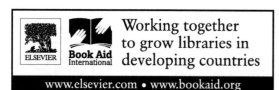

Dedication

For the many patients and colleagues who have taught us so much.

Contents

16 Cancer in Renal Transplant Patients
ALEKSANDRA M. DE GOLOVINE, HORACIO E. ADROGUE

Preface

We frequently encounter patients with renal disease and cancer, and hope this book will help clinicians optimize their management to provide them with lives that are not only long but of high quality. We welcome feedback from readers to facilitate future improvements in content, delivery, and relevance for patient care.

Foreword

Like many other disciplines in medicine, the care of patients with kidney disease has become increasingly complex and requires sub-specialization. For example, in the past general nephrologists provided care to recipients of renal transplants. However, given the rising co-morbidities of the transplant population and the increasing armamentarium of immunosuppressive medications, it is now common for centers to rely on transplant nephrologists. In a similar way a new sub-specialty has emerged related to kidney disease in patients with cancer: "Onco-Nephrology." There are several reasons for its development. First is the recognition that both acute and chronic kidney disease increases the morbidity and mortality in all patient populations including those with cancer. Since many oncology practices are associated with a comprehensive care center, nephrologists have become an integral part of the treatment team. Second, in addition to the kidney diseases seen in the general population, cancer patients develop unique disorders related to malignancy itself or its treatment. It requires nephrologists to develop a specialized knowledge related to these specific clinical problems. Third, since the prevalence of both cancer and chronic kidney disease are high, nephrologists must be familiar with an array of new chemotherapeutic agents and their potential effects on kidney function. They must also be knowledgeable about the effects of various dialytic modalities on drug clearance. Finally, as cancer patients are surviving longer with aggressive treatment protocols, there is a need for long-term management of patients who develop chronic kidney disease from their cancer treatment.

Who is the audience for this book? We believe it will serve well those who provide care to patients with cancer whether they are oncologists, nephrologists, or cancer hospitalists. Each chapter is meant to "stand alone" and allow the reader to review a specific topic related to what they encounter clinically.

The field of Onco-Nephrology is being promoted in several ways. There is an International and an American Society of Cancer Nephrology, an annual Onco-Nephrology Forum during the American Society of Nephrology's annual Kidney Week, a chapter on Renal Disease in Cancer Patients in a premier nephrology textbook [1], and a series of review articles in several journals. It is to that field *Renal Diseases in Cancer Patients* is dedicated.

Kevin W. Finkel, MD, FACP, FASN, FCCM
Scott C. Howard, MD

References

[1] Finkel K, Lahoti A, Foringer J. Renal disease in cancer patients. In Taal MW, Chertow GM, Marsden PA, Skorecki K, Yu ASL, Brenner BM, editors. Brenner & Rector's The Kidney 9th ed. Philadelphia, Pennsylvania: Elsevier Saunders; 2012. p. 1536–52.

Acknowledgement

Megan and Mara for their invaluable help and persistence to bring this book to fruition.

Contributors

Maen Abdelrahim MD, PhD Department of Internal Medicine, Baylor College of Medicine and Institute of Biosciences and Technology, Texas A&M Health Science Center, Houston, TX, USA

Ala Abudayyeh MD Assistant Professor, General Internal Medicine, Section of Nephrology, The University of Texas MD Anderson Cancer Center, Houston, TX, USA

Horacio E. Adrogue MD Associate Professor of Medicine, Division of Renal Diseases and Hypertension, Department of Internal Medicine, The University of Texas Medical School at Houston, Houston, TX, USA and Medical Director of Kidney and Pancreas Transplant at Memorial Hermann Hospital, Texas Medical Center, Houston, TX, USA

Robert J. Amato D.O. Division of Oncology, Department of Internal Medicine, UTHealth Science Center at Houston, Houston, TX, USA and University of Texas Memorial Hermann Cancer Center, Houston, TX, USA

Mark J. Amsbaugh MD The University of Texas Medical School at Houston, Houston, TX, USA

Joseph R. Angelo MD Assistant Professor, Department of Pediatrics, Division of Pediatric Nephrology and Hypertension, The University of Texas Health Science Center at Houston, Houston, TX, USA and The University of Texas MD Anderson Cancer Center, Houston, TX, USA

Putao Cen MD Division of Oncology, Department of Internal Medicine, UTHealth Science Center at Houston, Houston, TX, USA

Jeffrey Dome MD, PhD Division Chief, Oncology, Children's National Medical Center, Professor, Department of Pediatrics George Washington University School of Medicine and Health Sciences, Washington, DC, USA

Marc Earl PharmD Taussig Cancer Center, Cleveland Clinic, Cleveland, OH, USA

Kevin W. Finkel MD, FACP, FASN, FCCM Professor and Director, Division of Renal Diseases & Hypertension, UTHealth Science Center- Medical School, Houston, TX, USA and Professor of Medicine, Section of Nephrology, University of Texas MD Anderson Cancer Center, Houston, TX, USA

William H. Fissell, IV MD Departments of Nephrology and Hypertension and Biomedical Engineering, Cleveland Clinic, Cleveland, OH, USA

Ilya G. Glezerman MD Memorial Sloan-Kettering Cancer Center, New York, NY, USA and Weill-Cornell Medical College, New York, NY, USA

Aleksandra M. De Golovine MD Assistant Professor of Medicine, Division of Renal Diseases and Hypertension, Department of Internal Medicine, The University of Texas Medical School at Houston, Houston, TX, USA

Sangeeta R. Hingorani MD, MPH Associate Professor of Pediatrics, Division of Nephrology, Seattle Children's Hospital/University of Washington, and Clinical Research Division, Fred Hutchinson Cancer Research Center, Seattle, WA, USA

Scott C. Howard MD Assistant Professor, Division of Pediatric Nephrology and Hypertension. UTHealth Science Center at Houston, TX, USA and University of Texas MD Anderson Cancer Center, Houston, TX, USA

Amit Lahoti MD Associate Professor and Chief, Section of Nephrology, MD Anderson Cancer Center, Houston, TX, USA

Benjamin L. Laskin MD, MS Instructor of Pediatrics, Division of Nephrology, The Children's Hospital of Philadelphia, Philadelphia, PA, USA

Sheron Latcha MD FASN Associate Clinical Member, Memorial Sloan-Kettering Cancer Center, Assistant Professor of Clinical Medicine, Weill-Cornell Medical College, New York, NY, USA

Nwabugwu S. Ochuwa MD University of Texas Memorial Hermann Cancer Center, Houston, TX, USA

Amber S. Podoll MD Assistant Professor and Associate Program Director, Division of Renal Disease and Hypertension, Department of Internal Medicine, The University of Texas Medical School at Houston, Houston, TX, USA

Ching-Hon Pui MD Member, Department of Oncology, St. Jude Children's Research Hospital, Professor, Department of Pediatrics, University of Tennessee Health Sciences Center, College of Medicine, Memphis, TN, USA

Raul C. Ribeiro MD Member, Department of Oncology, St. Jude Children's Research Hospital, Professor, Department of Pediatrics, University of Tennessee Health Sciences Center, College of Medicine, Memphis, TN, USA

Abdulla Salahudeen MD Professor of Medicine, General Internal Medicine, Section of Nephrology, The University of Texas MD Anderson Cancer Center, Houston, TX, USA

Joshua A. Samuels MD, MPH Department of Pediatrics, Division of Pediatric Nephrology and Hypertension, The University of Texas Health Science Center at Houston and The University of Texas MD Anderson Cancer Center, Houston, TX, USA

Surya V. Seshan MD Professor of Clinical Pathology, Weill-Cornell Medical College, Chief, Division of Renal Pathology, New York-Presbyterian Medical Center, New York, NY, USA

Mika Stepankiw MS Division of Oncology, The University of Texas Health Science Center at Houston, Houston, TX, USA

Brett Stephens MD Assistant Professor, Division of Renal Diseases and Hypertension, The University of Texas Medical School at Houston, Houston, TX, USA

Kelly L. Vallance MD, MPH Department of Hematology/Oncology, Cook Children's Medical Center, Fort Worth, TX, USA

Carl Walther MD Division of Renal Diseases & Hypertension, Department of Internal Medicine, UTHealth Science Center at Houston, Houston, TX, USA and The University of Texas MD Anderson Cancer Center, Houston, TX, USA

1

Introduction

Scott C. Howard[1], Kevin W. Finkel[2]

[1]St. Jude Children's Research Hospital, Memphis, TN, USA and University of Tennessee Health Sciences Center, College of Medicine, Memphis, TN, USA
[2]UTHealth Science Center at Houston, Houston, TX, USA and University of Texas MD Anderson Cancer Center, Houston, TX, USA

Like many other disciplines in medicine, the care of patients with kidney disease has become increasingly complex and requires sub-specialization. For example, in the past, general nephrologists provided care to recipients of renal transplants. However, because of the extensive co-morbidities of patients after renal transplantation and the increasing armamentarium of immunosuppressive medications used to manage them, it is now common for transplant nephrologists to provide their care. Similarly, "onco-nephrology" has emerged as a new sub-specialty dedicated to management of kidney diseases in patients with cancer. There are several reasons for its development. First is the recognition that both acute and chronic kidney disease increase the morbidity and mortality in all patient populations including those with cancer. Since many oncology practices are associated with a comprehensive care center, nephrologists have become an integral part of the treatment team. Second,

in addition to the kidney diseases seen in the general population, cancer patients develop unique disorders related to malignancy itself or its treatment. It requires nephrologists to develop a specialized knowledge related to these specific clinical problems. Third, since the prevalence of both cancer and chronic kidney disease are high, a growing number of patients need the services of onco-nephrologists, who must be familiar with an array of new chemotherapeutic agents and their potential effects on kidney function. They must also be knowledgeable about the effects of various dialytic modalities on drug clearance. Finally, as cancer patients survive longer, there is a need for long-term management of patients who develop chronic kidney disease from their cancer treatment.

Who is the audience for this book? We believe it will serve well those who provide care to patients with cancer whether they are oncologists, nephrologists, or cancer hospitalists. Each chapter is meant to stand alone and allow the reader to review a specific topic related to what they encounter clinically, and all chapters have a clinical focus.

The field of onco-nephrology is being promoted in several ways. There is an International and an American Society of Cancer Nephrology, an annual Onco-Nephrology Forum during the American Society of Nephrology's annual Kidney Week, a chapter on renal disease in cancer patients in a premier nephrology textbook [1], and a series of review articles in several journals [2–5]. It is to this emerging field that *Renal Disease in Cancer Patients* is dedicated.

References

[1] Finkel K, Lahoti A, Foringer J. Renal disease in cancer patients. In: Taal Chertow, Marsden Skorecki, Yu Brenner, editors. Brenner & Rector's The Kidney. 9th ed. Philadelphia, Pennsylvania: Elsevier Saunders; 2012. p. 1536–52.

[2] Salahudeen AK, Bonventre JV. Onconephrology: the latest frontier in the war against kidney disease. J Am Soc Nephrol 2013;24:26–30.

[3] Bern JS, Rosner MH. Onco-nephrology: what the nephrologist needs to know about cancer and the kidney. Clin J Am Soc Nephrol 2012;7:1691.

[4] Lam LQ, Humpheys BD. Onco-nephrology: AKI in the cancer patient. Clin J Am Soc Nephrol 2012;7:1692–700.

[5] Humphreys BD. Onco-nephrology: kidney disease in the cancer patient: introduction. Semin Nephrol 2010;30:531–3.

Acute Kidney Injury in Cancer Patients

Joseph R. Angelo, Joshua A. Samuels

University of Texas Health Science Center at Houston and
University of Texas MD Anderson Cancer Center, Houston, TX, USA

INTRODUCTION

Acute kidney injury (AKI), characterized by an abrupt decrease in renal glomerular filtration rate (GFR), occurs commonly among all hospitalized patients and even more commonly in those patients admitted to the intensive care unit (ICU). The reported incidence of AKI in all hospitalized patients is approximately 5% and has been reported to be as high as 30% in ICU patients with an associated mortality approaching 60–80% in these patients [1–3]. In addition, there are data supporting increases in hospital length of stay and medical cost related to AKI [4,5]. This increase in length of stay has also been demonstrated in cancer patients in an ICU setting [2]. For all of these reasons, AKI presents a significant problem for physicians caring for patients in the hospital.

Cancer patients are a group particularly at risk for AKI secondary to exposure to chemotherapeutic agents [6] and other potential nephrotoxins [7], infection risks and sepsis, tumor lysis syndrome [8], hematopoietic stem cell transplantation [9] and direct effects from their primary malignancy [10]. In addition to having rates of morbidity and mortality at least as high as other patient populations with AKI, a decrease in renal function can have negative consequences unique to patients undergoing treatment for malignancy. A decline in renal function often requires delay in treatment or an adjustment of chemotherapy dosing and can preclude the use of certain chemotherapeutic agents which may reduce the overall effectiveness of the cancer treatment. In addition, those patients with the most severe cases of AKI will require acute dialytic therapy leading to unpredictable serum concentrations of both chemotherapeutics and antibiotics, both of which are crucial therapies for cancer patients and often have narrow therapeutic windows. Finally, those surviving the initial renal insult from AKI may later develop chronic kidney problems including proteinuria, hypertension and chronic kidney disease [11,12]. These chronic problems can adversely affect future cancer therapy, and thus lead to long-term morbidity and mortality, decreased quality of life and greatly increased health care costs. This chapter will review several aspects of AKI with focus on those issues specific to cancer patients.

DEFINING ACUTE KIDNEY INJURY

Current definitions of acute kidney injury are based on increases in serum creatinine (SCr) and decreased urine output. Prior to 2004, there was little consensus of the magnitude of changes in these parameters, and there were over 30 proposed criteria for defining AKI [13]. Since then, two systems have been developed and are widely used in clinical studies of AKI. These are the RIFLE [14] (Risk, Injury, Failure, Loss, ESRD) and Acute Kidney Injury Network [15] (AKIN) scoring systems which stratify AKI by progressively worsening levels of Cr and/or urine production. The RIFLE criteria stage severity of AKI into three distinct categories (Risk, Injury and Failure) based on incremental increases in SCr or progressive decline in urine output during a 48-hour time period from the onset of AKI. RIFLE also includes two additional categories (Loss, End-stage renal disease) describing two post-AKI clinical outcomes [16]. The more recent AKIN criteria also use changes in SCr and urine output to define three categories (I, II, III) of AKI and is similar to the first three stages of the RIFLE classification [17]. These scoring systems have proven useful for standardizing definitions of AKI across many clinical and research populations, and several studies have now shown a correlation between these scores and clinical outcomes [14], including those in cancer patients [5,18]. While these standardized AKI criteria have clear utility, one potential shortcoming in the clinical setting is inherent in the properties of SCr as a functional biomarker of AKI. There is a significant lag between kidney injury and an increase in SCr, and there is increasing evidence that SCr is notably elevated only after the development of AKI is well established. Thus, as a biomarker, SCr does not provide the earliest

possible window for intervention [19]. In addition, SCr can be affected by factors such as age, muscle mass, gender and hydration status. This issue is particularly relevant for cancer patients who often have poor nutritional status and muscle wasting. It is important to keep this in mind when using SCr as a measure of AKI in cancer, as even small changes in SCr in this population may represent significant decline in renal function [20] and have significant impact on outcomes [2]. Changes in SCr levels during the progression of AKI also present a problem as methods of estimating GFR, including 24-hour urine collection, are dependent on steady-state values of SCr. These dynamic changes in SCr make it impossible to estimate GFR while SCr is still rising and can result in overestimation of GFR, leading to inaccurate dosing of medications and the potential to hasten the progression of AKI. Recent research aimed at overcoming these shortcomings of SCr has focused on the development of AKI biomarkers that are more sensitive to the development of AKI, more specific to the underlying AKI etiology, appear earlier in the course and will mirror the dynamic changes in the onset and resolution of AKI [19]. While these biomarkers are not yet available for clinical use, the goal of their development is analogous to the utilization of troponins in the early detection and treatment of myocardial infarction. Some of these biomarkers are discussed in the following chapter.

CLASSIFICATION OF ACUTE KIDNEY INJURY

The next step in the evaluation of a patient with acute kidney injury is to determine the underlying etiology of kidney failure. The many potential causes of AKI typically fall into three broad categories: prerenal azotemia, intrinsic AKI and post-renal or obstructive AKI. Clinically, the classification of AKI into one of these categories helps narrow the differential diagnosis of AKI etiology and can allow for more targeted therapeutic intervention.

There are several easily obtainable indices which are useful in determining the type of AKI which is present. An accurate history provides data on the temporal relationship between inciting events, such as hypotension or administration of medication, and the onset of AKI. The physical exam provides clues to other signs which can be specific to systemic diseases that also involve the kidney. While urinary output changes can be present in all types of AKI, it is often readily available data which in combination with other markers can be helpful in distinguishing between AKI etiologies. Significantly decreased urine output, or oliguria, is defined as less than 400 ml/24-hour period. This can be important, since the management of non-oliguric and oligo-anuric renal failure is quite different. Important initial laboratory studies in the evaluation of AKI should include: serum electrolytes, blood urea nitrogen (BUN), serum creatinine (SCr) and complete blood count. Urine studies should include: urinalysis, urine specific gravity, urinary sediment analysis, urine electrolytes, urine creatinine, urine protein, urine osmolality and, in cases of drug-related renal toxicity, urine eosinophils can also be useful.

In addition to directly providing important pieces of data, these initial laboratory values can also be utilized to determine other useful indices for classifying AKI. These indices are fairly straightforward to calculate and thus are readily available at the bedside.

One important step in assessing AKI is distinguishing between AKI from decreased renal perfusion (pre-renal) and AKI directly related to intrinsic renal tubular dysfunction. As noted above, measurement of urine output is a useful tool but can be altered in most etiologies of AKI. Therefore, several indices have been developed to answer the question of whether a decline in kidney function has occurred due to decreased renal perfusion or if intrinsic dysfunction within the renal parenchyma itself is present. The basic concept behind these indices is the determination of whether the kidney has retained the ability to appropriately respond to decreases in renal perfusion. Under conditions of hypoperfusion the healthy kidney responds by increasing tubular reabsorption of both sodium and water through the actions of hormones such as aldosterone and antidiuretic hormone (ADH or vasopressin). One index which points to an appropriate renal response mechanism, and therefore intact tubular function, is an increase in BUN/creatinine ratio which typically is >20:1 in states of reduced renal perfusion. The fractional excretion of sodium (FENa) is a similar indicator of a decline in renal perfusion pressure and is based on the ability of the proximal and distal tubule to reabsorb sodium as renal perfusion falls. When this function is intact, sodium reabsorption by the renal tubular increases significantly, urine sodium falls to <20 mEq/L and the FENa is <1%, indicating the presence of prerenal AKI. In contrast, the FENa in acute tubular necrosis (ATN) or intrinsic forms of AKI is typically >3% [21]. Calculation of the FENa requires simultaneous measurements of the plasma sodium (PNa) and plasma creatinine (PCr), urine sodium (UNa) and urine creatinine (UCr) in mg/dL, and entering these values into the following formula:

$$\text{FENa (\%)} = (\text{UNa} \times \text{PCr})/(\text{PNa} \times \text{UCr}) \times 100$$

In certain clinical situations when urinary Na is affected by extrinsic factors, such as a patient on diuretic therapy, it may be beneficial to use the fractional excretion of urea (FEurea) [22]. The formula for this calculation is the same as that for the FENa with the substitution of plasma and urine urea for plasma and urine Na.

$$\text{FEurea (\%)} = (\text{Uurea} \times \text{PCr})/(\text{Purea} \times \text{UCr})$$
$$\times 100$$

In prerenal AKI, the FEurea is typically <35%.

Examination of the urine with urinalysis and microscopic evaluation of the urinary sediment can also provide clues to the underlying etiology of AKI. Urinalysis in prerenal azotemia is typically normal except for occasional fine granular and hyaline casts. Microscopic evaluation in intrinsic tubular injury, or acute tubular necrosis (ATN), shows epithelial cell casts and coarse granular casts. The presence of white blood cells and white blood cell casts is indicative of active inflammatory processes such as glomerulonephritis, infection, or acute tubulo-interstitial nephritis (TIN). Urine eosinophils are classically thought of as associated with TIN but can be seen in many other causes of AKI such as glomerulonephritis and cystitis. Albuminuria and red blood cell casts indicate underlying glomerular disease while the presence of proteins other than albumin in the urine can indicate damage to the renal tubule. In cases where distinguishing these types of proteinuria are important, urine protein electrophoresis (UPEP) can be performed [23–25].

Radiologic imaging of the kidney is also important in the evaluation of a patient with AKI. Of the imaging modalities available for assessing the kidney in AKI, renal ultrasound (RUS) is the most commonly used. RUS is particularly useful when obstructive AKI is suspected. Typical findings in urinary tract obstruction in cancer patients include hydronephrosis, ureteral dilatation, bladder dilation and changes in bladder wall contour. Specific to patients with retroperitoneal malignancy is the possibility of obstruction without hydronephrosis or hydroureter. Tumor can encase the ureters or kidneys, leading to obstruction without the classic radiologic signs. RUS is also an effective way to measure renal length which can provide information on such processes as kidney infiltration by leukemic cells, acute inflammatory processes within the kidney and can sometimes suggest underlying chronic kidney disease if small, atretic kidneys are noted [26].

Finally, by allowing direct visualization of renal tissue, renal biopsy can provide valuable information regarding the underlying pathogenesis of AKI. Biopsy is particularly helpful when proteinuria is present on urinalysis and urinary sediment analysis shows dysmorphic red blood cells and red blood cell casts raising suspicion for glomerulonephritis. An important consideration for renal biopsy in cancer patients is the presence of underlying bleeding diathesis related to their oncologic disease and/or cancer treatment. Therefore, biopsy should only be considered when the patient is clinically stable to tolerate the procedure and when the results of the biopsy will provide data which might guide therapy.

While all of these indices provide useful methods in the evaluation of AKI, all have limitations and should be considered as pieces of data to be applied in conjunction with the other available information. Many of the findings are not always unique to a particular etiology of AKI. In addition, laboratory values can be significantly affected by a patient's past medical history, such as underlying chronic kidney disease, evolving changes in clinical status and administration of medications. For example, in a patient receiving diuretic therapy, urinary sodium is altered, and the FENa is no longer a reliable marker of prerenal AKI versus ATN. Similarly, changes in BUN can result from pathologies other than AKI such as gastrointestinal bleeding and a catabolic state [27]. These examples highlight the importance of considering all tests and calculations in the context of the patient's recent history leading up to the onset of AKI.

The following sections focus more specifically on each of the three broad classifications of AKI and the causes related to each in cancer patients.

Prerenal Acute Kidney Injury

Prerenal AKI or prerenal azotemia is a consequence of renal hypoperfusion resulting in a subsequent reduction of GFR. The decrease in renal perfusion pressure can result from true loss of intravascular volume and systemic hypotension or can be secondary to states of decreased effective circulating volume such as congestive heart failure, liver failure and from capillary leak in sepsis. In response, the kidney employs several physiologic mechanisms in an attempt to maintain GFR in the face of a decline in glomerular perfusion pressure. The goal of these responses is to restore renal perfusion pressure through both systemic and local changes at the level of the glomerulus. The renin−angiotensin−aldosterone (RAA) axis acts on the systemic arteriolar smooth muscle to cause vasoconstriction and raise systemic blood pressure. Similarly, the RAA system exerts local effects on GFR by increasing vasomotor tone at the level of the glomerular efferent arteriole in coordination with other vasodilatory systems, such as nitric oxide and vasodilatory prostaglandins, which decreases afferent arteriolar vasomotor tone. This differential vasodilatation−vasoconstriction increases hemodynamic pressure within the glomerulus, and thus increases GFR. Additionally, the RAA results in increased renal tubular reabsorption of both sodium and water to restore systemic effective circulating volume. This process was alluded to above in discussion of the FENa, and is the reason why low urinary sodium and a FENa <1% are typically associated with prerenal AKI. Another key feedback system which aims to restore intravascular volume is the release of ADH from the posterior pituitary gland. Control of ADH secretion is highly sensitive to changes in serum osmolality and therefore is able to tightly regulate intravascular volume in states of volume depletion. After release from the posterior pituitary, ADH reaches the kidney, binds to vasopressin receptors (V2) in the distal collecting duct and stimulates trafficking of aquaporin channels to the apical surface of tubular epithelial cells resulting in the increased reabsorption of water into the vascular compartment. In addition to the ADH response, hypoperfusion also triggers the release of

norepinephrine (NE) in the sympathetic nervous system resulting in increases in cardiac output and systemic vascular resistance.

The ability of these physiologic feedback mechanisms to effectively restore and maintain renal perfusion is dependent on the severity and duration of the inciting event. Normal kidney function involves many highly energy dependent processes. Without rapid application of therapy targeted at resolution of the underlying cause of reduced effective circulating volume, decreased renal perfusion will result in significant and possibly irreversible hypoxic−ischemic renal injury with progression of prerenal AKI to frank ischemic damage and ATN. This highlights the importance of early detection of AKI and identification of the underlying cause.

Common Causes of Prerenal AKI in Cancer Patients

Volume Depletion

As noted above, true loss of intravascular volume is a common cause of prerenal AKI. Cancer patients are particularly susceptible to this problem due to gastrointestinal (GI) problems related to their underlying oncologic disease. The most common cause of volume depletion in these patients stems from poor oral intake, nausea, vomiting and diarrhea caused by chemotherapeutic agents [28]. While these issues typically occur in the period immediately following the receipt of chemotherapy, they can also persist for prolonged periods making it difficult for patients to maintain adequate fluid intake to match the increases in output from vomiting and diarrhea. Patients with either primary or metastatic intra-abdominal tumors are also at increased risk of volume depletion. Obstructive GI processes from either compression by an intra-abdominal mass or related to post-surgical adhesions can make oral intake difficult and also increase emesis in these patients. In addition, surgical diversions of the GI tract, such as ileostomies and colostomies, are sometimes necessary in these cases and can also result in less easily detectable increases in GI output. Graft-versus-host-disease (GVHD) is a problem unique to the stem cell transplant population. It attacks the GI mucosa and can cause significant difficulty for these patients in maintaining adequate fluid intake due to painful oral lesions and increased GI losses via vomiting and watery diarrhea [29]. A less common cause of volume depletion in cancer patients is the development of diabetes insipidus due to the presence of brain lesions. While these patients often have an increased thirst mechanism which pushes them to maintain large volumes of fluid intake to match increased urine output, they lack the normal physiologic activity of ADH to maintain intravascular volume, and any interruption in their ability to maintain this oral intake puts them at increased risk of developing volume depletion. Given the high risk of GI-associated losses in intravascular volume in cancer patients, treatment with anti-emetic medications and early initiation of intravenous fluids cannot be underestimated.

Loss of Effective Circulating Volume

Owing to either purposeful suppression of the immune system or as a side-effect of chemotherapy, sepsis is a common cause of morbidity and mortality in cancer patients. A major feature of sepsis is hypotension caused by inflammatory signals which lead to increased capillary permeability and intravascular fluid leak into the interstitium. This shift of fluid from the intravascular to extravascular space results in a state of total body volume overload and anasarca while significantly depleting the effective circulating volume and end organ perfusion [30]. The ongoing and persistent processes in sepsis often overwhelm the kidney's ability to auto-regulate perfusion pressure, making sepsis a common cause of AKI. In addition, the effects of sepsis are typically disseminated throughout the body resulting in a picture of multi-organ dysfunction of which the kidney is a major target.

Hepatorenal syndrome (HRS) or hepatic venoocclusive disease (VOD) is another cause of prerenal AKI in cancer patients due to decreased effective circulating volume. HRS is caused by decreased resistance in the systemic and splanchnic vasculature leading to renal hypoperfusion and compensatory increase in renal salt and water avidity reabsorption via the mechanisms described previously, such as the RAA axis, ADH and increased sympathetic tone. Clinically, HRS presents as oligo-anuric prerenal AKI with progressively worsening edema and low urinary sodium [31,32]. It is important to note that HRS is a diagnosis of exclusion. It must occur in the setting of acute or chronic liver failure, in the absence of septic shock, and other causes of prerenal, intrinsic or obstructive AKI must be ruled out.

Vascular Compression

One cause of prerenal AKI which is not directly related to loss of intravascular volume but rather physical compression of renal vasculature is intra-abdominal hypertension (IAH) or abdominal compartment syndrome (ACS). Normal intra-abdominal pressure is between 5 and 7 mmHg. IAH is defined as sustained IAP $\geq$12, while ACS is characterized by sustained IAP $\geq$20 mmHg with associated organ dysfunction [33]. Although the renal effects of ACS were first described in 1876 by Wendt, seminal work on this was done by Bradley and Bradley in the 1940s, and more recently in an important paper by Kron in 1984 [34,35]. For cancer patients, an increase in IAP generally results from intra-abdominal tumor burden or from postoperative and sepsis-associated ascites. The renal consequences of ACS are a reduction in renal blood flow and resultant ischemia, as well as increased renal venous back pressure due to direct compression of the renal veins and increased systemic venous congestion related to decreased venous return to the right heart [33]. As with the other causes of prerenal AKI, this reduction in normal blood flow through the kidney results in the clinical findings of prerenal AKI including oligo-anuria, azotemia and the characteristic laboratory findings consistent with the activation of the compensatory renal response to poor perfusion.

Intrinsic Acute Kidney Injury

Intrinsic acute kidney injury is associated with damage to the renal parenchyma itself and has multiple potential etiologies including ischemic or nephrotoxic injury, malignant or infectious infiltration of the kidney, cancer-associated glomerulonephritis or a combination of these factors. Of these etiologies, ischemic and nephrotoxic intrinsic renal injury (ATN) is the most common, accounting for 30–40% of AKI in the non-ICU setting and up to 80% in the ICU setting [1,36]. Intrinsic AKI differs from prerenal AKI in that there is specific pathologic change within the kidney and loss of renal tubular functions, including the renal protective compensatory mechanisms described above. These differences are reflected in the laboratory investigations which are used to distinguish intrinsic AKI from prerenal AKI. Since intact tubular function is required for sodium reabsorption, intrinsic AKI with tubular necrosis will typically have a lower urine specific gravity, higher urine sodium (>40 mEq/L) and higher FENa (>3%). Intrinsic AKI is similar to prerenal AKI in that it is a progressive process with distinct phases of initiation, maintenance and recovery, which means that there is a potential window for early intervention prior to averting permanent renal damage. Clinically, intrinsic AKI resembles prerenal AKI, with eventual development of decreased urine output and a fall in GFR.

Causes of Intrinsic AKI in Cancer Patients

Nephrotoxic Medications

CHEMOTHERAPEUTIC AGENTS

CISPLATIN Cisplatin is a commonly used chemotherapeutic agent which inhibits DNA synthesis by forming DNA crosslinks. Short-term renal toxicity from cisplatin appears approximately 3–5 days following administration of the drug, and typically results in non-oliguric AKI, commonly accompanied by salt-losing nephropathy and hypomagnesemia due to direct renal tubular toxicity. Other electrolyte abnormalities can include hypokalemia, hypocalcemia and depressed serum bicarbonate [37]. An important feature of cisplatin nephrotoxicity is its dose dependency. This is true for both immediate post-treatment AKI as well as longer-term effects on GFR seen with cumulative doses exceeding 120 mg/m^2. Repeated administration of doses ≤850 mg has been associated with a 9% reduction in GFR in a 5-day period while doses >850 mg were associated with a 40% reduction in GFR over the same time period [37]. Therefore, prevention of cisplatin-related renal toxicity requires keeping record of the cumulative of the course of treatment and use of the minimum dose necessary for adequate response whenever possible. In addition to dose dependence, increased risk of cisplatin nephrotoxicity has been associated with a low local chloride environment, making isotonic saline hydration a mainstay of preventive therapy during cisplatin administration [38]. Amifostine, inorganic triophosphate, administration is another therapy that should be considered for renal protection from cisplatin toxicity particularly in patients who are required to have repeated exposures [39].

ALKYLATING AGENTS

Ifosfamide and cyclophosphamide are two common alkylating agents which are classically associated with hemorrhagic cystitis. In addition, chloractealdehyde, an ifosfamide metabolite, has a well-documented association with renal tubular damage, particularly the proximal renal tubule. The outcome of this effect on the proximal tubule is the development of Fanconi syndrome with significant renal wasting of potassium, phosphorous, magnesium and bicarbonate [40]. The urinalysis in ifosfamide tubular toxicity classically shows glucosuria and tubular proteinuria, detected by the presence of urinary beta-2-microglobulin [41]. While recovery of proximal tubular dysfunction can be expected following discontinuation of ifosfamide therapy, this problem can sometimes become more chronic resulting in a clinical picture of hypophosphatemic rickets and osteomalacia [42,43]. In addition to aggressive replacement of electrolyte losses, supplementation with ergocalciferol may also help alleviate these sequelae of long-standing Fanconi syndrome.

METHOTREXATE (MTX) Methotrexate is an antimetabolite drug that irreversibly binds to dihydrofolate reductase, inhibiting the formation of reduced folates resulting in inhibition of purine synthesis. It is commonly used in the treatment of certain malignancies and often is given at high doses in combination with other chemotherapeutic agents (high-dose MTX is $>1\,g/m^2$), increasing the risk of AKI [44]. MTX induces AKI through the precipitation of both MTX itself and its metabolite, 7-hydroxymethotrexate, in the tubular lumen resulting in direct tubular toxicity as well as intrarenal tubular obstruction [45–47]. Given this, maintenance of high urinary flow rates (often >100 ml/hr) by giving isotonic saline prior to and during MTX administration is a critical component of renal protection. As low urine pH (<5.5) increases the likelihood of precipitation of these compounds, urinary alkalinization with saline plus bicarbonate can also provide renal protection. Recovery of folate stores using folinic acid (leucovorin) has also been shown to reduce MTX-related toxicity [48]. Maintaining adequate MTX clearance not only provides reno-protective effects but also can reduce the systemic toxicities of MTX, such as neutropenia, mucocytis and neurologic toxicity. Finally, there should be close monitoring of MTX levels to track drug clearance and guide subsequent dosing. In some cancer populations, implementation of all of these measures has been shown to reduce the incidence of MTX-related AKI to as low as 2% [47].

ANTIBIOTICS

VANCOMYCIN Vancomycin is a common frontline antibiotic for the empiric treatment of cancer patients presenting with fever and neutropenia. Such patients are at high risk for bacteremia and rapid progression to full-blown sepsis. While the reported incidence of vancomycin nephrotoxicity is typically ~5%, its concomitant use with other potential nephrotoxins can increase this rate to as high as 35% [49]. The mechanism of vancomycin-related nephrotoxicity is not known; however, recent animal data suggest an association with oxidative stress [50]. The key to prevention of vancomycin nephrotoxicity is both dose adjustment based on a patient's current level of GFR and close pharmacokinetic monitoring through trough levels of the drug.

AMPHOTERICIN B Along with their increased risk of bacterial infection, cancer patients also have increased risk of fungal infections, making the use of amphotericin B common in the oncology setting [51]. Incidence rates of nephrotoxicity as high as 80% have been reported in patients following treatment with amphotericin B [52]. Increased risk of amphotericin nephrotoxicity is associated with higher total accumulated dose, duration of therapy, dehydration, underlying renal dysfunction and concurrent use with other nephrotoxins [53]. Amphotericin-associated nephrotoxicity results from components of both ischemic prerenal AKI as well as direct injury [54–58] (94, 95). As expected with disruption in tubular structure and function, this results in electrolyte losses, metabolic acidosis and can also cause nephrogenic diabetes insipidus [59]. Reduction in the risk of amphotericin nephrotoxicity can be achieved through the maintenance of adequate hydration and also with the preferential use of liposomal forms of the drug which are now available [60]. Though somewhat protected, patients receiving the liposomal form of amphotericin are still at risk for acute kidney injury and should also be closely monitored [61].

ANTIVIRALS

Antiviral medications, such as acyclovir, cidofovir and foscarnet, are another class of drugs used frequently in cancer patients. They, too, have been associated with drug-induced nephrotoxicity [62]. AKI related to antiviral drugs has been shown to occur in 10–15% of overall treated patients [63]. However, exposure to foscarnet can cause changes in GFR in as many as 20–60% of patients [54–56,63]. Suggested mechanisms of renal toxicity from foscarnet, as well as other antivirals, include direct tubular toxicity and glomerular toxicity related to crystallization within glomerular capillaries [63]. Isotonic hydration prior to drug administration might reduce this risk.

While the medications described above represent only a small sample of the potential nephrotoxic drugs to which cancer patients are exposed, they demonstrate several important general principles regarding the risk and prevention of AKI when their use is necessary. Recognition of the initial renal function and appropriate dosing is critical to minimize toxicity, as is following renal function during therapy. Additionally, in nearly all cases of drug exposure, the maintenance of adequate hydration and high urinary flow prior to and during treatment is an important component of reducing drug-related AKI. Moreover, the risk of toxicity is significantly increased when potential nephrotoxins are used concurrently with other high-risk drugs. Similarly, the risk of toxicity is increased in those patients with underlying chronic morbidities, particularly chronic kidney disease. Finally, diligent monitoring of drug levels, during both the immediate post-exposure period as well as with cumulative dosing, is critically important to minimize exposure. In addition, changes in drug metabolism and clearance due to reductions in GFR must be considered in order to make appropriate dose adjustments. These changes are dynamic and therefore regular measures of renal function are required to avoid drug accumulation related to poor clearance. In addition to being a significant co-morbidity for cancer patients with other complex medical problems, nephrotoxic AKI often requires changes in drug dose and/or discontinuation of the medication, ultimately diminishing optimal delivery of the most effective treatment regimen.

Contrast-induced Nephropathy (CIN)

Contrast-induced AKI, or CIN, is typically defined as either a 0.5 mg/dL or a 25% rise in SCr within 48 hours following exposure to iodinated radiocontrast [64]. The condition occurs in 5–15% of contrast-exposed patients [65], though the risk is higher in some well-defined populations. Specifically, the risk of CIN is increased in those patients with pre-exposure eGFR <60 ml/min/1.73 m^2, diabetic patients, when used in conjunction with other nephrotoxic drugs, and in the setting of volume depletion. While even small volumes of contrast can result in CIN, risk is increased when higher volumes (>100 ml) are used and with repeated exposures [66,67]. Both of these risks are common in cancer patients, who often undergo multiple sequential imaging studies as part of an initial evaluation or re-staging workup. As renal vasoconstriction is the initiating AKI insult, concomitant use of other vasoconstrictive medications, NSAIDs, ACE-inhibitors and calcineurin inhibitors can be particularly problematic. Additional renal toxicity comes from stasis of contrast material within the renal tubule and direct tubular injury. With these two pathophysiologic mechanisms in mind, volume expansion has become a mainstay in prevention of CIN. There is some evidence that 0.9% normal saline is more efficacious than one containing 0.45% sodium chloride in preventing CIN [68]. Data on the use of bicarbonate containing solutions are variable, and thus require further investigation [69]. Regarding pharmacologic prophylaxis for the prevention of CIN, probably the most studied is N-acetylcysteine (NAC). To date there is no strong evidence supporting a definitive reduction in CIN risk with NAC [70–73]. However, use of NAC may have some efficacy and given that the risk of negative side-effects from NAC is fairly low, its use should be considered as an adjunct to volume expansion. Similar to NAC, there is currently no strong data to support the use of post-contrast dialysis in prevention of CIN. However, one study did show some benefit in a group of very high-risk subjects with severe chronic kidney disease (CKD) [74]. As with nephrotoxic medications, the prevention of CIN requires a multidisciplinary approach which weighs the risk of exposure against the importance of the data that will be provided, and the utilization of measures shown to be effective in reducing risk of CIN.

Other Causes of Intrinsic AKI

There are several other causes for intrinsic AKI which are common in cancer patients. These are discussed in detail in subsequent chapters, and therefore will only be listed briefly here. Tumor lysis syndrome (TLS) occurs in those patients with high tumor burden and can arise from high tumor growth rate, but is more commonly seen with tumor cell death following the induction phase of chemotherapy. It is characterized by hyperphosphatemia, hypocalcemia, hyperuricemia, hyperkalemia and hyperurecemia. The main mechanism of AKI in TLS is tubular obstruction due to intratubular precipitation of compounds such as uric acid. Chemotherapy-associated immunosuppression increases cancer patients' risk of many renal infections including bacterial pyelonephritis, invasive fungal infections and viral infections such as BK and adenovirus. Finally, kidney infiltration by leukemia and lymphoma cells can cause AKI through both parenchymal damage and an obstructive component.

Obstructive AKI

Cancer-related obstruction of the urinary tract (UTO) can occur at all levels from the renal pelvis to bladder outlet, can be either unilateral or bilateral and either complete or partial. In cancer patients, it is most commonly caused by large local tumor burden from gynecologic or other pelvic lesions. The symptoms of urinary tract obstruction vary based on the site of obstruction. By definition, complete obstruction will lead to anuria but this most extreme case occurs rarely and thus the obstruction can go unnoticed until it progresses and other symptoms appear. These symptoms can include pain, abdominal distension and hematuria. Tumors in close approximation to the bladder can result in voiding dysfunction, such as enuresis, urgency, hesitancy or dysuria. Other common clinical signs include hypertension, urinary tract infection and electrolyte disturbances related both to the onset of AKI and also secondary to direct renal tubular damage caused by the obstruction. Renal injury in obstructive AKI is caused by increasing back pressure from the point of obstruction to the tubular lumen [75,76]. Initially, this back pressure may cause an increase in renal blood flow (RBF) through the release of vasoactive substances, such as angiotensin and vasopressin. This increase in RBF works to temporarily maintain GFR. However, the increased RBF also further contributes to the increased tubular pressure and fairly quickly after obstruction GFR begins to fall. With persistence of pressure within the tubular lumen, irreversible tubular damage, atrophy and fibrosis will occur and with this permanent loss of renal function. This progressive nature of obstructive kidney injury underscores the importance of early diagnosis and intervention of urinary tract obstruction.

Definitive diagnosis of obstruction of the urinary tract is achieved through radiologic imaging. Ultrasound is non-invasive and can be obtained quickly and therefore is an excellent first-line tool. Typical ultrasonographic findings in urinary tract obstruction would include hydronephrosis and hydroureter. Computed tomography and magnetic resonance imaging are two other imaging techniques which can be particularly useful in assessing the cause, site and extent of the obstruction. This information can be of significant benefit in deciding on the most effective treatment plan to relieve the obstruction [77,78]. It is worth noting that not every obstructing lesion will lead to hydronephrosis and/or hydroureter. Tumors encasing the kidney or ureters will preclude the typical hydronephrosis. In these instances nuclear studies such as a MAG-3 renal scan or direct evaluation by either anterograde or retrograde cystoureteroscopy might be indicated.

While surgical removal of the obstructing mass would be the most definitive treatment, this is not always possible; therefore, other means of decompressing the urinary tract must be used. The placement of nephrostomy or ureterostomy tubes can achieve this by diverting and restoring urinary flow. For cancer patients, the insertion of these devices can protect the kidney from chronic damage while specific treatment aimed at decreasing tumor burden is administered. Less invasive than percutaneously placed nephrostomy tubes, the placement of internal ureteral stents can also be used to maintain urinary tract patency. When the malignant lesion is in the bladder or prostate, internal stenting might not be possible.

An important nephrologic consideration following decompression of the obstructed urinary tract is post-obstructive diuresis. Following relief of the obstruction the renal tubules may remain insensitive to ADH and thus be unable to adequately concentrate the urine. This will result, at least temporarily, in a clinical picture of nephrogenic diabetes insipidus. High urinary flow and the persistence of renal tubular dysfunction in this situation also can result in loss of electrolytes including sodium, potassium, phosphorous and bicarbonate [79]. Particularly important for cancer patients who, as previously discussed, have an increased susceptibility to volume depletion, is the diligent monitoring of urine output and appropriate replacement of that volume to maintain euvolemia.

Acute Kidney Injury Prevention and Treatment

Though many agents have shown both *in vitro* promise and success in animal studies, there is currently no specific therapy which has been clinically proven to effectively treat AKI in humans. Therefore, existing interventions are directed at the prevention of AKI and providing support after the onset of AKI. When these are unsuccessful, the AKI patient will require some form of renal replacement therapy.

Fluid Volume Management

As noted above, the mainstay of preventing many of the most common causes of AKI in cancer patients is the maintenance of renal perfusion through adequate hydration and possibly vasoactive medications [80]. This is particularly true for cases of prerenal AKI and with the administration of nephrotoxic drugs, but also for keeping patients euvolemic during post-obstructive diuresis. However, despite its presumed importance for the prevention of AKI, the proper administration of this therapy has many potential difficulties.

Assessing fluid status is clearly a key to guiding accurate administration of fluid therapy. This is particularly true for cancer patients who may be prone to fluid extravasation into extravascular spaces due to their high risk of systemic inflammatory processes, such as sepsis. There is evidence that fluid overload in itself is a predictor of mortality in critically ill patients. Two studies, one by Murphy et al. in 2009 and another by Boyd et al. in 2011, suggest an association between cumulative fluid balance volume and mortality in critically ill patients [81,82]. Stem cell transplant recipients are a population that may be particularly sensitive to these kinds of fluid issues [83]. In addition, fluid balance is a dynamic state making it even more difficult to accurately monitor with static measures, which currently are employed. As discussed previously, clinical markers in the history, physical exam, lab values and several formulas are commonly used to assess fluid status. Some methods of more dynamic monitoring, such as central venous pressure and cardiac output monitoring devices, are available but often require more invasive techniques and have limitations of their own [84,85]. In addition to usefulness in direct patient care, the development of more accurate and dynamic measures of fluid balance is important in establishing more definitive clinical outcomes which can be used for research assessing the best fluid management strategies.

Other Therapies

Low-dose dopamine is a treatment for AKI that has been used and studied for many years. Despite this, no clear evidence exists for its effectiveness in the treatment of AKI. At low infusion rates $(1-3\,\mu g/kg/min)$, dopamine causes renal vasodilatation, increased GFR and also acts as a proximal tubular diuretic. Studies of dopamine's use in the setting of AKI are quite homogeneous in terms of design, size and clinical outputs; therefore limiting their utility in assessing dopamine as a therapy for AKI [86]. In addition, dopamine is not without significant side-effects, such as cardiac arrhythmias and decreased intestinal blood flow [87]. This coupled with the limited data of dopamine's effectiveness preclude its use as a specific treatment for AKI.

Fenoldopam is a pure dopamine agonist with similar effects on the renal vasculature but without extensive α- and β-adrenergic effects. While some early evidence suggests that fenoldopam can reduce AKI risk in specific populations, no solid evidence from randomized-control studies support this, and thus fenoldopam is not currently a recommended therapy for the treatment of AKI [88].

As with dopamine and fenoldopam, data on the use of diuretics for treatment of AKI are unavailable and/or have not shown the drugs to be effective. In fact, a PICARD group study from 2002 showed an association between diuretic use and increased risk of death and non-recovery of renal function in critically ill patients [89]. Though the prognosis of oliguric AKI is worse than in non-oliguric forms, no benefit has been demonstrated in converting oliguric to non-oliguric AKI through the use of diuretics. The use of diuretics also has the potential to further complicate the fluid management issues just discussed. Therefore, in the absence of more compelling evidence diuretic use should be limited to specific clinical situations.

The lack of data supporting the use of most currently available treatments demonstrates the need for the development of novel interventions for the treatment of AKI. Ideally, these interventions will become coupled with earlier diagnosis of AKI through newly emerging biomarkers and will more specifically target the mechanisms involved in the pathogenesis of AKI. A more detailed discussion of these potential therapies is beyond the scope of this chapter.

When AKI cannot be prevented, and as there is not a universally successful treatment for AKI, dialysis is currently used as supportive therapy for the medically unresponsive fluid and metabolic problems associated with AKI. There are several modes of dialysis available. In intermittent hemodialysis (IHD) a patient receives treatment during a prescribed period of hours and then is off therapy for the remainder of that day. The finite period of time the patient is on dialysis in IHD requires that solute and fluid removal occur fairly rapidly. In some instances this does not notably affect hemodynamics and may even be desirable. However, for those patients with hemodynamic instability or with large volumes of fluid overload, fluid and solute removal at a slower rate using a continuous renal replacement therapy (CRRT) is more appropriate. In CRRT, the patient remains on dialysis continuously for 24 hours a day. Regulation of fluid removal is much slower and can be adjusted as needed throughout the treatment based on changes such as hypotension and changes in fluid input or output. This can be particularly helpful for critically ill patients who are more likely to be hypotensive and also have more dynamic changes in both clinical status and required interventions. Although no direct comparisons of IHD and CRRT have shown CRRT to be superior in terms of better clinical outcomes, the advantages described above often make it the treatment of choice in the critically ill [90–93]. A third, hybrid option is slow low efficiency dialysis, or SLED. In this modality, blood and dialysate are circulated more slowly than in IHD, but treatments extend beyond the few hours allotted for IHD [94]. In the extreme, some programs utilize continuous-SLED in a manner similar to CRRT.

One important issue for patients on dialysis is drug dosing. In addition to the clearance of unwanted solutes and fluid, dialysis can also remove medications including the potential to remove continuously infusing drugs such as vasopressors. In addition, the pharmacokinetics of drug clearance on dialysis can be quite variable and has not been worked out for many drugs.

This requires vigilant monitoring of drug levels when they are available and adjustment of dosing based on clinical response [95–97].

Outcomes following AKI in Cancer Patients

Prior to the use of dialysis, mortality from AKI was nearly universal. With the ability to dialyze patients starting in the 1950s, mortality is reported to have dropped to around 50% [98,99]. However, since that time there has been little to no significant reduction in mortality related to AKI. While there is much variability in the reported mortality rates for patients with AKI, a 2005 systemic review by Ympa et al. estimated that mortality rates in patients with AKI have remained near 50% [100]. Other findings support the impact of AKI on patient survival. In a study of 183 patients receiving radiocontrast, those developing AKI had a mortality of 34% compared to 7% for those without AKI [101]. Importantly, there are recent data supporting the idea that even small increases in SCr of between 0.3 and 0.5 mg/dL can increase mortality risk significantly [2,4,20,101,102]. For patients admitted to the ICU and particularly for those requiring renal replacement therapy (RRT), these mortality numbers can approach 70% [103]. For cancer patients with AKI, similarly high mortality rates have been seen. Classifying subjects into three categories (R, I, F) of AKI using the RIFLE criteria, a recently published study of AKI in critically ill patients with cancer showed adjusted odds ratio for 60-day mortality of 2.3, 3.0 and 14.0 for each of the respective categories [5].

TABLE 2.1 Urinary Indices in Acute Kidney Injury

AKI classification	Urine volume	BUN/Cr ratio	Urine specific gravity	FENa	FEurea
Prerenal AKI	≤0.5 ml/kg/hr	>20	>1.020	<1%	<35%
Intrinsic AKI	Variable	Variable	1.010–1.020	>3%	>35%
Obstructive AKI	Variable; high post-obstruction	Variable	Variable	Variable	Variable

TABLE 2.2   Common Causes of AKI in Cancer Patients

PRERENAL

Volume depletion

    Diarrhea

    Emesis

    Poor PO intake

Sepsis

Ascites

Hepatorenal syndrome

Cardiac failure

Abdominal compartment syndrome

Drugs

    ACE inhibitors

    NSAIDs

    Calcineurin inhibitors

INTRINSIC AKI

ATN

    Ischemia/progressive prerenal AKI

    Exogenous nephrotoxins

        Acyclovir

        Aminoglycosides

        Amphotericin B

        Cisplatin

        Cyclosporine

        Foscarnet

        Ifosfamide

        Pentamidine

        Radiocontrast

    Intrinsic nephrotoxins

        Myoglobinuria

        Hemoglobinuria

        Hyperuricosuria

Pyelonephritis

TABLE 2.2   Common Causes of AKI in Cancer Patients—(cont'd)

Viral infection

Cancer infiltration

Tumor lysis syndrome

Glomerulonephritis

    Thrombotic microangiopathy

    Amyloidosis

    Membranous GN

OBSTRUCTIVE AKI

Tumor

Surgical adhesions

Hemorrhagic cystitis

Nephrolithiasis

One cohort analysis followed 975 patients admitted to a cancer ICU. Roughly one-third of the patients developed AKI, of whom one-third required renal replacement therapy. Survival among those on dialysis was poor, with only 27% 6-month survival. Among survivors, renal recovery was good, with only 6% on chronic dialysis [104]. However, as with their high risk of developing kidney dysfunction in the acute setting, multiple factors related to their primary oncologic diagnosis can also make cancer patients particularly susceptible to long-term effects of AKI. The development of CKD following AKI may become a more significant clinical problem as cancer patients get older and sicker. Chronic kidney disease, and especially the need for regular dialysis, has significant effects on quality of life which is an important issue to consider and discuss with patients and their families prior to offering acute dialysis therapy.

CONCLUSION

Due to the nature of their underlying disease and the drug regimens that are required for treatment of malignancy, cancer patients have a high risk of AKI. Abrupt changes in kidney function necessitate many changes in treatment plans and also increase the cancer patient's overall morbidity and mortality both in the short and long term. This emphasizes the importance of early detection, differentiation of the etiology and intervention directed at alleviating the cause of AKI while providing supportive therapy for the physiologic disruptions associated with AKI. The high incidence and complexity of renal issues that occur related to malignancy gives nephrologists an essential role in the multidisciplinary care of cancer patients.

References

[1] Liano F, Junco E, Pascual J, Madero R, Verde E. The spectrum of acute renal failure in the intensive care unit compared with that seen in other settings. The Madrid Acute Renal Failure Study Group. Kidney Int Suppl 1998;66:S16−24.

[2] Samuels J, Ng CS, Nates J, Price K, Finkel K, Salahudeen A, et al. Small increases in serum creatinine are associated with prolonged ICU stay and increased hospital mortality in critically ill patients with cancer. Support Care Cancer 2011;19(10):1527−32.

[3] Uchino S, Kellum JA, Bellomo R, Doig GS, Morimatsu H, Morgera S, et al. Acute renal failure in critically ill patients: a multinational, multicenter study. JAMA 2005;294(7):813−8.

[4] Chertow GM, Burdick E, Honour M, Bonventre JV, Bates DW. Acute kidney injury, mortality, length of stay, and costs in hospitalized patients. J Am Soc Nephrol 2005;16(11):3365−70.

[5] Lahoti A, Nates JL, Wakefield CD, Price KJ, Salahudeen AK. Costs and outcomes of acute kidney injury in critically ill patients with cancer. J Support Oncol 2011;9(4):149−55.

[6] Lameire N, Kruse V, Rottey S. Nephrotoxicity of anticancer drugs − an underestimated problem? Acta Clin Belg 2011;66(5):337−45.

[7] Naughton CA. Drug-induced nephrotoxicity. Am Fam Physician 2008;78(6):743−50.

[8] Howard SC, Jones DP, Pui CH. The tumor lysis syndrome. N Engl J Med 2011;364(19):1844−54.

[9] Kogon A, Hingorani S. Acute kidney injury in hematopoietic cell transplantation. Semin Nephrol 2010;30(6):615−26.

[10] Benoit DD, Hoste EA, Depuydt PO, Offner FC, Lameire NH, Vandewoude KH, et al. Outcome in critically ill medical patients treated with renal replacement therapy for acute renal failure: comparison between patients with and those without haematological malignancies. Nephrol Dial Transplant 2005;20(3):552−8.

[11] Hingorani S. Chronic kidney disease in long-term survivors of hematopoietic cell transplantation: epidemiology, pathogenesis, and treatment. J Am Soc Nephrol 2006;17(7):1995−2005.

[12] Hingorani S, Guthrie KA, Schoch G, Weiss NS, McDonald GB. Chronic kidney disease in long-term survivors of hematopoietic cell transplant. Bone Marrow Transplant 2007;39(4):223−9.

[13] Kellum JA, Levin N, Bouman C, Lameire N. Developing a consensus classification system for acute renal failure. Curr Opin Crit Care 2002;8(6):509−14.

[14] Hoste EA, Clermont G, Kersten A, Venkataraman R, Angus DC, De Bacquer D, et al. RIFLE criteria for acute kidney injury are associated with hospital mortality in critically ill patients: a cohort analysis. Crit Care 2006;10(3):R73.

[15] Ronco C, Levin A, Warnock DG, Mehta R, Kellum JA, Shah S, et al. Improving outcomes from acute kidney injury (AKI): report on an initiative. J Artif Organs 2007;30(5):373−6.

[16] Bellomo R, Ronco C, Kellum JA, Mehta RL, Palevsky P. Acute Dialysis Quality Initiative workgroup. Acute renal failure − definition, outcome measures, animal models, fluid therapy and information technology needs: the Second International Consensus Conference of the Acute Dialysis Quality Initiative (ADQI) Group. Crit Care 2004;8(4):R204−12.

[17] Mehta RL, Kellum JA, Shah SV, Molitoris BA, Ronco C, Warnock DG, et al. Acute Kidney Injury Network: report of an initiative to improve outcomes in acute kidney injury. Crit Care 2007;11(2):R31.

[18] Lopes JA, Jorge S, Silva S, de Almeida E, Abreu F, Martins C, et al. Prognostic utility of the acute kidney injury network (AKIN) criteria for acute kidney injury in myeloablative haematopoietic cell transplantation. Bone Marrow Transplant 2007;40(10):1005−6.

[19] Devarajan P. Emerging biomarkers of acute kidney injury. Contrib Nephrol 2007;156:203−12.

[20] Lassnigg A, Schmidlin D, Mouhieddine M, Bachmann LM, Druml W, Bauer P, et al. Minimal changes of serum creatinine predict prognosis in patients after cardiothoracic surgery: a prospective cohort study. J Am Soc Nephrol 2004;15(6):1597−605.

[21] Varghese SA, Powell TB, Janech MG, Budisavljevic MN, Stanislaus RC, Almeida JS, et al.

Identification of diagnostic urinary biomarkers for acute kidney injury. J Investig Med 2010;58(4):612–20.

[22] Gotfried J, Wiesen J, Raina R, Nally Jr JV. Finding the cause of acute kidney injury: which index of fractional excretion is better? Cleve Clin J Med 2012;79(2):121–6.

[23] Miller TR, Anderson RJ, Linas SL, Henrich WL, Berns AS, Gabow PA, et al. Urinary diagnostic indices in acute renal failure: a prospective study. Ann Intern Med 1978;89(1):47–50.

[24] Singri N, Ahya SN, Levin ML. Acute renal failure. JAMA 2003;289(6):747–51.

[25] Esson ML, Schrier RW. Diagnosis and treatment of acute tubular necrosis. Ann Intern Med 2002;137(9):744–52.

[26] Barozzi L, Valentino M, Santoro A, Mancini E, Pavlica P. Renal ultrasonography in critically ill patients. Crit Care Med 2007;35(Suppl. 5):S198–205.

[27] Bonventre JV. Diagnosis of acute kidney injury: from classic parameters to new biomarkers. Contrib Nephrol 2007;156:213–9.

[28] Berk L, Rana S. Hypovolemia and dehydration in the oncology patient. J Support Oncol 2006;4(9):447–54. discussion 55–7.

[29] Pidala J. Graft-vs-host disease following allogeneic hematopoietic cell transplantation. Cancer Control 2011;18(4):268–76.

[30] Wan L, Bagshaw SM, Langenberg C, Saotome T, May C, Bellomo R. Pathophysiology of septic acute kidney injury: what do we really know? Crit Care Med 2008;36(Suppl. 4):S198–203.

[31] Angeli P, Morando F, Cavallin M, Piano S. Hepatorenal syndrome. Contrib Nephrol 2011;174:46–55.

[32] Kramer L, Horl WH. Hepatorenal syndrome. Semin Nephrol 2002;22(4):290–301.

[33] De Waele JJ, De Laet I, Kirkpatrick AW, Hoste E. Intra-abdominal hypertension and abdominal compartment syndrome. Am J Kidney Dis 2011;57(1):159–69.

[34] Kron IL, Harman PK, Nolan SP. The measurement of intra-abdominal pressure as a criterion for abdominal re-exploration. Ann Surg 1984;199(1):28–30.

[35] Bradley SE, Bradley GP. The effect of increased intra-abdominal pressure on renal function in man. J Clin Invest 1947;26(5):1010–22.

[36] Lameire N, Van Biesen W, Vanholder R. Acute renal failure. Lancet 2005;365(9457):417–30.

[37] Arany I, Safirstein RL. Cisplatin nephrotoxicity. Semin Nephrol 2003;23(5):460–4.

[38] Ries F, Klastersky J. Nephrotoxicity induced by cancer chemotherapy with special emphasis on cisplatin toxicity. Am J Kidney Dis 1986;8(5):368–79.

[39] Schuchter LM, Hensley ML, Meropol NJ, Winer EP. 2002 update of recommendations for the use of chemotherapy and radiotherapy protectants: clinical practice guidelines of the American Society of Clinical Oncology. J Clin Oncol 2002;20(12):2895–903.

[40] Suarez A, McDowell H, Niaudet P, Comoy E, Flamant F. Long-term follow-up of ifosfamide renal toxicity in children treated for malignant mesenchymal tumors: an International Society of Pediatric Oncology report. J Clin Oncol 1991;9(12):2177–82.

[41] Lee BS, Lee JH, Kang HG, Hahn H, Shin HY, Ha IS, et al. Ifosfamide nephrotoxicity in pediatric cancer patients. Pediatr Nephrol 2001;16(10):796–9.

[42] Church DN, Hassan AB, Harper SJ, Wakeley CJ, Price CG. Osteomalacia as a late metabolic complication of ifosfamide chemotherapy in young adults: illustrative cases and review of the literature. Sarcoma 2007;2007:91586.

[43] Fujieda M, Matsunaga A, Hayashi A, Tauchi H, Chayama K, Sekine T. Children's toxicology from bench to bed – drug-induced renal injury (2): nephrotoxicity induced by cisplatin and ifosfamide in children. J Toxicol Sci 2009;34(Suppl. 2):SP251–7.

[44] Abelson HT, Fosburg MT, Beardsley GP, Goorin AM, Gorka C, Link M, et al. Methotrexate-induced renal impairment: clinical studies and rescue from systemic toxicity with high-dose leucovorin and thymidine. J Clin Oncol 1983;1(3):208–16.

[45] Smeland E, Fuskevag OM, Nymann K, Svendesn JS, Olsen R, Lindal S, et al. High-dose 7-hydromethotrexate: acute toxicity and lethality in a rat model. Cancer Chemother Pharmacol 1996;37(5):415–22.

[46] Widemann BC, Adamson PC. Understanding and managing methotrexate nephrotoxicity. Oncologist 2006;11(6):694–703.

[47] Widemann BC, Balis FM, Kempf-Bielack B, Bielack S, Pratt CB, Ferrari S, et al. High-dose methotrexate-induced nephrotoxicity in patients with osteosarcoma. Cancer 2004;100(10):2222–32.

[48] Bender JF, Grove WR, Fortner CL. High-dose methotrexate with folinic acid rescue. Am J Hosp Pharm 1977;34(9):961–5.

[49] Downs NJ, Neihart RE, Dolezal JM, Hodges GR. Mild nephrotoxicity associated with vancomycin use. Arch Intern Med 1989;149(8):1777–81.

[50] Nishino Y, Takemura S, Minamiyama Y, Hirohashi K, Ogino T, Inoue M, et al. Targeting superoxide dismutase to renal proximal tubule cells attenuates vancomycin-induced nephrotoxicity in rats. Free Radic Res 2003;37(4):373–9.

[51] Kullberg BJ, Oude Lashof AM. Epidemiology of opportunistic invasive mycoses. Eur J Med Res 2002;7(5):183–91.

[52] Deray G. Amphotericin B nephrotoxicity. J Antimicrob Chemother 2002;49(Suppl. 1):37–41.

[53] Fisher MA, Talbot GH, Maislin G, McKeon BP, Tynan KP, Strom BL. Risk factors for Amphotericin B-associated nephrotoxicity. Am J Med 1989;87(5): 547–52.

[54] Cacoub P, Deray G, Baumelou A, Le Hoang P, Rozenbaum W, Gentilini M, et al. Acute renal failure induced by foscarnet: 4 cases. Clin Nephrol 1988; 29(6):315–8.

[55] Chatelain E, Deminiere C, Lacut JY, Potaux L. Severe renal failure and polyneuritis induced by foscarnet. Nephrol Dial Transplant 1998;13(9):2368–9.

[56] Deray G, Martinez F, Katlama C, Levaltier B, Beaufils H, Danis M, et al. Foscarnet nephrotoxicity: mechanism, incidence and prevention. Am J Nephrol 1989;9(4):316–21.

[57] Sawaya BP, Briggs JP, Schnermann J. Amphotericin B nephrotoxicity: the adverse consequences of altered membrane properties. J Am Soc Nephrol 1995;6(2): 154–64.

[58] Sawaya BP, Weihprecht H, Campbell WR, Lorenz JN, Webb RC, Briggs JP, et al. Direct vasoconstriction as a possible cause for amphotericin B-induced nephrotoxicity in rats. J Clin Invest 1991;87(6):2097–107.

[59] Fanos V, Cataldi L. Amphotericin B-induced nephrotoxicity: a review. J Chemother 2000;12(6):463–70.

[60] Saliba F, Dupont B. Renal impairment and amphotericin B formulations in patients with invasive fungal infections. Med Mycol 2008;46(2):97–112.

[61] Safdar A, Ma J, Saliba F, Dupont B, Wingard JR, Hachem RY, et al. Drug-induced nephrotoxicity caused by amphotericin B lipid complex and liposomal amphotericin B: a review and meta-analysis. Medicine 2010;89(4):236–44.

[62] Becker BN, Schulman G. Nephrotoxicity of antiviral therapies. Curr Opin Nephrol Hypertens 1996;5(4): 375–9.

[63] Patzer L. Nephrotoxicity as a cause of acute kidney injury in children. Pediatr Nephrol 2008;23(12): 2159–73.

[64] Palevsky PM. Defining contrast-induced nephropathy. Clin J Am Soc Nephrol 2009;4(7):1151–3.

[65] McCullough PA, Soman SS. Contrast-induced nephropathy. Crit Care Clin 2005;21(2):261–80.

[66] McCullough PA, Adam A, Becker CR, Davidson C, Lameire N, Stacul F, et al. Risk prediction of contrast-induced nephropathy. Am J Cardiol 2006;98(6A): 27K–36K.

[67] McCullough PA, Adam A, Becker CR, Davidson C, Lameire N, Stacul F, et al. Epidemiology and prognostic implications of contrast-induced nephropathy. Am J Cardiol 2006;98(6A):5K–13K.

[68] Mueller C, Buerkle G, Buettner HJ, Petersen J, Perruchoud AP, Eriksson U, et al. Prevention of contrast media-associated nephropathy: randomized comparison of 2 hydration regimens in 1620 patients undergoing coronary angioplasty. Arch Intern Med 2002;162(3):329–36.

[69] Merten GJ, Burgess WP, Gray LV, Holleman JH, Roush TS, Kowalchuk GJ, et al. Prevention of contrast-induced nephropathy with sodium bicarbonate: a randomized controlled trial. JAMA 2004;291(19):2328–34.

[70] Birck R, Krzossok S, Markowetz F, Schnulle P, van der Woude FJ, Braun C. Acetylcysteine for prevention of contrast nephropathy: meta-analysis. Lancet 2003;362(9384):598–603.

[71] Alonso A, Lau J, Jaber BL, Weintraub A, Sarnak MJ. Prevention of radiocontrast nephropathy with N-acetylcysteine in patients with chronic kidney disease: a meta-analysis of randomized, controlled trials. Am J Kidney Dis 2004;43(1):1–9.

[72] Isenbarger DW, Kent SM, O'Malley PG. Meta-analysis of randomized clinical trials on the usefulness of acetylcysteine for prevention of contrast nephropathy. Am J Cardiol 2003;92(12):1454–8.

[73] Kshirsagar AV, Poole C, Mottl A, Shoham D, Franceschini N, Tudor G, et al. N-acetylcysteine for the prevention of radiocontrast induced nephropathy: a meta-analysis of prospective controlled trials. J Am Soc Nephrol 2004;15(3):761–9.

[74] Marenzi G, Lauri G, Campodonico J, Marana I, Assanelli E, De Metrio M, et al. Comparison of two hemofiltration protocols for prevention of contrast-induced nephropathy in high-risk patients. Am J Med 2006;119(2):155–62.

[75] Chevalier RL. Pathogenesis of renal injury in obstructive uropathy. Curr Opin Pediatr 2006;18(2): 153–60.

[76] Klahr S. Obstructive nephropathy. Intern Med 2000;39(5):355–61.

[77] Coleman BG. Ultrasonography of the upper genitourinary tract. Urol Clin North Am 1985;12(4): 633–44.

[78] Riccabona M. Obstructive diseases of the urinary tract in children: lessons from the last 15 years. Pediatr Radiol 2010;40(6):947–55.

[79] Atamer T, Artim-Esen B, Yavuz S, Ecder T. Massive post-obstructive diuresis in a patient with Burkitt's lymphoma. Nephrol Dial Transplant 2005;20(9): 1991–3.

[80] Bellomo R, Wan L, May C. Vasoactive drugs and acute kidney injury. Crit Care Med 2008;36(Suppl. 4): S179–86.

[81] Boyd JH, Forbes J, Nakada TA, Walley KR, Russell JA. Fluid resuscitation in septic shock: a positive fluid balance and elevated central venous

pressure are associated with increased mortality. Crit Care Med 2011;39(2):259−65.

[82] Murphy CV, Schramm GE, Doherty JA, Reichley RM, Gajic O, Afessa B, et al. The importance of fluid management in acute lung injury secondary to septic shock. Chest 2009;136(1):102−9.

[83] Michael M, Kuehnle I, Goldstein SL. Fluid overload and acute renal failure in pediatric stem cell transplant patients. Pediatr Nephrol 2004;19(1):91−5.

[84] Heenen S, De Backer D, Vincent JL. How can the response to volume expansion in patients with spontaneous respiratory movements be predicted? Crit Care 2006;10(4): R102.

[85] Mehta RL, Clark WC, Schetz M. Techniques for assessing and achieving fluid balance in acute renal failure. Curr Opin Crit Care 2002;8(6):535−43.

[86] Patel NN, Rogers CA, Angelini GD, Murphy GJ. Pharmacological therapies for the prevention of acute kidney injury following cardiac surgery: a systematic review. Heart Fail Rev 2011;16(6):553−67.

[87] Denton MD, Chertow GM, Brady HR. "Renal-dose" dopamine for the treatment of acute renal failure: scientific rationale, experimental studies and clinical trials. Kidney Int 1996;50(1):4−14.

[88] Tumlin JA, Finkel KW, Murray PT, Samuels J, Cotsonis G, Shaw AD. Fenoldopam mesylate in early acute tubular necrosis: a randomized, double-blind, placebo-controlled clinical trial. Am J Kidney Dis 2005;46(1):26−34.

[89] Mehta RL, Pascual MT, Soroko S, Chertow GM, Group PS. Diuretics, mortality, and nonrecovery of renal function in acute renal failure. JAMA 2002;288(20):2547−53.

[90] Bagshaw SM, Berthiaume LR, Delaney A, Bellomo R. Continuous versus intermittent renal replacement therapy for critically ill patients with acute kidney injury: a meta-analysis. Crit Care Med 2008;36(2): 610−7.

[91] Rabindranath K, Adams J, Macleod AM, Muirhead N. Intermittent versus continuous renal replacement therapy for acute renal failure in adults. Cochrane Database Syst Rev 2007;(3): CD003773.

[92] Kellum JA, Angus DC, Johnson JP, Leblanc M, Griffin M, Ramakrishnan N, et al. Continuous versus

intermittent renal replacement therapy: a meta-analysis. Intensive Care Med 2002;28(1):29−37.

[93] Tonelli M, Manns B, Feller-Kopman D. Acute renal failure in the intensive care unit: a systematic review of the impact of dialytic modality on mortality and renal recovery. Am J Kidney Dis 2002;40(5):875−85.

[94] D'Intini V, Ronco C, Bonello M, Bellomo R. Renal replacement therapy in acute renal failure. Best Pract Res Clin Haematol 2004;18(1):145−57.

[95] Keller F, Bohler J, Czock D, Zellner D, Mertz AK. Individualized drug dosage in patients treated with continuous hemofiltration. Kidney Int Suppl 1999;72: S29−31.

[96] Bohler J, Donauer J, Keller F. Pharmacokinetic principles during continuous renal replacement therapy: drugs and dosage. Kidney Int Suppl 1999;72:S24−8.

[97] Bugge JF. Influence of renal replacement therapy on pharmacokinetics in critically ill patients. Best Pract Res Clin Haematol 2004;18(1):175−87.

[98] Bywaters EG. 50 years on: the crush syndrome. BMJ 1990;301(6766):1412−5.

[99] Kolff WJ. First clinical experience with the artificial kidney. Ann Intern Med 1965;62:608−19.

[100] Ympa YP, Sakr Y, Reinhart K, Vincent JL. Has mortality from acute renal failure decreased? A systematic review of the literature. Am J Med 2005;118(8): 827−32.

[101] Levy EM, Viscoli CM, Horwitz RI. The effect of acute renal failure on mortality. A cohort analysis. JAMA 1996;275(19):1489−94.

[102] Lassnigg A, Schmid ER, Hiesmayr M, Falk C, Druml W, Bauer P, et al. Impact of minimal increases in serum creatinine on outcome in patients after cardiothoracic surgery: do we have to revise current definitions of acute renal failure? Crit Care Med 2008;36(4):1129−37.

[103] Mehta RL, Pascual MT, Soroko S, Savage BR, Himmelfarb J, Ikizler TA, et al. Spectrum of acute renal failure in the intensive care unit: the PICARD experience. Kidney Int 2004;66(4):1613−21.

[104] Soares M, Salluh JI, Carvalho MS, Darmon M, Rocco JR, Spector N. Prognosis of critically ill patients with cancer and acute renal dysfunction. J Clin Oncol 2006;24(24):4003−10.

3

Biomarkers in Oncology and Nephrology

Putao Cen[1], Carl Walther[1,2], Kevin W. Finkel[1,2], Robert J. Amato[1,3]

[1]UTHealth Science Center at Houston, Houston, TX, USA [2]University of Texas MD Anderson Cancer Center, Houston, TX, USA [3]University of Texas Memorial Hermann Cancer Center, Houston, TX, USA

INTRODUCTION

The term biological marker (biomarker) was first introduced in 1989 as a term in the US National Library of Medicine's controlled vocabulary thesaurus Medical Subject Headings. It was defined as "measurable and quantifiable biological parameters which serve as indices for health- and physiology-related assessments." Later the Federal Drug Administration defined a biomarker as a "characteristic that is objectively measured and evaluated as an indicator of normal biological processes, pathogenic processes, or pharmacologic responses to therapeutic intervention."

Biomarkers can serve a wide range of roles including disease detection, response to therapy, drug development and disease prognosis. Biomarkers can be measured in tissue, cells and body fluids. They may be composed of proteins, lipids, genomic or proteomic patterns, or cell surface markers. The ideal biomarker is easily measurable and interpretable, and is present in readily available specimens.

The development of a biomarker should proceed in a systematic fashion through several phases. This process of development was first described in the early diagnosis of cancer [1,2]. *Phase 1* refers to preclinical studies using various techniques and technologies to detect differences in tissues and body fluid between diseased and normal animals or humans. In *Phase 2*, the sensitivity and specificity of the potential biomarker is determined. This step includes development and optimization of the measuring assay as well as its reproducibility. *Phase 3* involves using the biomarker in previously conducted clinical trials to determine its diagnostic potential. *Phase 4* examines the sensitivity and specificity of the potential biomarker in a prospective cohort allowing for determination of its false-positive rate. Finally, *Phase 5* addresses whether or not the biomarker impacts current clinical care by either changing physician practice or improving mortality and morbidity.

The use of biomarkers has remarkably changed the practice of oncology. Biomarkers have been developed in several cancers that define the molecular mechanisms of pathogenesis and metastases, predict prognosis and response to therapy, and guide drug development. On the other hand, nephrology has long relied on non-specific biomarkers such as serum creatinine levels and urinary protein excretion. Although still in its infancy, novel biomarkers are now being explored as a means to better understand the pathogenesis and prognosis of kidney disease and lead to new therapeutic regimens. In this chapter we review the field of biomarkers in both specialties.

BIOMARKERS IN ONCOLOGY

Tumor biomarkers are biomolecules produced by cancer cells or by other cells of the body in response to cancer or a noncancerous condition such as inflammation. These biomolecules can be identified in the blood, urine, stool, tumor tissue, or other tissues or bodily fluids of some patients with cancer.

The anatomically based TNM Classification of Malignant Tumors staging system, a combination of tumor size or depth (T), lymph node spread (N) and presence or absence of metastases (M), remains useful for predicting survival, choice of initial treatment, stratification of patients in clinical trials, accurate communication among health care providers and uniform reporting of outcomes. Novel biomarkers provide additional new opportunities to the TNM staging system for risk assessment, screening, diagnosis, prognosis, and selection and monitoring of therapy. For example, individual biomarkers are successfully subdividing traditional tumor classes into subsets that behave differently from each other;

chemotherapeutic and biological agents could be more effective when their respective molecular markers are mutated or expressed at sufficient levels. The use of novel biomarkers for cancer differential diagnosis and personalization of therapy should theoretically improve patient care.

The ability of malignant cells to proliferate and metastasize is complex and can involve activation of proto-oncogenes, inactivation of tumor-suppressor genes or DNA repair mechanisms, epigenetic modulation of mRNA expression or differences in protein expression, post-translational modification, or function. Advances in genomics, proteomics and molecular pathology have generated many candidate biomarkers with potential clinical value (Table 3.1) [3].

Humoral Biomarkers

Alpha Fetoprotein

Alpha fetoprotein (AFP) is a glycoprotein that is normally produced during gestation by the fetal liver and yolk sac. Many tissues regain the ability to produce this oncofetal protein when they undergo malignant degeneration.

[1] **Hepatocellular carcinoma (HCC):** AFP and liver ultrasonography are the most widely used methods of screening for HCC. A rise in serum AFP in a patient with cirrhosis should raise concerns that HCC has developed; however, serum AFP can be normal in up to 40% of small HCCs. Furthermore, AFP can also be elevated in intrahepatic cholangiocarcinoma, liver metastases from colon cancer, or liver damage (e.g. cirrhosis, hepatitis, or drug or alcohol abuse). Therefore, its utility as a screening biomarker is limited. The updated American Association for the Study of Liver Diseases guidelines no longer recommend AFP testing as part of diagnostic evaluation. If no liver mass is detected following

TABLE 3.1   Biomarkers in Oncology

Humoral biomarkers	Tumor marker	Cancer type	Clinical application
	Alpha-fetoprotein (AFP)	Liver cancer; Germ cell tumors	Assist in diagnosis, staging, assessment of prognosis and treatment response
	Beta-2-microglobulin (B2M)	Multiple myeloma; Chronic lymphocytic leukemia; Some lymphomas	Prognosis and follow treatment response
	Beta-human chorionic gonadotropin (Beta-hCG)	Germ cell tumor	Assess stage, prognosis and treatment response
	CA 15-3/CA 27.29	Breast cancer	Assess treatment response and recurrence
	CA 19-9	Pancreatic cancer; Gallbladder cancer; Bile duct cancer; Gastric cancer	Assess treatment response
	CA 125	Ovarian cancer	For diagnosis, evaluation of recurrence and to assess treatment response
	Carcinoembryonic antigen (CEA)	Colorectal cancer; Breast cancer	Assess tumor burden, recurrence and treatment response
	Chromogranin A (CgA)	Neuroendocrine tumors	Assist in diagnosis, evaluation of recurrence and assessment of treatment response
	Prostate-specific antigen (PSA)	Prostate cancer	Assist in diagnosis, evaluate recurrence and assess treatment response
	Serotonin and 5-hydroxyindoleacetic acid (HIAA)	Neuroendocrine tumors	Monitor progression and treatment response
	21-Gene signature (oncotype DX)	Breast cancer	Evaluate risk of recurrence and predict chemotherapy benefit
	ALK gene rearrangements	Non-small cell lung cancer; Anaplastic large cell lymphoma	Assess prognosis and to select a targeted agent
	BCR-ABL	Chronic myeloid leukemia	Assist in diagnosis; monitor recurrence and treatment response
	BRAF mutation V600E	Cutaneous melanoma; colorectal cancer	Predict response to targeted therapies

(Continued)

TABLE 3.1   Biomarkers in Oncology—(*cont'd*)

Humoral biomarkers	Tumor marker	Cancer type	Clinical application
	CD20	Non-Hodgkin lymphoma	Select targeted therapies
	Chromosomes 3, 7, 17 and 9p21	Bladder cancer; Cholangiocarcinoma	Monitor tumor recurrence; to assist in diagnosis
	Chromosomes 1p and 19q co-deletions	Low-grade anaplastic oligodendrogliomas and oligoastrocytomas	Predict response to chemotherapy
	Circulating tumor cell	Various cancers	Assist in prognosis, to monitor progression and treatment response
	DNA mismatch repair (MMR) gene	Lynch syndrome; Colorectal cancers	Assist in diagnosis, prognosis and to predict response to chemotherapy
	EGFR mutation analysis	Non-small cell lung cancer	Select targeted therapies
	ERCC1 and RRM1	Non-small cell lung cancer	Assess prognosis and predict response to chemotherapy
	Estrogen receptor (ER)/ progesterone receptor (PR)	Breast cancer; Gynecology cancer	Select hormonal therapy
	HER2/neu	Breast cancer; Gastric cancer; Esophageal cancer	Select targeted therapies
	Human papillomavirus (HPV) and P16	Head and neck cancer	Assess prognosis and predict response to treatment
	Ki67 and mitotic index	Various cancers	Assess tumor aggressiveness in clinical course
	KIT	Gastrointestinal stromal tumor; Melanoma	Assist in diagnosis and select targeted therapies
	KRAS mutation analysis	Colorectal cancer; Non-small cell lung cancer	Select targeted therapies
	MicroRNAs (miRNAs)	Various cancers	Assist in diagnosis and evaluate prognosis
	Cell-free nucleic acids (cfNA)	Various cancers	Evaluate prognosis, predict treatment response

measurement of an elevated AFP level, the patient should be followed with AFP testing and liver imaging every 3 months [4,5].

[2] **Nonseminomatous germ cell tumor (NSGCT):** AFP is not elevated in patients with pure seminomas, therefore, it is an important biomarker to help in the differential diagnosis of NSGCTs. The extent of elevation of AFP is an important prognostic marker and this information has

been incorporated into the International Germ Cell Cancer Collaborative Group risk stratification system and the Tumor Node Metastasis (TNM) staging system. AFP should be measured prior to orchiectomy, following orchiectomy and prior to each chemotherapy cycle. Following effective therapy, normalization of the serum AFP concentration occurs over 25 to 30 days [6].

Beta-human Chorionic Gonadotropin (Beta-hCG)

Beta-hCG is a family of pituitary and placental glycoprotein hormones that share the same alpha subunit and differ in the beta subunit from follicle stimulating hormone, luteinizing hormone and thyroid stimulating hormone. Because the alpha subunit is common to several pituitary hormones, serum assays measure the beta subunit.

[1] **Germ cell tumor (GCT):** Beta-hCG elevation can be seen in pure seminomas or nonseminomatous germ cell tumor (mixed embryonal carcinoma or choriocarcinoma). The extent of elevation of beta-hCG is prognostic and has been incorporated into the staging system. Beta-hCG should be measured prior to and following surgery, and prior to each chemotherapy cycle. Although persistent elevation in serum beta-hCG after treatment implies the presence of residual disease, it should be interpreted with caution since several factors can contribute to false-positive elevation of beta-hCG including hypogonadism and marijuana use. Clinical hyperthyroidism can develop in patients with markedly elevated beta-hCG due to ligand-receptor cross-reactivity between beta-hCG and thyroid stimulating hormone [6].

[2] **Gestational trophoblastic disease (GTD):** This is a proliferative disorder of trophoblastic cells, including hydatidiform mole (complete or partial), persistent/ invasive gestational trophoblastic neoplasia, choriocarcinoma and placental site trophoblastic tumors. The serum beta-hCG concentration is always elevated in gestational trophoblastic disease.

Beta-2-microglobulin (B2M)

Beta-2 microglobulin levels correlate with disease stage, tumor burden and response to therapy in *lymphoma*, *chronic lymphocytic leukemia* and *plasma cell dyscrasias* (monoclonal gammopathy of undetermined significance (MGUS), solitary plasmacytoma of bone, extramedullary plasmacytoma, multiple myeloma, lymphoplasmacytic lymphoma, primary amyloidosis, and light- and heavy-chain deposition disease). High beta-2 microglobulin levels are also correlated with worsening renal function.

CA 15-3 and CA 27.29

CA 15-3 and CA 27.29 are soluble forms of the glycoprotein Mucin 1 (MUC1) antigen in peripheral blood, and have been shown to correlate with tumor burden in *breast cancer*. However, they are neither sensitive nor specific for breast cancer. Elevated levels can also be seen in other adenocarcinomas.

CA 19-9

CA 19-9 is a sialylated Lewis antigen of the MUC1 protein. Elevated CA 19-9 can be seen in *pancreatic adenocarcinoma, cholangiocarcinoma, ampullary cancer* and other gastrointestinal cancer. CA 19-9 may also be positive in patients with non-malignant diseases such as cirrhosis, chronic pancreatitis, cholangitis and biliary obstruction [7]. Perioperative CA 19-9 is prognostic for survival in pancreatic cancer [8]. Patients with blood type of Lewis a- and b-genotype (5—10% of the Caucasian population) are incapable of synthesizing the CA19-9 epitope.

CA 125

The serum CA 125 is elevated in 50% of women with early stage and in over 80% of women with advanced *epithelial ovarian cancer*. However, it is non-specific. Patients with ascites or pleural fluid of any cause can have an elevated serum level of CA 125, probably from shear forces on mesothelial cells. When ascites is controlled, the serum CA 125 level decreases. CA 125 levels can increase with age, and are elevated in women with benign gynecologic conditions as well as in 1% of healthy women and fluctuate during the menstrual cycle [9].

CEA Antigen

Serum CEA levels should be obtained in patients with *colorectal cancer* before surgery, chemotherapy planning and during post-treatment follow-up [10]. However, CEA is not a sensitive tool for diagnosis. Also, elevated CEA can be seen in other gastrointestinal cancers, gastritis, peptic ulcer disease, diverticulitis, liver disease, chronic obstructive pulmonary disease, diabetes and any acute or chronic inflammatory state.

Chromogranin A

Chromogranin A is a protein stored and released with peptides and amines in a variety of neuroendocrine tissues. The plasma level of chromogranin A in patients with *neuroendocrine tumors* has a sensitivity and specificity of 75% and 84%, respectively. Chromogranin A levels increase with tumor burden. False-positive elevations can be found in patients who are taking a proton pump inhibitor, or who have concurrent medical conditions such as renal or hepatic insufficiency. It is used as a tumor marker in patients with an established diagnosis in order to assess disease progression, response to therapy and recurrence after surgical resection [11].

Neuron-specific Enolase

Neuron-specific enolase is a glycolytic enzyme that is present almost exclusively in the cytoplasm of neurons and neuroendocrine cells. In cancers with neuroendocrine tumor differentiation (for example, in renal cell carcinoma, prostate cancer, or lung cancer), neuron-specific enolase can be used to assist in differential diagnosis, assess prognosis and predict treatment response [12–15].

Prostate-specific Antigen (PSA)

Prostate-specific antigens are glycoproteins expressed by both normal and neoplastic prostate tissue. The absolute value of serum PSA is useful for determining the extent of prostate cancer and assessing the response to prostate cancer treatment. Its use as a screening method to detect prostate cancer is common although controversial. A PSA level lower than 4 ng/mL has historically been considered normal. However, 15% of men with this "normal" PSA will have prostate cancer and 2% will have high-grade cancer. As prostate size increases with age the PSA concentration also rises. Age-specific reference ranges have been suggested to improve the accuracy of screening for prostate cancer [16]. An elevated serum PSA that continues to rise over time is more likely to reflect prostate cancer than one that is consistently stable (PSA velocity) [17,18]. Taking 5-alpha-reductase inhibitors, non-steroidal anti-inflammatory drugs, acetaminophen, statins and thiazide diuretic can decrease serum PSA levels [19]. Besides benign prostate hypertrophy, elevated PSA level can be seen in prostatitis and perineal trauma.

Serotonin and 5-hydroxyindoleacetic Acid (HIAA)

Urinary excretion of 5-hydroxyindoleacetic acid (HIAA) is the end product of serotonin metabolism. False-positive blood serotonin tests may occur due to release of platelet serotonin as well as by ingestion of tryptophan/serotonin-rich foods. Blood serotonin levels are not recommended as a standard diagnostic test for *neuroendocrine tumors*. Measurement of the 24-hour urinary excretion of HIAA is generally most useful in patients with primary midgut (jejunoileal, appendiceal, ascending colon) carcinoid tumors. Foregut (gastroduodenal, bronchus) and hindgut (transverse, descending and sigmoid colon, rectum, genitourinary) carcinoids rarely secrete serotonin, because they lack the enzyme DOPA decarboxylase and cannot convert 5-hydroxytryptophan (5-HT) to serotonin, and therefore to 5-HIAA into urine. A patient with symptoms may still have a carcinoid tumor even if the 5-HIAA level is normal. In patients treated for a carcinoid tumor, decreasing levels of 5-HIAA indicate a response to treatment, while increasing or excessive levels indicate a non-response.

Cellular Biomarkers

21-gene Signature (Oncotype Dx®)

Oncotype Dx® is a reverse-transcriptase-polymerase-chain-reaction (RT-PCR) assay of 21 prospectively selected genes examined in paraffin-embedded tumor tissue, which is recommended by the American Society of Clinical Oncology for use in women with *node-negative, hormonal receptor (ER/PR)-positive breast cancer* [20]. Gene expression profiling has identified molecular signatures that not only predict the likelihood of tumor recurrence after receiving hormonal therapy but also can predict the magnitude of chemotherapy benefit for patients.

ALK Gene Rearrangements

An inversion in chromosome 2 [Inv(2) (p21p23)] that juxtaposes the 5′ end of the echinoderm microtubule-associated protein-like 4 (*EML4*) gene with the 3′ end of the anaplastic lymphoma kinase (*ALK*) gene results in the novel fusion oncogene and chimeric protein EML4-ALK. This fusion oncogene rearrangement leads to the development of a subset of *non-small cell lung cancer*, which accounts for 2–7% of the total lung cancer population. This subset of lung cancer has distinct clinicopathologic features including no or light smoking history, younger age, male gender, adenocarcinoma with signet ring or acinar histology, and high sensitivity to therapy with the ALK tyrosine kinase inhibitor crizotinib. *ALK* gene rearrangements or the resulting fusion proteins may be detected in tumor specimens using immunohistochemistry, RT-PCR and fluorescence *in situ* hybridization (FISH). ALK positivity must be demonstrated by the FDA-approved FISH test (Vysis Probes) [21]. ALK expression also defines more than half of primary *systemic anaplastic large cell lymphomas*. This subset has significantly better prognosis than ALK-negative tumors. There are rare cases of ALK$^+$ diffuse large B-cell lymphoma, retinoblastoma, melanoma and breast carcinoma.

BCR-ABL

The Philadelphia chromosome t(9;22)(q34;q11), which juxtaposes a 5′ segment of a breakpoint cluster region (BCR) at 22q11 and the 3′ segment of the ABL oncogene (ABL) at 9q34, results in the formation of a fusion gene (*BCR-ABL*). The *BCR-ABL* encodes a constitutively active tyrosine kinase [22]. The diagnostic test of choice for Ph-positive leukemia is RT-PCR for *BCR-ABL*, including *chronic myeloid leukemia and B-cell acute lymphoblastic leukemia*, and is a predictor of response to tyrosine kinase inhibitors imatinib, dasatinib and nilotinib [23]. Drug resistance is generally a consequence of reactivation of *BCR-ABL* signaling, most commonly by the development of single nucleotide mutations in *BCR-ABL* which results in amino acid substitutions. Cytogenetic response is determined by the decrease in the number of Ph-positive metaphases, as determined by bone marrow aspirate and cytogenetic evaluation. FISH using 5′-BCR and 3'-*ABL* probes can be performed on peripheral blood specimens or bone marrow aspirates. Molecular response is determined by the decrease in the amount of *BCR-ABL* chimeric mRNA as assessed by quantitative RT-PCR on peripheral blood specimens.

BRAF Mutation V600E

The BRAF proteins are serine−threonine kinases, a component of the RAS-RAF-MAPK signaling pathway. Activating mutations in BRAF are present in 40−60% of advanced *melanoma* and consist of the substitution of glutamic acid for valine at amino acid 600 (V600E mutation) in 80−90% of the cases. The tyrosine kinase inhibitor vemurafenib produces rapid tumor regressions in patients with V600 mutant melanoma [24,25]. BRAF mutations are found in about 5−10% of metastatic *colorectal cancer*. BRAF mutations have been associated with poor prognosis in colorectal cancer and potential resistance to EGFR-targeted agents. Somatic mutations in BRAF are present in 3% of patients with *non-small cell lung cancer* and 50% of these are V600E mutations. *BRAF* mutations (mostly V600E mutations) also occur in 30−69% of *papillary thyroid cancers*, but not in benign or follicular neoplasms, and may confer a worse prognosis.

CD20 (Cluster of Differentiation 20)

CD20 is an activated-glycosylated phosphoprotein expressed on the surface of all stages of B-cell development except early pro-B-cells (the first stage) and plasma cells (the last stage). CD20 can be determined by immunohistochemistry and is found expressed by most of *B-cell non-Hodgkin lymphomas and chronic lymphocytic leukemia*. Expression of CD20 on tumor cells is the target of the monoclonal antibodies rituximab, ofatumumab, ibritumomab tiuxetan and tositumomab treatment for lymphoma and leukemia [26,27].

Chromosomes 3, 7, 17 and 9p21 (Vysis® UroVysion)

This set of FISH analyses can help in monitoring *bladder cancer* recurrence [28] and assist in the diagnosis of *cholangiocarcinoma* [29].

Chromosomes 1p and 19q Co-deletions

This abnormality arises from an unbalanced translocation of the short arm of chromosome 19 (19p) to the long arm of chromosome 1 (1q), after which the derivative chromosome with the short arm of 1 and the long arm of 19 is lost. Co-deletions of chromosomes 1p and 19q have been reported in 60−70% of classical *anaplastic oligodendrogliomas* and predict a better prognosis. In *low-grade anaplastic oligodendrogliomas* and *oligoastrocytomas*, co-deletions of chromosomes 1p and 19q are associated with good response to chemotherapy [30,31].

Circulating Tumor Cells

Circulating tumor cells (CTCs) (also known as circulating cancer cells) circulate via normal vessels and capillaries formed through tumor-induced angiogenesis. CTCs from patients' blood samples can be prognostic for tumor staging, disease relapse and overall survival, as well as predictive for tumor response to therapy in patients with a variety of cancers. The CellSearch® system (Veridex LLC) using antibodies directed against cell surface antigens, epithelial cell adhesion molecule (EpCAM), has received FDA approval to aid in monitoring patients with *metastatic breast, prostate* and *colon cancer* [32,33]. However, its sensitivity is low and it has not been widely accepted into routine clinical practice. Numerous novel assays for detecting CTCs have been developed and clinical trials are ongoing.

DNA Mismatch Repair (MMR) Gene

The role of the DNA MMR system is to maintain genomic integrity by correcting base substitution mismatches and small insertion–deletion mismatches that are generated by errors in base pairing during DNA replication. *Lynch syndrome* (hereditary nonpolyposis colorectal cancer) results from a germline mutation in one allele of a DNA MMR gene. There are two groups of *microsatellite instability-high (MSI-H) colorectal cancers*: sporadic and Lynch-associated MSI-H cancers [1]. The sporadic groups can be differentiated by direct measurement for hypermethylation of MLH1 in the tumor, or by genetic analysis for BRAF gene mutation [34]. The National Comprehensive Cancer Network panel recommends that MMR testing should be strongly considered for all colon cancer patients less than 50 years of age based on an increased likelihood of *Lynch syndrome* in this population. The biomarker of microsatellite instability predicts more favorable outcome and decreased metastasis, but decreased benefit from 5FU-alone adjuvant chemotherapy in patients with stage II lymph node-negative disease [35].

Epidermal Growth Factor Receptor (EGFR) Mutation

Epidermal growth factor receptor (also called HER1 or erbB-1) is a transmembrane receptor that controls the intracellular signal transduction pathways regulating proliferation, apoptosis, angiogenesis, adhesion and motility. It is detectable in 80–85% of patients with *non-small cell lung cancer*. The most commonly found activating mutations in the tyrosine kinase domain of the EGFR in patients with non-small cell lung cancer are exon 19 deletions (45% of patients) and exon 21 point mutation (in another 45%). These mutations result in activation of the tyrosine kinase domain and are predictive of responsiveness to the EGFR tyrosine kinase inhibitors erlotinib and gefitinib. Other drug-sensitive mutations include point mutations at exon 21 and exon 18. The T790M mutation is associated with resistance to tyrosine kinase inhibitor therapy and has been reported in 50% of patients with disease progression. DNA mutational analysis and direct

sequencing of DNA corresponding to exons 18–21 are reasonable approaches in clinical practice [36–41].

ERCC1 and RRM1

ERCC1 is the 5′ endonuclease of the nucleotide excision repair complex and RRM1 is the regulatory subunit of ribonucleotide reductase. High ERCC1 level and high RRM1 levels are prognostic of better survival for patients with *non-small cell lung cancer* when compared to low levels of expression, independent of therapy [42]. High levels of ERCC1 expression are predictive of poor response to platinum-based chemotherapy [43]. High levels of RRM1 expression are also predictive of poor response to chemotherapy [44].

Estrogen Receptor (ER)/Progesterone Receptor (PR)

ER and PR are both members of the nuclear hormone receptor superfamily, located in the cytosol of target cells and operate as ligand-dependent transcription. Attachment of a lipid-soluble hormone to the ligand-binding domain results in unmasking of the DNA-binding sites on the receptor, followed by migration into the nucleus and transcription of messenger RNA and ribosomal RNA. Immunohistochemistry is the predominant method for measuring ER and PR status, which should be determined on all invasive breast cancers and breast cancer recurrences. ER and PR assays are considered positive if there are at least 1% positive tumor nuclei in the sample on testing based on the National Comprehensive Cancer Network (NCCN) Task Force and American Society of Clinical Oncology (ASCO) guideline recommendation [45,46]. Receptor positivity is predictive of response to endocrine therapy in *breast cancer* and *endometrial cancer*.

Human Epidermal Growth Factor Receptor 2 (HER2)

The HER2 receptor (also called HER2/neu, or erbB-2) is a transmembrane glycoprotein receptor with intracellular tyrosine kinase activity. Amplification of HER2 oncogene or overexpression of its protein product is observed in 20% of *breast cancers* [47]. HER2 positivity predicts survival benefit from receiving HER-targeted agents, such as trastuzumab and lapatinib. A positive HER2 is also found in 25% of *adenocarcinoma of esophagogastric junction*, *lower esophagus* and *stomach*. Overexpression of HER2 is more common in the intestinal type of gastric cancers than in diffuse type of gastric cancers (32% versus 6%). A positive HER2 predicts a survival benefit from receiving trastuzumab [48].

Human Papillomavirus (HPV)

Human papillomavirus-related cancers include *squamous cancer of cervix*, *vulvar*, *anus* and *penis*. Recent studies have documented a rapid increase in the incidence of HPV-related *head and neck cancer*, which comprises up to 60–70% of newly diagnosed squamous cancer of oropharynx in the West, particularly *cancers of the lingual*, *palatine tonsils* and *base of tongue* [49,50]. Patients with HPV-positive head and neck cancer have improved response to treatment and improved survival when compared to those with HPV-negative tumors [51].

Ki67 and Mitotic Index

Ki67 is a large nuclear protein (395 kDa) that is closely associated with the nucleolus and heterochromatin. Ki67 is expressed in G1, S, G2 and M phases, with a peak level during mitosis. Increased mitotic rate and high Ki67 index are associated with a more aggressive clinical course in *neuroendocrine tumors, lymphoma* and *breast cancer*.

KIT

In 80% of *gastrointestinal stromal tumors (GISTs)* cases, a mutation in the KIT (also denoted c-kit) protooncogene leads to a structural variant of the KIT protein that is abnormally activated. The CD117 antigen is part of the KIT transmembrane receptor tyrosine kinase

(RTK). Overexpression of CD117 or KIT protein is found in 90% cases of GISTs arising in adults. The uncontrolled oncogenic signaling through KIT predicts response to orally active tyrosine kinase inhibitors such as imatinib and sunitinib [52]. Activation of the c-kit receptor tyrosine kinase has been identified in *lung cancer, melanoma* and *acute myeloid leukemia*. Mutations of the KIT gene can be detected in 20–30% of patients with acute myeloid leukemia and either confer a higher risk of relapse or adversely affect overall survival.

K-ras Mutation

The RAS/RAF/MAPK pathway is downstream of EGFR. The ras oncogene exists as three cellular variants, H-ras, K-ras and N-ras. K-ras is a GTP-binding protein and involved in G-protein coupled receptor signaling. In its mutated form, K-ras is constitutively active, able to transform immortalized cells and promote cell proliferation and survival. K-ras mutations are found in 25% of *adenocarcinomas of the lung* in North American populations, and they are associated with cigarette smoking. It is prognostic of shorter survival and predicts resistance to the EGFR tyrosine kinase inhibitors erlotinib or gefitinib [53,54]. K-ras mutation is also found in 40% of *colorectal cancer* and its codon 12 or 13 mutations predict resistance to the EGFR tyrosine kinase inhibitors cetuximab or panitumumab [55–57].

MicroRNAs (miRNAs)

MicroRNAs are small, non-coding RNAs that repress gene expression through interaction with 3′ untranslated regions (3′ UTRs) of mRNAs [58]. MicroRNAs are predicted to target over 50% of all human protein-coding genes, enabling them to have numerous regulatory roles in many physiological and developmental processes. MicroRNA expression profiles have since been shown to have signatures that are related to tumor classification, diagnosis and disease progression. For example, patients with advanced staged breast cancer had significantly more miR-34a in their blood than patients at early tumor stages, and changes in miR-10b, miR-34a and miR-155 serum levels correlated with the presence of metastases [59].

Cell-free Nucleic Acids (cfNA)

DNA, mRNA and microRNA are released and circulate in the blood of cancer patients. Changes in the levels of circulating nucleic acids have been associated with tumor burden and malignant progression. The release of DNA from tumor cells can be through various cell physiological events such as apoptosis, necrosis and secretion. Tumors usually represent a mixture of different cancer cell clones, which account for the genomic and epigenomic heterogeneity of tumors and other normal cell types, such as hematopoietic and stromal cells. Thus, during tumor progression and turnover, both tumor-derived and wild-type (normal) cfNA can be released into the blood. Nucleic acids are cleared from the blood by the liver and kidney, and they have a variable half-life in the circulation. Mutations, methylation, DNA integrity, microsatellite alterations, loss of heterozygosity and viral DNA can be detected in cell-free DNA (cfDNA) in blood. For example, circulating BRAF DNA mutation in patients with different stages of *melanoma* and cfDNA mutation detection has clinical utility for monitoring patient responses before and after therapy [60]. However, the levels of cfDNA might also reflect physiological and pathological processes that are not tumor specific. Cell-free DNA yields are higher in patients with malignant lesions than in patients without tumors, but increased levels have also been quantified in patients with benign lesions, inflammatory diseases and tissue trauma. As metastatic and primary tumors from the same patient can vary at the genomic, epigenomic and transcriptomic levels, such assays allow the repetitive monitoring of blood samples to assess cancer progression in patients from whom tumor tissue is not available [61].

BIOMARKERS IN NEPHROLOGY

The field of biomarkers in nephrology remains in its infancy compared to oncology. Traditional biomarkers can be broadly categorized as markers of function (serum creatinine) or markers of pathology (urinary protein), or both. Current research is focused on developing and characterizing new biomarkers that: (1) provide more accurate assessments of renal function; (2) predict the development of acute kidney injury and its prognosis; (3) identify the site of renal injury; (4) predict the progression of chronic kidney disease; and (5) lead to development of novel therapies.

Traditional Biomarkers

Creatinine

Serum creatinine, a surrogate marker for glomerular filtration rate (GFR), is the most commonly used biomarker in clinical medicine. Since Colls identified a "small but ponderable amount" of this molecule in blood in the late 19th century its use remains exceedingly common [62]. An ideal biomarker for assessing GFR would be produced at a constant rate, freely filtered by the glomerulus, neither secreted nor reabsorbed by the renal tubules, and cleared solely by the kidney. Although creatinine, a 113 dalton product of muscle metabolism, meets some of these criteria, it has several shortcomings. The rate of production varies greatly depending on muscle mass, diet, age, gender, race and the presence of sepsis. Serum levels of creatinine are also influenced by fluid administration and various medications. Finally, tubular secretion and extra-renal elimination increase with decreasing renal function, further limiting accuracy of GFR estimations. Although several investigators have developed various formulae to account for this degree of inaccuracy, none have proven exact.

Proteinuria and Albuminuria

Proteinuria develops in several kidney diseases and is an important biomarker. The degree of proteinuria correlates with the prognosis of both kidney and cardiovascular disease [63]. Urinary protein level is the strongest predictor of decline in renal function in chronic kidney disease (CKD) [64]. The benefit of blockade of the renin—angiotensin system in CKD and cardiovascular disease is due to reduction in the degree of proteinuria independent of blood pressure control. Specific characteristics of proteinuria, such as relative concentrations of albumin and total protein, can also be used for determining specific pathophysiologic states [65]. Microalbuminuria, undetectable by normal dipstick analysis (urine albumin to creatinine ratios of 30 to 300 mg/g), is associated with higher rates of cardiovascular events and suggests it is a marker of overall endothelial dysfunction rather than of renal dysfunction alone [66].

Biomarkers in Acute Kidney Injury

Cystatin C

Cystatin C is a 13 kDa protein which is produced by all nucleated cells and freely filtered by the glomerulus. There has been significant interest in using serum cystatin C levels to improve GFR estimation. It has been evaluated for use as a prognostic marker in CKD and acute kidney injury (AKI), and higher levels are associated with several adverse effects including mortality in trauma patients, development of the metabolic syndrome and risk of hip fracture [67—69]. Although initial hopes that cystatin C levels would be less affected by variations in clinical variables compared to serum creatinine, investigations have shown that cystatin C levels are influenced by lean body mass, gender, smoking, inflammation, thyroid dysfunction and steroid use [70—72]. Additionally, standardizing assays has been challenging. Nonetheless, interest in serum cystatin C has remained strong.

The utility of using increased levels of cystatin C to detect AKI prior to the traditional rise in serum creatinine levels has been intensely investigated. A 2011 meta-analysis of studies in critical care and postoperative settings found that cystatin C elevation occurred earlier in AKI than a rise in the serum creatinine level [73]. Cystatin C elevation occurring as early as 8 hours postoperatively has been shown to predict subsequent development of AKI in children undergoing cardiac surgery [74]. However, in a large prospective study of adults undergoing cardiac surgery, cystatin C elevation was less sensitive than serum creatinine for predicting development of AKI [75].

Neutrophil Gelatinase Associated Lipocalin (NGAL)

A 25 kDa protein originally isolated from neutrophils, NGAL is one of the most extensively studied renal biomarkers. Rodent ischemia-reperfusion AKI models have shown that NGAL mRNA and protein are upregulated in the kidney following an insult, and urine concentrations rapidly reach detectable levels [76]. Cisplatin-induced injury has the same effect, and in vitro work shows ischemia increases expression of NGAL in cultured human tubular cells [76]. Subsequent studies have suggested a role for NGAL in iron transport and regeneration of damaged renal tubular cells, and exogenous NGAL has been shown to mitigate ischemic AKI in animal models [77—79].

In the clinical setting, NGAL has been primarily studied in the setting of cardiac surgery. NGAL levels increase in both serum and urine early after cardiac surgery in children who later develop AKI [80]. Urinary NGAL levels early after cardiac surgery in children correlate with AKI, need for dialysis and mortality [81].

In adults, serum NGAL levels after cardiac surgery predict development of AKI independently of serum cystatin C, suggesting a complementary role for the two biomarkers [82]. A large cohort study of adult patients undergoing cardiac surgery showed that both serum and urine NGAL reached their highest levels within 6 hours after surgery. Peak serum levels in the highest 20% of the cohort were associated with five-fold odds of developing AKI [83].

In other studies, NGAL modestly predicted the development of AKI in critical illness. Among critically ill patients those with AKI from sepsis had significantly higher serum and urine NGAL levels compared to other causes of AKI [84]. However, NGAL provided modest prognostic information.

In a study of over 600 adult patients presenting to the emergency department at a large academic medical center, an elevated urinary NGAL concentration had very high sensitivity and specificity for the subsequent diagnosis of AKI [85].

Kidney Injury Molecule-1 (KIM-1)

KIM-1 is a 90-kDa transmembrane protein with immunoglobulin and mucin homology. It is overexpressed in rat proximal tubules after ischemic kidney injury and is thought to play a role in tubular epithelial repair [86,87]. KIM-1 is also expressed in human proximal tubule cells in biopsy-proven acute tubular necrosis (ATN) and soluble KIM-1 is detectable in the urine [88].

Small clinical trials assessing the utility of KIM-1 as a biomarker for early AKI have been reported. KIM-1 levels have been shown to predict adverse clinical outcomes (need for dialysis or death) in patients with established AKI [89]. In a prospective study evaluating patients undergoing cardiac surgery, postoperative KIM-1 levels showed modest power in discriminating patients who would later develop AKI [90]. Furthermore, in another group of patients undergoing cardiac surgery, preoperative KIM-1

levels were associated with higher risk of developing postoperative AKI leading to speculation that KIM-1 may be useful for predicting risk before surgery [91].

Interleukin-18 (IL-18)

IL-18 is a pro-inflammatory cytokine that was first characterized in the mid-1990s and originally named interferon-γ (IFN-γ) inducing factor [92]. Its use as a renal biomarker was demonstrated in an early murine model which found that urine IL-18 levels doubled after induction of ischemic AKI. Mice deficient in an enzyme necessary for the cleavage of an IL-18 precursor to its final form have less severe kidney injury by functional and histological measures, and less tubular neutrophil infiltration [93]. The proximal tubule seems to be both an important site of IL-18 production and IL-18-induced damage [94].

Human studies on urinary IL-18 as a biomarker have assessed a variety of kidney diseases including AKI, nephrotic syndrome and renal transplantation [95]. It was found that urine IL-18 levels are significantly higher in patients with clinically defined ATN than in those with prerenal AKI, the nephrotic syndrome, or CKD. In recently transplanted patients, lower urine IL-18 levels were associated with less tubular debris on urine microscopy and more rapid improvement in renal function. In a study of 400 critically ill patients, an increased urinary IL-18 level on admission was independently associated with an increased mortality rate although it performed poorly in predicting AKI [96].

N-acetyl-b-D-glucosaminidase (NAG)

NAG is a large enzyme (approximately twice the molecular weight of albumin) and has been investigated for use in monitoring renal dysfunction for several decades. Initial investigation was primarily in the diagnosis of drug-related renal injury, but later work has focused on a more general use in AKI. The large size of the enzyme prevents filtration by intact glomeruli so elevated urinary levels are thought to reflect release from damaged tubular epithelial cells [97]. Investigations have suggested that NAG is reliably elevated in a variety of disease states resulting in AKI, but utility has been somewhat limited because diseases affecting glomerular permeability increase urinary levels irrespective of tubular injury [98].

Biomarkers in Glomerular Disease

Soluble Urokinase Receptor (suPAR)

The existence of a so-called circulating permeability factor in primary focal segmental glomerulosclerosis (FSGS) has long been suspected because of the rapid reoccurrence in kidney allografts transplanted into some patients with the disease, and induction of disease remission with plasmapheresis [99]. SuPAR has subsequently been isolated from the serum of patients with FSGS, and has been shown to lead to FSGS-like histological and functional changes in animal studies. In the clinical setting, suPAR levels currently can be measured with commercially available assays. Levels in patients with FSGS have been shown to be significantly higher than in patients with other proteinuric glomerular diseases or healthy controls [100]. Some centers are using suPAR levels to guide therapy in patients with primary FSGS undergoing renal transplant but further work must be done to better establish the proper role of this biomarker.

Biomarker Panels in Lupus Nephritis

Nephritis is a common and morbid complication of systemic lupus erythematosis, and currently requires renal biopsy for determination of the specific variant of lupus nephritis to guide treatment. Investigations into using panels of multiple biomarkers have led to some promising findings. Urine levels of several molecules, including lipocalin-like prostaglandin D synthase

(L-PGDS), α(1)-acid glycoprotein (AAG), transferrin (TF), ceruloplasmin (CP), NGAL and monocyte chemotactic protein 1 (MCP-1) were found to correlate in different combinations with nephritis activity, chronicity and presence of the membranous nephritis subtype [101].

Proteomics

This technique has been applied to the study of urine proteins in renal disease. A model developed to determine cause of nephrotic syndrome based on analysis of urine protein components in patients with FSGS, lupus nephritis, membranous nephropathy and diabetic nephropathy found that the pattern of the various proteins, including orosomucoid, transferrin α-1 antitrypsin, haptoglobin and transthyretin, were different among the diseases allowing significant discrimination [102]. Study of urine proteins in patients with anti-neutrophil cytoplasmic antibody-associated (ANCA) vasculitis enabled development of a model with approximately 90% sensitivity and specificity for ANCA vasculitis compared to controls with other renal diseases [103].

SUMMARY

In the age of personalized medicine the use of specific biomarkers is the next step to individualize therapy at a molecular or mechanistic level. Oncology has played a pivotal role in advancing this field by identification of molecules or mutations that have led to specific drug development and targeted therapies. In addition, many of these biomarkers can be used to improve risk assessment and the likelihood of responding to treatment. On the other hand, the role of biomarkers in nephrology is still in its infancy. Although numerous molecules have been identified and studied, they have yet to enter the realm of clinical practice and are still undergoing validation. In this area of medicine nephrology should follow the lead of their oncology colleagues.

Acknowledgments

The authors would like to thank Mika Stepankiw for her editorial support.

References

[1] Pepe MS, et al. Phases of biomarker development for the early detection of cancer. J Natl Cancer Int 2001;93:1054–61.

[2] Srivastvas S, Gopal-Srivastvas R. Biomarkers in cancer screening: a public health perspective. J Nutr 2002;132:2471S–5S.

[3] Ludwig JA, Weinstein JN. Biomarkers in cancer staging, prognosis and treatment selection. Nat Rev Cancer 2005;5(11):845–56.

[4] Bruix J, Sherman M. Management of hepatocellular carcinoma: an update. Hepatology 2011;53(3): 1020–2.

[5] Gilligan TD, et al. American Society of Clinical Oncology Clinical Practice Guideline on uses of serum tumor markers in adult males with germ cell tumors. J Clin Oncol 2010;28(20):3388–404.

[6] Duffy MJ, et al. Tumor markers in pancreatic cancer: a European Group on Tumor Markers (EGTM) status report. Ann Oncol 2010;21(3):441–7.

[7] Berger AC, Garcia Jr M, Hoffman JP, Regine WF, Abrams RA, Safran H, et al. Postresection CA 19-9 predicts overall survival in patients with pancreatic cancer treated with adjuvant chemoradiation: a prospective validation by RTOG 9704. J Clin Oncol 2008;26(36):5918–22.

[8] Bast Jr RC, et al. A radioimmunoassay using a monoclonal antibody to monitor the course of epithelial ovarian cancer. N Engl J Med 1983;309(15): 883–7.

[9] Rodriguez-Moranta F, et al. Postoperative surveillance in patients with colorectal cancer who have undergone curative resection: a prospective, multicenter, randomized, controlled trial. J Clin Oncol 2006;24(3):386–93.

[10] Yao JC, et al. Daily oral everolimus activity in patients with metastatic pancreatic neuroendocrine tumors after failure of cytotoxic chemotherapy: a phase II trial. J Clin Oncol 2010;28(1):69–76.

[11] Flechon A, et al. Phase II study of carboplatin and etoposide in patients with anaplastic progressive metastatic castration-resistant prostate cancer (mCRPC) with or without neuroendocrine differentiation: results of the French Genito-Urinary Tumor Group (GETUG) P01 trial. Ann Oncol 2011;22(11):2476–81.

[12] Ronkainen H, Soini Y, Vaarala MH, Kauppila S, Hirvikoski P. Evaluation of neuroendocrine markers in renal cell carcinoma. Diagn Pathol 2010;5:28.

[13] Yao JC, et al. Chromogranin A and neuron-specific enolase as prognostic markers in patients with advanced pNET treated with everolimus. J Clin Endocrinol Metab 2011;96(12):3741–9.

[14] Hirose T, et al. Are levels of pro-gastrin-releasing peptide or neuron-specific enolase at relapse prognostic factors after relapse in patients with small-cell lung cancer? Lung Cancer 2011;71(2):224–8.

[15] Catalona WJ, Smith DS, Ornstein DK. Prostate cancer detection in men with serum PSA concentrations of 2.6 to 4.0 ng/mL and benign prostate examination. Enhancement of specificity with free PSA measurements. JAMA 1997;277(18):1452–5.

[16] Catalona WJ, et al. Use of the percentage of free prostate-specific antigen to enhance differentiation of prostate cancer from benign prostatic disease: a prospective multicenter clinical trial. JAMA 1998;279(19):1542–7.

[17] Oesterling JE, et al. Serum prostate-specific antigen in a community-based population of healthy men. Establishment of age-specific reference ranges. JAMA 1993;270(7):860–4.

[18] D'Amico AV, Chen MH, Roehl KA, Catalona WJ. Preoperative PSA velocity and the risk of death from prostate cancer after radical prostatectomy. N Engl J Med 2004;351(2):125–35.

[19] Vickers AJ, Till C, Tangen CM, Lilja H, Thompson IM. An empirical evaluation of guidelines on prostate-specific antigen velocity in prostate cancer detection. J Natl Cancer Inst 2011;103(6):462–9.

[20] Chang SL, Harshman LC, Presti Jr JC. Impact of common medications on serum total prostate-specific antigen levels: analysis of the National Health and Nutrition Examination Survey. J Clin Oncol 2010;28(25):3951–7.

[21] Paik S, et al. A multigene assay to predict recurrence of tamoxifen-treated, node-negative breast cancer. N Engl J Med 2004;351(27):2817–26.

[22] Choi YL, et al. EML4-ALK mutations in lung cancer that confer resistance to ALK inhibitors. N Engl J Med 2010;363(18):1734–9.

[23] Faderl S, Talpaz M, Estrov Z, O'Brien S, Kurzrock R, Kantarjian HM. The biology of chronic myeloid leukemia. N Engl J Med 1999;341(3):164–72.

[24] Kantarjian H, Sawyers C, Hochhaus A, Guilhot F, Schiffer C, Gambacorti-Passerini C, et al. Hematologic and cytogenetic responses to imatinib mesylate in chronic myelogenous leukemia. N Engl J Med 2002;346(9):645–52.

[25] Flaherty KT, et al. Inhibition of mutated, activated BRAF in metastatic melanoma. N Engl J Med 2010;363(9):809–19.

[26] Chapman PB, et al. Improved survival with vemurafenib in melanoma with BRAF V600E mutation. N Engl J Med 2011;364(26):2507–16.

[27] Cheson BD, Leonard JP. Monoclonal antibody therapy for B-cell non-Hodgkin's lymphoma. N Engl J Med 2008;359(6):613–26.

[28] Kaminski MS, et al. 131I-tositumomab therapy as initial treatment for follicular lymphoma. N Engl J Med 2005;352(5):441–9.

[29] Sokolova IA, et al. The development of a multitarget, multicolor fluorescence in situ hybridization assay for the detection of urothelial carcinoma in urine. J Mol Diagn 2000;2(3):116–23.

[30] Kipp BR, et al. A comparison of routine cytology and fluorescence in situ hybridization for the detection of malignant bile duct strictures. Am J Gastroenterol 2004;99(9):1675–81.

[31] Hoang-Xuan K, et al. Temozolomide as initial treatment for adults with low-grade oligodendrogliomas or oligoastrocytomas and correlation with chromosome 1p deletions. J Clin Oncol 2004;22(15):3133–8.

[32] Kaloshi G, et al. Temozolomide for low-grade gliomas: predictive impact of 1p/19q loss on response and outcome. Neurology 2007;68(21):1831–6.

[33] Allard WJ, et al. Tumor cells circulate in the peripheral blood of all major carcinomas but not in healthy subjects or patients with nonmalignant diseases. Clin Cancer Res 2004;10(20):6897–904.

[34] Cristofanilli M, et al. Circulating tumor cells, disease progression, and survival in metastatic breast cancer. N Engl J Med 2004;351(8):781–91.

[35] Markowitz SD, Bertagnolli MM. Molecular origins of cancer: molecular basis of colorectal cancer. N Engl J Med 2009;361(25):2449–60.

[36] Ribic CM, et al. Tumor microsatellite-instability status as a predictor of benefit from fluorouracil-based adjuvant chemotherapy for colon cancer. N Engl J Med 2003;349(3):247–57.

[37] Paez JG, et al. EGFR mutations in lung cancer: correlation with clinical response to gefitinib therapy. Science 2004;304(5676):1497–500.

[38] Lynch TJ, et al. Activating mutations in the epidermal growth factor receptor underlying responsiveness of non-small-cell lung cancer to gefitinib. N Engl J Med 2004;350(21):2129–39.

[39] Tsao MS, et al. Erlotinib in lung cancer — molecular and clinical predictors of outcome. N Engl J Med 2005;353(2):133–44.

[40] Sequist LV, et al. First-line gefitinib in patients with advanced non-small-cell lung cancer harboring somatic EGFR mutations. J Clin Oncol 2008;26(15):2442–9.

[41] Maemondo M, et al. Gefitinib or chemotherapy for non-small-cell lung cancer with mutated EGFR. N Engl J Med 2010;362(25):2380–8.

[42] Maheswaran S, et al. Detection of mutations in EGFR in circulating lung-cancer cells. N Engl J Med 2008;359(4):366–77.

[43] Zheng Z, Chen T, Li X, Haura E, Sharma A, Bepler G. DNA synthesis and repair genes RRM1 and ERCC1 in lung cancer. N Engl J Med 2007;356(8):800–8.

[44] Olaussen KA, et al. DNA repair by ERCC1 in non-small-cell lung cancer and cisplatin-based adjuvant chemotherapy. N Engl J Med 2006;355(10):983–91.

[45] Reynolds C, et al. Randomized phase III trial of gemcitabine-based chemotherapy with in situ RRM1 and ERCC1 protein levels for response prediction in non-small-cell lung cancer. J Clin Oncol 2009;27(34):5808–15.

[46] Allred DC, et al. NCCN Task Force Report: estrogen receptor and progesterone receptor testing in breast cancer by immunohistochemistry. J Natl Compr Canc Netw 2009;7(Suppl. 6):S1–21. quiz S22–3.

[47] Hammond ME, et al. American Society of Clinical Oncology/College of American Pathologists guideline recommendations for immunohistochemical testing of estrogen and progesterone receptors in breast cancer. J Clin Oncol 2010;28(16):2784–95.

[48] Carlson RW, et al. HER2 testing in breast cancer: NCCN Task Force report and recommendations. J Natl Compr Canc Netw 2006;4(Suppl. 3):S1–22. quiz S23–4.

[49] Bang YJ, et al. Trastuzumab in combination with chemotherapy versus chemotherapy alone for treatment of HER2-positive advanced gastric or gastro-oesophageal junction cancer (ToGA): a phase 3, open-label, randomised controlled trial. Lancet 2010;376(9742):687–97.

[50] D'Souza C, et al. Case–control study of human papillomavirus and oropharyngeal cancer. N Engl J Med 2007;356(19):1944–56.

[51] Chaturvedi AK, Engels EA, Anderson WF, Gillison ML. Incidence trends for human papillomavirus-related and -unrelated oral squamous cell carcinomas in the United States. J Clin Oncol 2008;26(4):612–9.

[52] Ang KK, et al. Human papillomavirus and survival of patients with oropharyngeal cancer. N Engl J Med 2010;363(1):24–35.

[53] Demetri GD, et al. Efficacy and safety of imatinib mesylate in advanced gastrointestinal stromal tumors. N Engl J Med 2002;347(7):472–80.

[54] Slebos RJ, et al. K-ras oncogene activation as a prognostic marker in adenocarcinoma of the lung. N Engl J Med 1990;323(9):561–5.

[55] Eberhard DA, et al. Mutations in the epidermal growth factor receptor and in KRAS are predictive and prognostic indicators in patients with non-small-cell lung cancer treated with chemotherapy alone and in combination with erlotinib. J Clin Oncol 2005;23(25):5900–9.

[56] Van Cutsem E, et al. Cetuximab and chemotherapy as initial treatment for metastatic colorectal cancer. N Engl J Med 2009;360(14):1408–17.

[57] Karapetis CS, et al. K-ras mutations and benefit from cetuximab in advanced colorectal cancer. N Engl J Med 2008;359(17):1757–65.

[58] Jonker DJ, et al. Cetuximab for the treatment of colorectal cancer. N Engl J Med 2007;357 (20):2040–8.

[59] Bartel DP. MicroRNAs: target recognition and regulatory functions. Cell 2009;136(2):215–33.

[60] Roth C, Rack B, Muller V, Janni W, Pantel K, Schwarzenbach H. Circulating microRNAs as blood-based markers for patients with primary and metastatic breast cancer. Breast Cancer Res 2010;12(6):R90.

[61] Schwarzenbach H, Hoon DS, Pantel K. Cell-free nucleic acids as biomarkers in cancer patients. Nat Rev Cancer 2011;11(6):426–37.

[62] Colls PC. Notes on creatinine. J Physiol 1896;20(2–3): 107–11.

[63] Myers VL, W.. The creatinin of the blood in nephritis. Its diagnostic value. Ann Intern Med 1915;xvi.

[64] Gerstein HC, et al. Albuminuria and risk of cardiovascular events, death, and heart failure in diabetic and nondiabetic individuals. JAMA 2001;286(4): 421–6.

[65] Peterson JC, et al. Blood pressure control, proteinuria, and the progression of renal disease. The Modification of Diet in Renal Disease Study. Ann Intern Med 1995;123(10):754–62.

[66] Ohisa N, et al. A comparison of urinary albumin-total protein ratio to phase-contrast microscopic examination of urine sediment for differentiating glomerular and nonglomerular bleeding. Am J Kidney Dis 2008;52(2):235–41.

[67] Glassock RJ. Is the presence of microalbuminuria a relevant marker of kidney disease? Curr Hypertens Rep 2010;12(5):364–8.

[68] Senturk GO, et al. The prognostic value of cystatin C compared with trauma scores in multiple blunt trauma: a prospective cohort study. J Emerg Med 2013;44(6):1070–6.

[69] Magnusson M, et al. High levels of cystatin C predict the metabolic syndrome: the prospective Malmo Diet and Cancer Study. J Intern Med Epub 2013; Feb 18.

[70] Ensrud KE, et al. Cystatin C and risk of hip fractures in older women. J Bone Miner Res 2013;28(6):1175–82.

[71] Knight EL, et al. Factors influencing serum cystatin C levels other than renal function and the impact on renal function measurement. Kidney Int 2004;65(4): 1416–21.

[72] MacDonald J, et al. GFR estimation using cystatin C is not independent of body composition. Am J Kidney Dis 2006;48(5):712–9.

[73] Inker LA, Okparavero A. Cystatin C as a marker of glomerular filtration rate: prospects and limitations. Curr Opin Nephrol Hypertens 2011;20(6):631–9.

[74] Zhang Z, et al. Cystatin C in prediction of acute kidney injury: a systemic review and meta-analysis. Am J Kidney Dis 2011;58(3):356–65.

[75] Hassinger AB, et al. Predictive power of serum cystatin C to detect acute kidney injury and pediatric-modified RIFLE class in children undergoing cardiac surgery. Pediatr Crit Care Med 2012;13(4):435–40.

[76] Spahillari A, et al. Serum cystatin C- versus creatinine-based definitions of acute kidney injury following cardiac surgery: a prospective cohort study. Am J Kidney Dis 2012;60(6):922–9.

[77] Mishra J, et al. Identification of neutrophil gelatinase-associated lipocalin as a novel early urinary biomarker for ischemic renal injury. J Am Soc Nephrol 2003;14(10):2534–43.

[78] Yang J, et al. Iron, lipocalin, and kidney epithelia. Am J Physiol Renal Physiol 2003;285(1):F9–18.

[79] Mori K, et al. Endocytic delivery of lipocalin-siderophore-iron complex rescues the kidney from ischemia-reperfusion injury. J Clin Invest 2005;115(3): 610–21.

[80] Mishra J, et al. Amelioration of ischemic acute renal injury by neutrophil gelatinase-associated lipocalin. J Am Soc Nephrol 2004;15(12):3073–82.

[81] Mishra J, et al. Neutrophil gelatinase-associated lipocalin (NGAL) as a biomarker for acute renal injury after cardiac surgery. Lancet 2005;365(9466):1231–8.

[82] Bennett M, et al. Urine NGAL predicts severity of acute kidney injury after cardiac surgery: a prospective study. Clin J Am Soc Nephrol 2008;3(3): 665–73.

[83] Haase-Fielitz A, et al. Novel and conventional serum biomarkers predicting acute kidney injury in adult cardiac surgery — a prospective cohort study. Crit Care Med 2009;37(2):553–60.

[84] Parikh CR, et al. Postoperative biomarkers predict acute kidney injury and poor outcomes after adult

cardiac surgery. J Am Soc Nephrol 2011;22(9): 1748–57.

[85] Nickolas TL, et al. Sensitivity and specificity of a single emergency department measurement of urinary neutrophil gelatinase-associated lipocalin for diagnosing acute kidney injury. Ann Intern Med 2008;148(11):810–9.

[86] Ichimura T, et al. Kidney injury molecule-1 (KIM-1), a putative epithelial cell adhesion molecule containing a novel immunoglobulin domain, is up-regulated in renal cells after injury. J Biol Chem 1998;273(7): 4135–42.

[87] Bailly V, et al. Shedding of kidney injury molecule-1, a putative adhesion protein involved in renal regeneration. J Biol Chem 2002;277(42): 39739–48.

[88] Han WK, et al. Kidney Injury Molecule-1 (KIM-1): a novel biomarker for human renal proximal tubule injury. Kidney Int 2002;62(1):237–44.

[89] Liangos O, et al. Urinary N-acetyl-beta-(D)-glucosaminidase activity and kidney injury molecule-1 level are associated with adverse outcomes in acute renal failure. J Am Soc Nephrol 2007;18(3):904–12.

[90] Han WK, et al. Urinary biomarkers in the early detection of acute kidney injury after cardiac surgery. Clin J Am Soc Nephrol 2009;4(5):873–82.

[91] Koyner JL, et al. Urinary biomarkers in the clinical prognosis and early detection of acute kidney injury. Clin J Am Soc Nephrol 2010;5(12):2154–65.

[92] Peralta CA, et al. Associations of urinary levels of kidney injury molecule 1 (KIM-1) and neutrophil gelatinase-associated lipocalin (NGAL) with kidney function decline in the Multi-Ethnic Study of Atherosclerosis (MESA). Am J Kidney Dis 2012;60(6): 904–11.

[93] Bhavsar NA, et al. Neutrophil gelatinase-associated lipocalin (NGAL) and kidney injury molecule 1

(KIM-1) as predictors of incident CKD stage 3: the Atherosclerosis Risk in Communities (ARIC) Study. Am J Kidney Dis 2012;60(2):233–40.

[94] Dinarello CA. Interleukin-18. Methods 1999;19(1): 121–32.

[95] Melnikov VY, et al. Impaired IL-18 processing protects caspase-1-deficient mice from ischemic acute renal failure. J Clin Invest 2001;107(9): 1145–52.

[96] Melnikov VY, et al. Neutrophil-independent mechanisms of caspase-1- and IL-18-mediated ischemic acute tubular necrosis in mice. J Clin Invest 2002;110(8):1083–91.

[97] Parikh CR, et al. Urinary interleukin-18 is a marker of human acute tubular necrosis. Am J Kidney Dis 2004;43(3):405–14.

[98] Siew ED, et al. Elevated urinary IL-18 levels at the time of ICU admission predict adverse clinical outcomes. Clin J Am Soc Nephrol 2010;5(8): 1497–505.

[99] Shankland SJ, Pollak MR. A suPAR circulating factor causes kidney disease. Nat Med 2011;17(8):926–7.

[100] Wei C, et al. Circulating urokinase receptor as a cause of focal segmental glomerulosclerosis. Nat Med 2011;17(8):952–60.

[101] Brunner HI, et al. Association of noninvasively measured renal protein biomarkers with histologic features of lupus nephritis. Arthritis Rheum 2012;64(8):2687–97.

[102] Varghese SA, et al. Urine biomarkers predict the cause of glomerular disease. J Am Soc Nephrol 2007;18(3):913–22.

[103] Haubitz M, et al. Identification and validation of urinary biomarkers for differential diagnosis and evaluation of therapeutic intervention in antineutrophil cytoplasmic antibody-associated vasculitis. Mol Cell Proteomics 2009;8(10):2296–307.

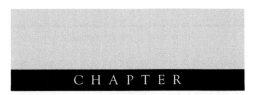

Tumor Lysis Syndrome

Scott C. Howard, Ching-Hon Pui, Raul C. Ribeiro

St. Jude Children's Research Hospital, Memphis, TN, USA and University of Tennessee Health
Sciences Center, College of Medicine, Memphis, TN, USA

INTRODUCTION

Tumor lysis syndrome (TLS) is the most common disease-related emergency of children or adults with hematologic cancers [1–4]. It develops most often in patients with acute leukemia (Figure 4.1) or non-Hodgkin lymphoma (Figure 4.2), and is the most common cause of

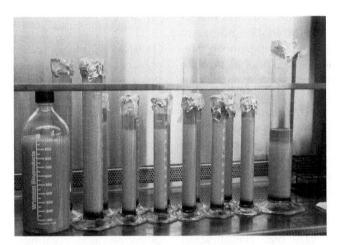

FIGURE 4.1 Leukemia cells removed by leukapheresis. The graduated cylinders contain leukemic cells removed by leukapheresis from a patient with T-cell acute lymphoblastic leukemia and hyperleukocytosis (white blood cell count 365,000 per cubic millimeter). Each cylinder contains straw-colored clear plasma at the top, a thick layer of white leukemic cells in the middle, and a thin layer of red cells at the bottom. This figure is reproduced in color in the color plate section. *Reprinted from Howard et al. [12] with the permission of the publisher.*

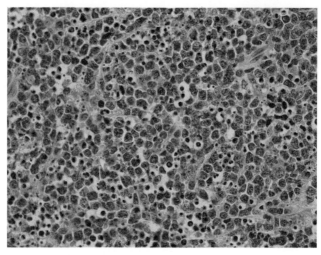

FIGURE 4.2 **Burkitt lymphoma of the appendix.** The highly cellular nature of Burkitt lymphoma is evident (hematoxylin and eosin). This figure is reproduced in color in the color plate section. *Reprinted from Howard et al. [12] with the permission of the publisher.*

acute kidney injury (AKI) in patients with these cancers. Furthermore, its frequency is increasing among patients whose tumors were once rarely associated with this complication, including chronic lymphocytic leukemia and solid tumors [5–11]. Classic TLS occurs when tumor cells lyse and release their contents into the bloodstream, leading to the characteristic findings of hyperuricemia, hyperkalemia, hyperphosphatemia and hypocalcemia [1–3]. These electrolyte and metabolic disturbances can progress to clinical toxicities, including acute kidney injury, cardiac arrhythmias, seizures and death due to multi-organ failure. New kinds of tumor lysis syndrome have been described, in which the predominant metabolic abnormalities result from the release of specific contents of cancer cells, such as cytoplasmic granules in eosinophilic leukemia. This chapter reviews the pathophysiology and epidemiology of TLS, provides recommendations for TLS risk classification for patients with newly diagnosed cancer, and suggests management strategies for each risk group. Recommendations are based on published guidelines for risk stratification, expert

panel recommendations, emerging literature and personal experience [2,12,13].

DEFINITION OF TUMOR LYSIS SYNDROME

TLS is classified as laboratory or clinical TLS (Table 4.1) [2,14,15]. Laboratory TLS requires the presence of two or more metabolic abnormalities (hyperuricemia, hyperkalemia, hyperphosphatemia, hypocalcemia) and clinical TLS is present when laboratory TLS is accompanied by an increased creatinine level that meets the definition of acute kidney injury, seizures, cardiac dysrhythmia or death attributed to hypocalcemia or hyperkalemia. Laboratory abnormalities should be present simultaneously because some patients may present with one abnormality but later develop another one unrelated to TLS, such as an elevated creatinine due to dehydration followed by hypocalcemia associated with sepsis or aggressive hydration with normal saline.

To establish the diagnosis of TLS, metabolic abnormalities should occur within 3 days before

TABLE 4.1 Definitions of Laboratory and Clinical Tumor Lysis Syndrome

Metabolic abnormality	Criteria to define laboratory TLS (two or more abnormalities must be present during the same 24-hour period from 3 days before starting therapy until 7 days afterwards)	Criteria to define clinical TLS (presence of laboratory TLS plus any one of the following clinical conditions)
Hyperuricemia	Uric acid >8.0 mg/dL (475.8 μmol/liter) in adults or > the upper limit of normal for age in children	
Hyper-phosphatemia	Phosphorus >4.5 mg/dL (1.5 mmol/L) in adults or >6.5 mg/dL (2.1 mmol/L) in children	
Hyperkalemia	Potassium >6.0 mmol/L	Cardiac dysrhythmia, sudden death probably or definitely caused by hyperkalemia
Hypocalcemia	Corrected calcium* <7.0 mg/dL or ionized calcium <1.12 mmol/L	Cardiac dysrhythmia, sudden death, seizure, neuromuscular irritability (tetany, paresthesias, muscle twitching, carpopedal spasm, Trousseau's sign, Chvostek's sign, laryngospasm or bronchospasm), hypotension, or heart failure probably or definitely caused by hypocalcemia
Acute kidney injury [79]**	Not present in laboratory TLS	Increase in the serum creatinine level of 0.3 mg/dL (or a single value >1.5 times the upper limit of the age-appropriate normal range if no baseline creatinine is available) or the presence of oliguria, defined as an average urine output less than 0.5 mL/kg body weight per hour for 6 hours

Corrected calcium concentration [mg/dL] = measured calcium concentration [mg/dL] + 0.8 × (4 − albumin [g/dL]).
** Acute kidney injury is defined as an increase in creatinine of at least 0.3 mg/dL or a period of oliguria lasting 6 hours or more. By definition, if acute kidney injury is present the patient has clinical TLS.
TLS, tumor lysis syndrome.
Reprinted from Howard et al. [12] with the permission of the publisher.

or up to 7 days after initiation of therapy. However, exceptions may occur, such as the patient who fails to respond to initial therapy, but has a brisk response to subsequent therapy, such that tumor lysis occurs within 7 days of initiation of the subsequent, more effective, treatment. This situation is most common in patients with acute lymphoblastic leukemia who are treated with an initial week of prednisone but have prednisone-resistant disease. The leukocyte count may increase during initial therapy with prednisone, but drop precipitously when standard four-drug remission induction therapy is initiated.

PATHOPHYSIOLOGY

When cancer cells lyse, they release potassium, phosphorus and nucleic acids, which are metabolized into hypoxanthine, then xanthine and finally uric acid, an end product in humans (Figure 4.3) [15,16]. Hyperkalemia can cause serious and occasionally fatal dysrhythmias. Hyperphosphatemia can cause secondary hypocalcemia leading to neuromuscular irritability (tetany), dysrhythmia and seizure. Hyperphosphatemia can also cause precipitation as calcium phosphate crystals in various organs

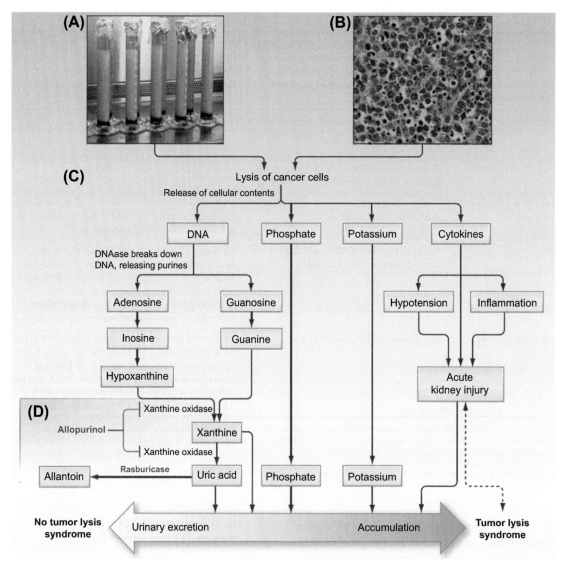

FIGURE 4.3 Lysis of tumor cells and the release of DNA, phosphate, potassium and cytokines. The graduated cylinders shown in Panel A contain leukemic cells removed by leukapheresis from a patient with T-cell acute lymphoblastic leukemia and hyperleukocytosis (white cell count, 365,000 per cubic millimeter). Each cylinder contains straw-colored clear plasma at the top, a thick layer of white leukemic cells in the middle and a thin layer of red cells at the bottom. The highly cellular nature of Burkitt lymphoma is evident in Panel B (Burkitt lymphoma of the appendix, hematoxylin and eosin). Lysis of cancer cells (Panel C) releases DNA, phosphate, potassium and cytokines. DNA released from the lysed cells is metabolized into adenosine and guanosine, both of which are converted into xanthine. Xanthine is then oxidized by xanthine oxidase, leading to the production of uric acid, which is excreted by the kidneys. When the accumulation of phosphate, potassium, xanthine, or uric acid is more rapid than excretion, the tumor lysis syndrome develops. Cytokines cause hypotension, inflammation and acute kidney injury, which increase the risk for the tumor lysis syndrome. The bidirectional dashed line between acute kidney injury and tumor lysis syndrome indicates that acute kidney injury increases

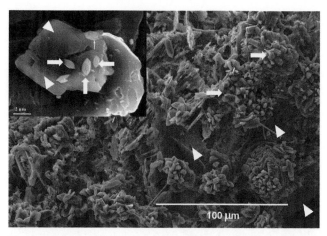

FIGURE 4.4 **Crystals of uric acid, calcium phosphate and calcium oxalate.** Crystallization of uric acid and calcium phosphate are the primary means of renal damage in the tumor lysis syndrome. The presence of crystals of one solute can promote crystallization of the other solutes. These scanning electron micrographs show large uric acid crystals (arrowheads), which served as seeds for the formation of calcium oxalate crystals (arrows). *Reprinted from Bouropoulos et al. [86] and Grases et al. [87] with the permission of the publishers.*

including kidneys with the potential to cause acute kidney injury (Figures 4.4, 4.5 and 4.6) [17]. Uric acid can induce acute kidney injury not only by intrarenal crystallization but also by crystal-independent mechanisms including renal vasoconstriction, impaired autoregulation, decreased renal blood flow, oxidation, and inflammation [18–20]. Tumor lysis also releases cytokines that cause a systemic inflammatory response syndrome and often multi-organ failure [21–23].

TLS occurs when the amount of potassium, phosphorus, nucleic acids and cytokines released from cell lysis exceeds the body's homeostatic mechanisms to deal with them. Renal excretion is the primary means of clearing urate, xanthine and phosphate which can precipitate in any part of the renal collecting system. The large

capacity of kidneys to excrete these solutes makes clinical TLS unlikely without first developing nephropathy and a consequent inability to excrete solutes quickly enough to cope with the metabolic load.

Crystal-induced tissue injury occurs in TLS when calcium phosphate, uric acid or xanthine precipitate in renal tubules and cause inflammation and obstruction (Figure 4.5) [24,25]. High solute concentration, low solubility, slow urine flow and high concentrations of co-crystallizing substances favor crystal formation and worsen TLS [26–28]. The presence of high concentrations of both uric acid and phosphate renders patients with TLS at particularly high risk of crystal-associated AKI because uric acid precipitates more readily in the presence of calcium phosphate and vice versa (Figure 4.5).

the risk of the tumor lysis syndrome by reducing the ability of the kidneys to excrete uric acid, xanthine, phosphate and potassium. By the same token, development of the tumor lysis syndrome can cause acute kidney injury by renal precipitation of uric acid, xanthine and calcium phosphate crystals and by crystal independent mechanisms. Allopurinol inhibits xanthine oxidase (Panel D) and prevents the conversion of hypoxanthine and xanthine into uric acid but does not remove existing uric acid. In contrast, rasburicase removes uric acid by enzymatically degrading it into allantoin, a highly soluble product that has no known adverse effects on health. This figure is reproduced in color in the color plate section. *Reprinted from Howard et al. [12] with the permission of the publisher.*

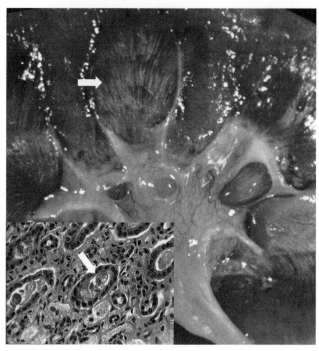

FIGURE 4.5 Renal findings in a child with fatal tumor lysis syndrome. The kidney shown was examined at the autopsy of a 4-year-old boy who had high-grade non-Hodgkin lymphoma and died of acute tumor lysis syndrome. Linear yellow streaks of precipitated uric acid in the renal medulla are shown (arrow); a single tubule containing a uric acid crystal (arrow) is shown in the panel. This figure is reproduced in color in the color plate section. *Reprinted from Howard et al. [17] with the permission of the publisher.*

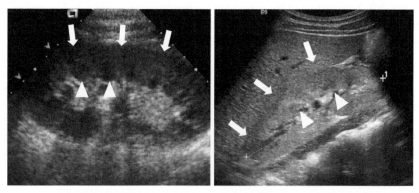

Normal kidney   **Kidney in a patient with TLS**

FIGURE 4.6 Sonographic appearance of a normal kidney and a kidney with acute kidney injury. In the normal kidney on the left, the medullary pyramids are visible deep in the kidney (arrowheads) and are surrounded by the renal cortex (arrows), which is darker than the collecting system and adjacent liver. The ultrasonographic image on the right shows a kidney from a patient with the tumor lysis syndrome, in which there is loss of the normal corticomedullary differentiation (arrowheads) and poor visualization of the renal pyramids. The brightness is similar to that of the adjacent liver (arrows), and the kidney is abnormally enlarged.

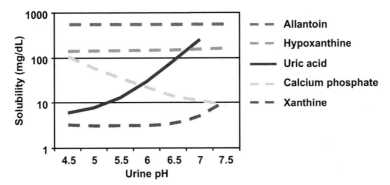

FIGURE 4.7 Solubility of metabolites important in tumor lysis syndrome over a range of physiologic urine pH values. Uric acid solubility is highly pH dependent. As urine pH rises from 5 to 7, the solubility increases 25-fold, from 8 to 200 mg/dL. This increased uric acid solubility and consequent decreased risk of crystal formation and acute kidney injury is the reason urine alkalinization was standard for patients at risk for tumor lysis syndrome prior to the advent of rasburicase. In contrast to uric acid, calcium phosphate becomes less soluble and more likely to crystallize as urine pH increases. Xanthine has low solubility and hypoxanthine relatively high solubility, regardless of urine pH. Note that the scale is logarithmic. This figure is reproduced in color in the color plate section. *Reprinted from Howard et al. [17] with the permission of the publisher.*

Also, higher urine pH increases the solubility of uric acid but decreases that of calcium phosphate (Figure 4.7). In patients treated with allopurinol, the accumulation of xanthine, a precursor of uric acid that has low solubility regardless of urine pH, could lead to xanthine nephropathy or urolithiasis (Figure 4.4) [24,29].

Calcium phosphate can precipitate throughout the body, particularly when the calcium × phosphate product is high (more than 60) (Figure 4.8). The risk of ectopic calcification is particularly high when patients require intravenous calcium [17]. When calcium phosphate precipitates in the cardiac conducting system, serious and occasionally fatal dysrhythmias can occur.

TUMOR LYSIS SYNDROME: ONE SYNDROME OR SEVERAL?

Tumor lysis syndrome is classically defined by elevations in phosphorus, potassium and uric acid that are associated with nephropathy and hypocalcemia in the context of rapid lysis of tumor cells [12,30]. However, patients with specific subtypes of leukemia, such as acute

myeloid leukemia FAB subtypes M4 or M5, may have a type of TLS in which hyperuricemia and hyperphosphatemia are not the major pathophysiologic abnormalities [21,31,32]. For example, acute myelomonoblastic leukemia

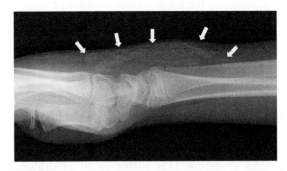

FIGURE 4.8 Soft-tissue calcification of the dorsum of the distal forearm. This soft tissue calcification of the dorsum of the distal forearm occurred in a 15-year-old boy with acute lymphoblastic leukemia and an initial white cell count of 283,000 per cubic millimeter in whom tumor lysis syndrome, hyperphosphatemia and symptomatic hypocalcemia developed. Several weeks after the treatment of hypocalcemia with multiple doses of intravenous calcium gluconate administered by means of a peripheral intravenous catheter in the dorsum of the hand, ectopic calcification was confirmed radiographically (arrows). *Reprinted from Howard et al. [17] with the permission of the publisher.*

cells contain lysozyme and granules that contain vasoactive substances, such as histamine and cytokines, that can cause inflammation and tissue damage when released [21,31,32]. Treatment for this form of TLS includes supportive care, suspension of chemotherapy and administration of high-dose glucocorticoids plus antihistamines; leukotriene receptor agonists may also aid in recovery. In some cases, renal tubular damage caused by lysozyme can result in hypokalemia [33]. Another syndrome that results from lysis of tumor cells occurs with acute promyelocytic leukemia, in which cell lysis causes coagulopathy and disseminated intravascular coagulation [34]. In all cases, the syndrome produced by tumor lysis depends on the contents of the cells lysed and the types of tissue damaged. Although clinicians should be aware of special cases that produce specific clinical manifestations, such as patients with acute promyelocytic leukemia or acute myeloid leukemia M4 or M5, by far the most common manifestations of tumor lysis are those of classically defined TLS, which is the focus of this chapter [2,35,36].

EPIDEMIOLOGY AND RISK FACTORS

The incidence and severity of TLS depend on the cancer mass, cell lysis potential, patient characteristics and supportive care (Table 4.2, Figure 4.9). The historical absence of standard criteria to define TLS, inclusion of laboratory TLS in some studies versus only clinical TLS in others, and variability of patient cohorts further contribute to a wide range of reported incidences (Table 4.3) [2,37].

Cancer Cell Mass and Lysis Potential

The greater the cancer cell mass, the greater the quantity of cellular contents released when effective anti-cancer therapy causes cell lysis [12]. By the same token, the greater the cancer cell lysis potential, the more rapidly the cells release their contents when exposed to effective therapy. Caution must be used when new therapies are introduced, since the term "effective therapy" changes when new agents are used in patients with a significant cancer cell mass (as opposed to use as part of consolidation therapy for those already in remission). Historically, cancers with high cell lysis potential included high-grade lymphomas, acute leukemias and other rapidly proliferating tumors, but examples of TLS in new cancer types have proliferated in recent years. For example, Krishnan and colleagues reported a case of fatal TLS after cetuximab treatment in an adult with metastatic colon carcinoma, a cancer in which TLS had not been previously reported [5], and Michels and colleagues documented TLS in renal cell carcinoma treated with sunitinib [38]. TLS has now been reported in neuroblastoma, endometrial cancer, colon carcinoma, renal cell carcinoma, hepatocellular carcinoma, chronic lymphocytic leukemia, chronic myelogenous leukemia and other cancers [5–8,39–44]. Indeed, TLS has been the dose-limiting toxicity in studies of patients with chronic lymphocytic leukemia treated with flavopiridol [9].

Patient Characteristics

High-risk patient characteristics include pre-existing chronic renal insufficiency, dehydration, hypotension, acidic urine and oliguria [2]. Patients with chronic renal insufficiency have less reserve and those who present with dehydration or hypotension have decreased renal perfusion, which puts them at higher risk for AKI. When the urine is acidic at presentation, increased uric acid crystals will have formed in the renal collecting system and initiated the inflammatory cascade that leads to renal tubular damage and AKI (Figure 4.5) [2,12].

TABLE 4.2 Risk Factors for Tumor Lysis Syndrome

Risk factor category	Risk factor	Comments
Cancer mass	Bulky tumor or extensive metastasis	The larger the cancer mass or the higher the number of cells that will lyse with treatment, the higher the risk of clinical TLS.
	Organ infiltration by cancer cells	Hepatomegaly, splenomegaly and nephromegaly generally represent tumor infiltration into these organs, and therefore a larger tumor burden than that of patients without these findings.
	Bone marrow involvement	Healthy adults have 1.4 kg of bone marrow. A marrow that has been replaced by leukemic cells contains a cancer mass greater than 1 kg and therefore represents bulky disease.
	Renal infiltration or outflow tract obstruction	Cancers that infiltrate the kidney or obstruct urine flow predispose to nephropathy from other causes, such as TLS.
Cell lysis potential	High cancer cell proliferation rate	Lactate dehydrogenase level is a surrogate for tumor proliferation. The higher the level, the greater the risk for TLS.
	Cancer cell sensitivity to anti-cancer therapy	Cancers that are inherently more sensitive to therapy have a higher rate of cell lysis and a greater risk for TLS than the other cancers.
	Intensity of initial anti-cancer therapy	The higher the intensity of initial therapy, the greater the rate of cancer cell lysis and the risk of TLS. For example, some protocols for acute lymphoblastic leukemia begin with a week of prednisone monotherapy, while others begin with prednisone, vincristine, asparaginase and/or daunorubicin. A patient treated on the latter protocol would have a higher risk for TLS.
Patient presenting features	Nephropathy prior to cancer diagnosis	A patient with pre-existing nephropathy from hypertension, diabetes, gout, or other causes has a greater risk for acute kidney injury and TLS.
	Dehydration or volume depletion	Dehydration decreases the rate of urine flow through renal tubules and increases the concentration of solutes (e.g. phosphorus, uric acid) that can crystallize and cause nephropathy.
	Acidic urine	Uric acid has a lower solubility in acidic urine and therefore crystallizes more rapidly. A patient who presents with acidic urine and hyperuricemia usually already has uric acid crystals or microcrystals in the renal tubules.
	Hypotension	Hypotension decreases urine flow and increases the concentration of solutes that can crystallize. Hypotension can also independently cause acute kidney injury.
	Nephrotoxin exposure	Vancomycin, aminoglycosides, contrast agents for diagnostic imaging, and other potential nephrotoxins increase the risk of acute kidney injury from cancer cell lysis.

(Continued)

TABLE 4.2 Risk Factors for Tumor Lysis Syndrome—(cont'd)

Risk factor category	Risk factor	Comments
Supportive care	Inadequate hydration	Initial boluses of normal saline until the patient is euvolemic followed by infusion of suitable intravenous fluids at two times maintenance rate (about 180 mL/hr in an adult who can tolerate hyperhydration) increases the rate of urine flow through renal tubules, decreases the concentration of solutes that can crystallize and cause acute kidney injury, and decreases the time that those solutes remain in the tubules so that even if microcrystals form they may not have time to aggregate into clinically important crystals prior to removal by the high flow of urine.
	Exogenous potassium	Unless the patient has severe hypokalemia or a dysrhythmia from hypokalemia, potassium should not be included in the intravenous fluids, and potassium (from food or medications) should be minimized until the risk period for TLS has passed.
	Exogenous phosphate	Restricting dietary phosphate and adding a phosphate binder reduce the exogenous load of phosphate so that the kidneys need only excrete the endogenous load of phosphate released by cancer cell lysis.
	Delayed uric acid removal	Allopurinol prevents formation of new uric acid by inhibiting *xanthine oxidase* and preventing conversion of xanthine to uric acid. It does not remove existing uric acid and does increase urinary excretion of xanthine, which can crystallize and cause nephropathy. Rasburicase is an enzyme that rapidly removes uric acid by converting it to allantoin, which is highly soluble and readily excreted in the urine. The longer the uric acid level remains high, the greater the risk of crystal formation and acute kidney injury.

TLS, tumor lysis syndrome.
Reprinted from Howard et al. [12] with the permission of the publisher.

Supportive Care

Supportive care also affects the development and severity of TLS. Thus, disastrous TLS cases have occurred in non-hematologic cancer patients who received effective anti-cancer treatment without intravenous fluids or monitoring because TLS was not anticipated [5,42]. By contrast, patients with a bulky Burkitt lymphoma with high lysis potential may have a low risk of clinical TLS when routinely managed with hyperhydration, rasburicase, phosphate-lowering agents and close monitoring. The five-fold decrease in dialysis use (3% instead of 15%) in children with Burkitt lymphoma who received rasburicase instead of allopurinol illustrates the dramatic difference that supportive care can make, even when other TLS risk factors are the same [45].

RISK ASSESSMENT

Acute kidney injury is the most common manifestation of clinical TLS, and is associated with significant morbidity and occasional mortality [12,46,47]. Prevention of clinical TLS and AKI therefore requires an awareness of the patient's *a priori* TLS risk and a monitoring and management strategy tailored to the *a priori* risk. TLS risk-predictive models have been developed for adults with acute myeloid leukemia [48,49], children with acute lymphoblastic leukemia treated with hydration and allopurinol (but not rasburicase) [50], adults with chronic lymphocytic leukemia [9] and other cancers [12]. However, models published to date suffer from lack of a standard definition of TLS, use of different primary endpoints (clinical versus any TLS), lack of standardized supportive care guidelines and complex scoring systems. Experts and professional societies have also issued TLS management guidelines [2,13,51], but the recommendations are controversial due to lack of randomized trials using clinical TLS as the primary outcome [51,52]. The medical community still needs a simple risk prediction model with a standardized TLS definition and uniform supportive care validated for each cancer type and each associated therapy, since even stratifying by cancer type is not sufficient to predict TLS when new therapies are employed [12,37]. In the meantime, Figure 4.9 presents a practical approach for clinicians [12].

GRADING OF TUMOR LYSIS SYNDROME SEVERITY

The National Cancer Institute Common Terminology Criteria for Adverse Events version 4 (CTCAE 4.03, http://evs.nci.nih.gov/ftp1/CTCAE/CTCAE_4.03_2010-06-14_Quick Reference_8.5x11.pdf) defines TLS as follows: a disorder characterized by metabolic abnormalities that result from a spontaneous or therapy-related cytolysis of tumor cells. It grades TLS as either absent (grade 0), present (grade 3), life-threatening (grade 4), or fatal (grade 5). Having an accepted grading system allows

researchers to more consistently report the results of studies and health care professionals to more accurately and uniformly diagnose and manage their patients with TLS. In conjunction with their classification scheme, Cairo and Bishop have also proposed a grading system for TLS that follows the format of the CTCAE [2]. In this grading system, the grade of the clinical symptom (renal, cardiac, or seizure) with the highest severity grade defines the grade of TLS [2].

MANAGEMENT

Optimal management of TLS reduces the risk of AKI and prevents symptomatic electrolyte abnormalities, such as dysrhythmias and neuromuscular irritability from hyperkalemia or hypocalcemia (Figure 4.9). Key components of management include maintaining high urine output, reducing uric acid levels and controlling phosphorus levels, thus preserving renal function and preventing hyperkalemia and hyperphosphatemia, which cause most of the symptoms of TLS.

Monitoring

Urine output is the key parameter to monitor patients at risk for TLS or after the syndrome develops. In patients whose risk of clinical TLS is non-negligible, urine output and fluid balance should be recorded and assessed frequently. High risk patients should also receive intensive nursing care with continuous cardiac monitoring and measurement of electrolytes, creatinine and uric acid every 4 to 6 hours after starting therapy. Those at intermediate risk should undergo laboratory monitoring every 8 to 12 hours and those at low risk daily. Monitoring should continue over the entire risk period for TLS, which depends on the therapeutic regimen. In one of our protocols for acute lymphoblastic leukemia, which featured upfront single-agent methotrexate treatment

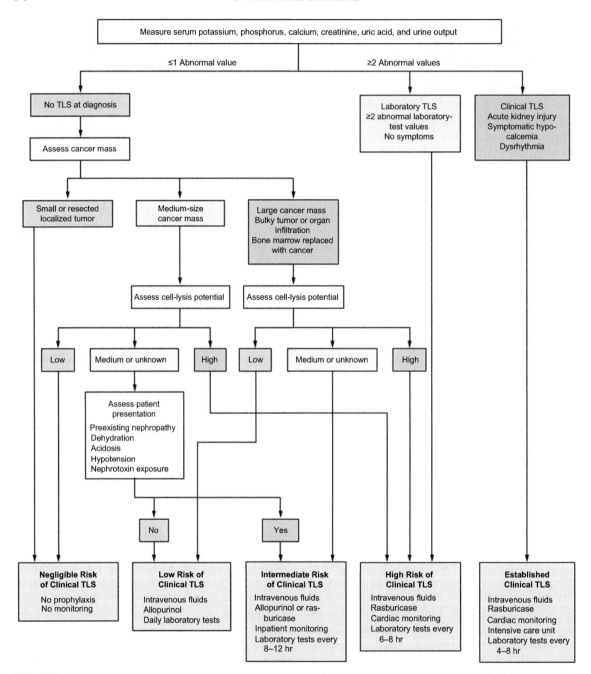

FIGURE 4.9 Assessment and initial management of tumor lysis syndrome. Assessment and initial management described in this algorithm are meant to guide care at the time of patient presentation. Subsequent management depends on how the patient progresses. Some low-risk patients unexpectedly develop tumor lysis syndrome (TLS) and require more aggressive management and some high-risk patients have no evidence of TLS after a few days of treatment and need less

[53], some patients developed new-onset TLS at day 6 or day 7 of remission induction therapy (after initiation of combination chemotherapy with prednisone, vincristine and daunorubicin on day 5 and asparaginase on day 6).

Hydration and Maintaining Urine Output

All patients at risk for TLS should receive intravenous hydration to rapidly improve renal perfusion and glomerular filtration, minimize acidosis and prevent oliguria. Acidosis lowers urine pH and increases uric acid crystallization, while oliguria increases the concentration of solutes in the urine and prolongs the time those solutes remain in the renal collecting system, thus increasing the risk of uric acid and calcium phosphate crystallization, with their associated nephrotoxic consequences (Figure 4.6). Hyperhydration consists of rapid fluid resuscitation with normal saline until the patient is euvolemic, followed by hydration with isotonic intravenous fluids at 2500 to 3500 mL/m^2 per day in patients at highest risk [2,12,30]. Hydration is the preferred method to increase urine output, but diuretics may be used once the patient is euvolemic or hypervolemic if urine output remains less than 2 mL/kg/hr (Table 4.2). In a rat model of urate nephropathy with elevated serum uric acid levels induced by continuous intravenous infusion of high doses of uric acid, high urine output due to treatment with high-dose furosemide or congenital diabetes insipidus (in the group of mice with this genetic modification)

protected the kidneys equally well, while acetazolamide (mild diuresis and urine alkalinization) and bicarbonate (urine alkalinization) provided only modest renal protection, but no more than low-dose furosemide without bicarbonate [54]. The best diuretic for patients with TLS is not known, and loop diuretics like furosemide not only promote diuresis, but also increase potassium secretion, so are preferred until further evidence indicates otherwise.

Urinary Alkalinization

Urinary alkalinization increases uric acid solubility, but decreases calcium phosphate solubility (Figure 4.7). Because it is more difficult to correct hyperphosphatemia than hyperuricemia, urinary alkalinization should be avoided in patients with TLS in countries in which rasburicase is available [17]. Whether urine alkalinization prevents or reduces the risk of acute kidney injury in patients without access to rasburicase is unknown, but an animal model of urate nephropathy suggested no benefit [54]. If alkalinization is used, it should be initiated when hyperuricemia develops and discontinued when hyperphosphatemia develops, since the increased solubility of uric acid at alkaline pH must be balanced against the decreased solubility of calcium phosphate (Figure 4.7) [12].

Reduction of Uric Acid

Uric acid reduction can preserve or improve renal function and reduce peak serum

---

intense management after the initial period. Assessment of TLS risk factors requires clinical judgment. It may not always be clear whether mild or transient dehydration should count, whether a cancer mass is medium or large, or whether cell lysis potential for a particular cancer with a particular treatment is medium or high. In equivocal cases, other criteria can be useful to clarify the degree of risk: an elevated lactate dehydrogenase level (greater than two times the upper limit of normal) and an elevated uric acid at presentation are associated with increased TLS risk, and can be used to help classify borderline cases into a suitable risk group. If in doubt between two categories, the patient should be managed in the higher-risk category. Because the algorithm presented is designed for use by both oncologists and non-oncologists, a conservative approach is presented to maximize safety.

*Tumor bulk includes the entire cancer cell mass from the primary site and all metastatic sites. Bone marrow can be a site of bulky disease if completely replaced with cancer cells.

TABLE 4.3   Incidence of Tumor Lysis Syndrome in Selected Studies with 100 Patients or More

Reference	Cancers included	Patients	TLS prevention used in addition to intravenous fluids	Incidence of TLS*	Incidence of dialysis	Death from TLS
COHORTS TREATED WITH ALLOPURINOL						
Montesinos et al., 2008 [48]	Acute myeloid leukemia	772 adults	Allopurinol	17%	0.9%	2.5%
Mato et al., 2006 [49]	Acute myeloid leukemia	194 adults	Allopurinol	9.8%	0.5%	0%
Truong et al., 2007 [50]	Acute lymphoblastic leukemia	326 children	Allopurinol (rasburicase in 6% of patients)	23%	Not reported	Not reported
Bowman et al., 1996 [80]	Advanced-stage, B-cell non-Hodgkin lymphoma	133 children	Allopurinol	Not reported	21%	2.2%
CLINICAL TRIAL IN WHICH RASBURICASE WAS USED WHERE AVAILABLE						
Cairo et al., 2007 [45]	Advanced-stage, B-cell non-Hodgkin lymphoma	101 children (USA)	Allopurinol	26%	15%	0%
		98 children (France)	Rasburicase	9%	3%	0%
Cortes et al., 2010 [81]	Hematologic malignancies	91 adults	Allopurinol	41% (4% clinical)	Not reported	0%
		92 adults	Rasburicase	21% (3% clinical)		0%
		92 adults	Rasburicase plus allopurinol	27% (3% clinical)		0%
COHORTS TREATED WITH RASBURICASE (OR A NON-RECOMBINANT URATE OXIDASE)						
Patte et al., 2002 [82]	Advanced-stage, B-cell non-Hodgkin lymphoma	410 children	Non-recombinant urate oxidase	Not reported (8.3% had metabolic problems)	1.7%	0%
Jeha et al., 2005 [64]	Mostly hematologic malignancies	1069 adults and children	Rasburicase	Not reported (4.2% had renal insufficiency)	2.8%	0%
Coiffier et al., 2003 [83]	Diffuse or bulky lymphoma (mostly diffuse large B-cell histology)	100 adults	Rasburicase	Not reported	0%	0%
Pui et al., 2001 [55]	Leukemia or lymphoma	131 children	Rasburicase	Not reported	0%	0%
Bosly et al., 2003 [84]	Mostly hematologic malignancies	278 adults and children	Rasburicase	Not reported	1.8%	0.4%

TABLE 4.3 Incidence of Tumor Lysis Syndrome in Selected Studies with 100 Patients or More—(cont'd)

Reference	Cancers included	Patients	TLS prevention used in addition to intravenous fluids	Incidence of TLS*	Incidence of dialysis	Death from TLS
Pui et al., 2001 [36]	Mostly hematologic malignancies	245 adults and children	Rasburicase	Not reported	4.1%	0.4%
Pui et al., 1997 [85]	Hematologic malignancies	134 children	Rasburicase	Not reported	0%	0%

* Includes both laboratory and clinical TLS. Unfortunately, many publications do not report these separately. Note that the definition of TLS and clinical TLS differed somewhat in different studies.

TLS, tumor lysis syndrome.

Reprinted from Howard et al. [12] with the permission of the publisher.

phosphorus levels as a secondary beneficial effect of renal protection [55]. Although allopurinol prevents uric acid formation, existing uric acid must still be renally excreted, and the level may take 2 days or more to decrease, a delay that allows urate nephropathy to develop (Figures 4.3 and 4.10). Moreover, despite allopurinol treatment, xanthine may accumulate, resulting in xanthine nephropathy [17,24,29]. Since serum xanthine level is not routinely measured, its impact on acute kidney injury development is uncertain. By directly breaking down uric acid and avoiding xanthine accumulation, rasburicase is more effective than allopurinol for the prevention and treatment of TLS (Figure 4.10).

In a randomized study of allopurinol versus rasburicase for patients at risk for TLS, the mean serum phosphorus concentration peaked at 7.1 mg/dL in the rasburicase group (whose mean uric acid levels decreased by 86% to 1 mg/dL at 4 hours) compared to 10.3 mg/dL in the allopurinol group (whose mean uric acid levels decreased by only 12% to 5.7 mg/dL at 48 hours) [56,57]. Serum creatinine improved by 31% in the rasburicase group, but worsened by 12% in the allopurinol group. Pui and colleagues [55] documented no increase in phosphorus levels and improved creatinine levels among 131 patients at high risk for TLS who were treated with rasburicase. In a multi-center

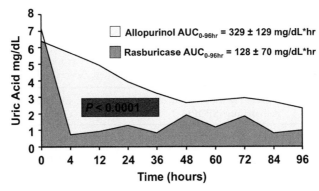

FIGURE 4.10 Uric acid levels during the first four days of treatment in patients at risk for tumor lysis syndrome randomized to receive rasburicase versus allopurinol. In patients at risk for tumor lysis syndrome, rasburicase was associated with a rapid decrease in uric acid and a corresponding lower area-under-the-concentration-time curve for uric acid, as measured over the first 4 days of therapy (128 ± 70 versus 329 ± 129 mg/dL*hr, $p < 0.0001$). This figure is reproduced in color in the color plate section. *Adapted from Goldman et al. [56].*

study of pediatric, advanced-stage, high-grade, B-cell non-Hodgkin lymphoma, patients at all sites received identical chemotherapy and aggressive hydration. However, patients treated in France all received rasburicase as part of routine supportive care; whereas, those at centers in the USA received allopurinol, since rasburicase was not yet available in the USA at the time of the study (Table 4.4). TLS occurred in 9% of 98 French patients who received rasburicase versus 26% of 101 US patients who received allopurinol ($p = 0.002$, Table 4.4) [45]. Dialysis was required in only 3% of French but 15% of the US patients ($p = 0.004$).

Rasburicase

Rasburicase is recommended as first-line treatment for patients at high risk of clinical TLS [13]. It is highly effective and reduces serum uric acid concentrations successfully in 99% of patients, and to undetectable levels in the vast majority. The efficacy of rasburicase is undisputed, but its use in patients at intermediate or low risk of clinical TLS has been restricted due to cost considerations, and there is no consensus on rasburicase use in patients at intermediate risk. Some have advocated use of a small dose of rasburicase in this setting (see below) [58,59]. Low-risk patients can usually be managed using intravenous fluids alone or with allopurinol, but should be monitored daily for signs of TLS [12].

Reduced Doses of Rasburicase

In an effort to reduce costs, some clinicians advocate use of lower doses of rasburicase than the 0.15−0.2 mg/kg/day approved by the US Food and Drug Administration (FDA). One way to reduce the amount of rasburicase used is to give a single dose (rather than consecutive daily doses) at the FDA-approved dose, with repeated doses if uric acid fails to decrease or rebounds after an initial decrease. This practice is widespread in the USA and was studied in a randomized trial of single-dose rasburicase 0.15 mg/kg with subsequent doses as needed versus five daily doses of 0.15 mg/kg in 82 adults at risk for TLS documented excellent efficacy of both strategies [60]. Meta-analysis showed equal efficacy to the daily strategy, provided that patients are carefully monitored and subsequent rasburicase doses are given to those who need them [61].

Another way to decrease dose is to give 0.1 mg/kg, 0.05 mg/kg, or a low fixed dose (e.g. 3 mg or 7.5 mg) and repeat in patients who fail to respond. This strategy has been reported in a number of retrospective studies

TABLE 4.4   Tumor Lysis Syndrome Outcomes for Pediatric Patients with Advanced Stage High-grade B-cell Lymphomas Treated on a Uniform Protocol with or without Access to Rasburicase [45]

	Société Française d'Oncologie Pédiatrique (SFOP)	Children's Cancer Group (CCG)	P-value
Number per group	98	101	
Supportive care	Rasburicase	Allopurinol	
Clinical outcomes			
Tumor lysis syndrome	9%	26%	0.002
Renal insufficiency	11%	27%	0.005
Dialysis	3%	15%	0.004

and case reports have been published in which lower doses of rasburicase have been used with mixed results. Lee and colleagues used a 4.5-mg, non-weight-adjusted dose to treat three children with acute lymphoblastic leukemia [62]. When the weight-adjusted dose was determined for the 4.5-mg dose, it was found that one patient received a higher quantity than the FDA-approved dose (0.26 mg/kg); one received the approved dose (0.17 mg/kg) and one received 50% of the approved dose (0.08 mg/kg). All three patients had a rapid reduction in uric acid. Another case series examined 11 adults with hematologic malignancies at risk for TLS [63]. Eight patients had renal impairment due to TLS at the time of presentation, and all of these patients were treated with a 6-mg, single dose of rasburicase (corresponding to a median weight-based dose of 0.08 mg/kg). In 10 of the 11 patients, single-dose rasburicase lowered and maintained normal uric acid levels; the mean pretreatment uric acid level, 11.7 mg/dL, was reduced to 2.0 mg/dL post-treatment. One morbidly obese patient required a second dose of rasburicase (12 mg; 0.0463 mg/kg, based on actual body weight) to control his uric acid levels. Among the eight patients with renal impairment, three had a return to baseline renal function after receiving rasburicase; one patient required hemodialysis and four patients had no subsequent renal function data reported. Although the authors conclude that use of a fixed, 6-mg dose of rasburicase appeared to be safe and effective, the fact that one patient required a large second dose and one required dialysis implies inadequate uric acid control, especially when compared to the 98 to 100% efficacy reported in large studies using the FDA-approved dose [64]. Another report describes an obese woman with chronic myelomonocytic leukemia in blast crisis who was treated with rasburicase 11 mg (a dose based on her ideal body weight), which adequately controlled her uric acid [65].

Four retrospective cohorts of patients treated with reduced-dose rasburicase have been reported recently [66–69]. A fixed, rasburicase 3-mg dose, with repeated doses as needed based on subsequent uric acid levels, was administered to 43 adult patients undergoing stem cell transplantation (51%) or receiving chemotherapy (49%) [66]. The total doses received were rasburicase 3 mg ($n = 37$), 4.5 mg ($n = 2$), or 6 mg ($n = 4$), and uric acid levels were all within normal limits 48 hours after the first dose. Although three patients were already receiving dialysis at the time of the study, no additional patients required dialysis. What is not clear from this study is whether the patients were at risk for TLS. Many patients undergoing stem cell transplantation already have a low bulk of disease and would not be expected to have TLS, and the disease status of the patients in the study cohort was not described. The second cohort in which use of reduced-dose rasburicase was evaluated included 46 adults with hematologic cancers and four with solid tumors [67]. Patients were eligible to receive rasburicase if they had bulky disease, elevated WBC count, elevated LDH in addition to elevated uric acid, or if they had a history of TLS after a prior course of chemotherapy. Rasburicase dosing was at the discretion of the treating clinician, and the initial dose ranged from 1.5 to 16.5 mg. Nine patients had uric acid levels above the normal range after the initial rasburicase dose, despite a mean decrease of 41% from their baseline levels. Because the cohort included patients with acute lymphoblastic leukemia, acute myeloid leukemia, chronic lymphoblastic leukemia, myeloma, solid tumors, both high- and low-grade lymphomas, and a wide range of rasburicase doses used, it is difficult to derive specific treatment recommendations from the data presented. However, the results do suggest that using doses of rasburicase that are lower than recommended may be effective for some patients.

Coutsouvelis and colleagues [72] reported 41 adults treated at a single institution in which a fixed dose of rasburicase 3 mg was given to patients considered to have high risk for TLS, including those with Burkitt lymphoma, acute lymphoblastic leukemia, bulky non-Hodgkin lymphoma, lymphoblastic lymphoma or acute myeloid leukemia with serum uric acid above the normal range, white cell count $>50,000/mm^3$ or LDH more than two times the upper limit of the normal range. Patient risk factors were not assessed. Of 42 episodes in the 41 patients, 34 required only one 3 mg dose of rasburicase to maintain normal uric acid; the remaining eight required multiple (two to six) doses. Clinical outcomes were not reported. Trifilio and colleagues [73] reported use of rasburicase 3 mg to treat 287 episodes of hyperuricemia in 247 adults with cancer, with normalization of uric acid in 72% of patients, with most of the responders in the group with uric acid levels of 7 to 12 mg/dL (only an 18% response rate for patients with uric acid >12 mg/dL). However, the relevance of this study to patients at risk for TLS is difficult to ascertain, since 122 of the episodes were given to patients during conditioning for stem cell transplantation, when most patients have little or no residual cancer mass (and therefore no risk for TLS). Furthermore, 40 of the patients had two episodes of rasburicase treatment, defined as that given at least 7 days apart from each other, which implies that many of the patients treated were not newly diagnosed patients at risk for TLS. In studies of healthy volunteers and patients with renal insufficiency, rasburicase even at low doses of 0.05 mg/kg was highly effective at reducing uric acid, but this situation differs from TLS, in which there can be extensive new uric acid formation as tumor cells lyse. Of note, reducing uric acid with a single dose of rasburicase has proven beneficial in patients with AKI from causes other than TLS, indicating that much remains to be learned about the complex pathophysiology of hyperuricemia and AKI [70–73].

In summary, the use of reduced doses of rasburicase should be studied in defined cohorts of patients with well-defined risk features who have an intermediate risk for developing TLS to determine the most cost-effective dose, defined as the dose at which no patient progresses to renal failure and at which the least amount of rasburicase is used. In patients receiving low-dose rasburicase to prevent TLS, serum uric acid levels must be measured frequently and precisely. In this regard, blood samples must be collected into chilled tubes, placed on ice immediately and assayed promptly to avoid *ex vivo* breakdown of uric acid by rasburicase, which produces artificially low levels of uric acid [64].

Rasburicase Side-effects

In patients treated with rasburicase, blood samples for uric acid concentration measurement must be placed on ice to prevent *ex vivo* breakdown of uric acid by rasburicase and thus a spuriously low level. Rasburicase should be avoided in patients with glucose-6-phosphate dehydrogenase (G6PD) deficiency because when it catalyzes conversion of uric acid to allantoin, hydrogen peroxide is produced, with a concomitant oxidative stress that can cause methemoglobinemia and hemolytic anemia (Figure 4.11) [64,74]. Patients with normal G6PD function can produce enough reduced glutathione to protect cells from oxidative damage, but patients with G6PD deficiency cannot produce sufficient reduced glutathione to remove free radicals, and are prone to hemolysis. Hemolysis preferentially affects old red blood cells, which have lower levels of G6PD (Figure 4.12A). After a hemolysis from an oxidative stress, remaining red blood cells have relatively high levels of G6PD activity, since otherwise they would have undergone

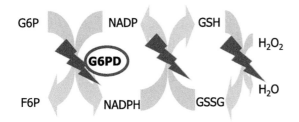

FIGURE 4.11 **Role of glucose-6-phosphate dehydrogenase deficiency during oxidative stress.** Reduced glutathione (GSH) is necessary to reduce hydrogen peroxide (H_2O_2) to water and remove the oxidative stress, forming oxidized glutathione (GSSG) in the process. However, for each molecule of hydrogen peroxide reduced, one molecule of GSH is needed. Oxidized glutathione is reduced by NADPH, which is oxidized to NADP, and requires glucose-6-phosphate dehydrogenase to reduce it back to its active form. Deficiency of G6PD inhibits reduction of NADP to NADPH, thereby inhibiting the reduction of GSSG back to GSH, and thus leaving hydrogen peroxide and other oxygen radicals free to damage red blood cell membranes and hemoglobin. G6P, glucose-6-phosphate; F6P, fructose-6-phosphate; G6PD, glucose-6-phosphate dehydrogenase; NADP, nicotinamide adenine dinucleotide phosphate; NADPH, reduced NADP; GSH, reduced glutathione; GSSG, oxidized glutathione; H_2O_2, hydrogen peroxide. This figure is reproduced in color in the color plate section.

hemolysis; therefore, measurement of G6PD activity after a hemolytic episode yields artificially high results (Figure 4.12A). Patients with African or Mediterranean ancestry are at risk for G6PD deficiency, and G6PD testing should be performed prior to administration of rasburicase if possible. If not possible, and the clinical situation is urgent, a low dose of rasburicase (0.05 mg/kg) can be used initially with careful monitoring for hemolysis, and repeated as necessary if no hemolysis occurs (Figure 4.12B).

Management of Hyperkalemia

Hyperkalemia can cause sudden death due to cardiac dysrhythmia, and is the most common cause of death due to TLS. Potassium and phosphorus intake must be limited in newly diagnosed cancer patients until the period of TLS

risk has passed [12,75]. Measurement of potassium every 4 to 6 hours (Figure 4.9), intravenous fluids without potassium, continuous cardiac monitoring and oral sodium polystyrene sulfate are recommended in patients with TLS who develop AKI. Renal replacement therapy should be readily available to such patients in case potassium levels rise rapidly despite all precautions. Glucose plus insulin or beta agonists may temporarily decrease serum potassium levels and calcium gluconate may stabilize the myocardium and thus reduce the risk of dysrhythmia, but these measures are only temporary, and prompt initiation of hemodialysis is paramount in oliguric or anuric patients with TLS.

Management of Hypocalcemia and Prevention of Neuromuscular Irritability

Like hyperkalemia, hypocalcemia can lead to life-threatening dysrhythmias and neuromuscular irritability. However, management is not straightforward, since the hypocalcemia that occurs in patients with TLS is secondary to hyperphosphatemia, such that administration of exogenous calcium can raise the calcium × phosphate product to dangerously high levels (>60 mg^2/dL^2, Figures 4.4 and 4.8), at which calcium phosphate can precipitate in tissues. Therefore, the key to controlling hypocalcemia is to reduce the serum phosphorus. Symptomatic hypocalcemia should be treated with calcium at the lowest dose required to relieve symptoms and asymptomatic hypocalcemia does not require treatment. Because they have few side-effects and may be helpful, phosphate binders are usually given to patients with TLS. Products that do not contain calcium or aluminum are preferred, such as lanthanum or sevelamer [76].

Renal Replacement Therapy

Despite optimal management, some patients with TLS develop severe AKI and require renal replacement therapy (Table 4.5). Patients with

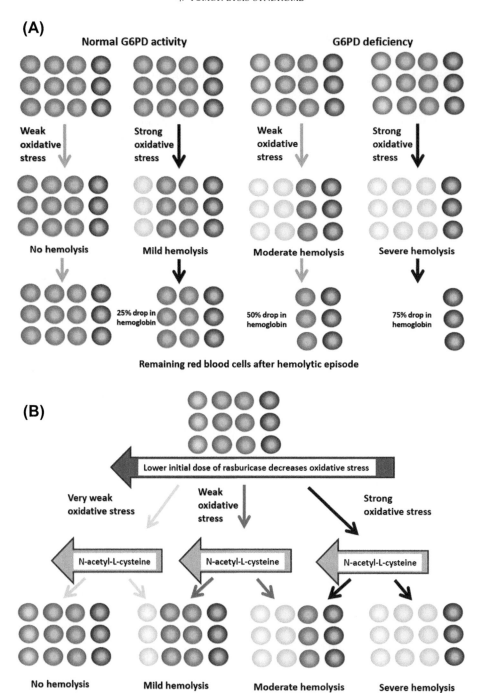

FIGURE 4.12   (A) Effect of oxidative stress on patients with normal and decreased glucose-6-phosphate dehydrogenase activity. (B) Potential mitigating strategies for patients with glucose-6-phosphate dehydrogenase activity who

TABLE 4.5 Comparison of Renal Replacement Methods

	Hemodialysis	Continuous veno-venous hemofiltration	Continuous veno-venous hemodialysis
Clearance mechanism			
Convection	+	++++	+
Diffusion	++++	−	++++
Hemodynamic stability	++	+++	+++
Blood flow rate (mL/min)	≥200	<200	<200
Dialysate flow rate (mL/min)	≥500	−	20−80
Fluid replacement rate (mL/min)	−	20−80	−
Ultrafiltration rate* (net, mL/hr)	0−1000	0−200	0−200
Solute clearance	Efficient	Less efficient	Less efficient
Typical duration	3−4 hours	24 hours	24 hours
Membrane size exclusion (daltons)	5000	50,000	50,000
Drug and nutrient clearance	+	++++	++++
Anticoagulant	Heparin or none	Citrate or heparin	Citrate or heparin

* The ultrafiltration rate refers to the volume of fluid removed per unit of time. Net ultrafiltration is the ultimate volume removed from the patient after total intake is subtracted from total output.

Information for this table was adapted from: Mehta RL, Supportive Therapies: Intermittent Hemodialysis, Continuous Renal Replacement Therapies, and Peritoneal Dialysis. From Atlas of Diseases of the Kidney, Ed. Robert Schrier, Volume One, Editors: T. Berl and J.V. Bonventre. Section II. Chapter 19, pages 19.0−19.16. http://www.kidneyatlas.org/toc.htm.

◀───

require rasburicase. Red blood cells circulate for 120 days, but gradually lose their glucose-6-phosphate dehydrogenase (G6PD) activity. In this figure, cells with the highest G6PD activity are shown in red and those with decreased activity in green. At any given age, circulating red blood cells have less G6PD activity in people with mutations in this enzyme, but the youngest cells of a G6PD deficient person may have more activity than the oldest cells of a normal person. In patients with tumor lysis syndrome, the higher the uric acid, the more hydrogen peroxide produced and the greater the oxidative stress when rasburicase is administered. A decrease of uric acid from 9.0 to 2.2 mg/dL, as occurred in the patient reported by Elinoff et al. [46], is associated with a production of 2 mmol of hydrogen peroxide, a quantity sufficient to hemolyze two-thirds of the patient's erythrocytes. (A) Effect of oxidative stress on patients with normal and decreased G6PD activity. Note that red blood cells that remain after a hemolytic episode are those that contain the highest G6PD activity; thus, measurement of G6PD activity immediately after an episode is not advisable, since it would yield falsely elevated activity levels. (B) Potential mitigating strategies for patients with G6PD deficiency who require rasburicase. Use of an initial small "test dose" of rasburicase (e.g. 1.5 mg) results in a smaller oxidative stress and potentially less hemolysis than use of the regular dose. N-acetyl-L-cysteine may partially protect red blood cells from oxidative damage and decrease the amount of hemolysis at any given degree of oxidative stress. This figure is reproduced in color in the color plate section. *Reprinted from Howard et al. [88] with the permission of the publisher.*

TLS have a lower threshold for dialysis because of potentially rapid potassium release and accumulation, particularly in oliguric patients. Some of the indications for renal replacement therapy are similar to those in patients with other causes of AKI (e.g. hyperkalemia, fluid overload), but in patients with TLS, severe hyperphosphatemia with refractory hypocalcemia may also warrant dialysis. Phosphate removal increases as treatment time increases, so continuous veno-venous hemofiltration, continuous veno-venous hemodialysis or continuous veno-venous hemodiafiltration have been used for TLS patients in whom hyperphosphatemia was the indication for renal replacement therapy [77]. These dialysis methods use filters with a larger pore size that allow more rapid clearance of molecules that are not efficiently removed by conventional hemodialysis (Table 4.5). Among adults with AKI, one study showed that continuous veno-venous hemodiafiltration reduced phosphate more effectively than conventional hemodialysis [78]. Hyperuricemia is virtually never an indication for dialysis in countries where rasburicase is available [36,55,64]. In patients who require renal replacement therapy, it should be continued until urine output resumes and the majority of the cancer cell mass is gone, indicating that the period of risk for worsening TLS has passed.

SEQUELAE OF TUMOR LYSIS SYNDROME

The most important consequences of TLS, such as AKI and sudden death, occur within days of developing the syndrome. However, patients who develop AKI often develop hypertension and a reduced glomerular filtration rate that can last weeks or months. They also remain at higher risk for subsequent kidney injury, which is common among cancer patients, who are exposed to multiple nephrotoxic drugs, and also at risk for infections that can affect renal function. Long-term consequences of TLS are unknown.

PREVENTION OF TUMOR LYSIS SYNDROME BY ALTERING INITIAL CANCER THERAPY

In addition to the management strategies described, the risk of TLS may also be reduced by altering initial anti-cancer therapy to reduce the cancer mass more slowly and thus allow more time for renal excretion of cell lysis products. Slower cancer cell lysis allows renal homeostatic mechanisms to clear metabolites before they accumulate and cause organ damage. In this regard, low-dose cyclophosphamide, vincristine and prednisone for a week prior to starting intense chemotherapy are routinely used for patients with high-grade, B-cell non-Hodgkin lymphomas or Burkitt leukemia. Similarly, for decades the Berlin–Frankfurt–Muenster group has treated childhood acute lymphoblastic leukemia patients with a week of prednisone monotherapy prior to starting standard remission induction therapy with multiple cytotoxic agents.

SUMMARY

Laboratory TLS is defined as the presence of two or more of the following abnormalities present on the same day: hyperuricemia, hyperkalemia, hyperphosphatemia, hypocalcemia secondary to hyperphosphatemia.

Clinical TLS is defined as laboratory TLS plus acute kidney injury, symptomatic hyperkalemia, or symptomatic hypocalcemia, and should be prevented whenever possible.

Clinical TLS can occur in any patient with newly diagnosed or relapsed cancer, and its incidence depends on cancer cell mass and lysis potential, patient risk factors (nephropathy, dehydration, acidosis, hypotension, nephrotoxin exposure) and the supportive care provided to patients potentially at risk. Therefore, all patients should be risk stratified and managed according to their risk for clinical TLS: negligible risk — no prophylaxis, no monitoring; low risk — hyperhydration, allopurinol, daily laboratory evaluation; intermediate risk — hyperhydration, rasburicase if hyperuricemic, inpatient monitoring and laboratory evaluation every 8—12 hours; and high risk or with established TLS at presentation — hyperhydration, rasburicase, inpatient with cardiac monitoring, laboratory evaluation every 4—8 hours and rapid access to hemodialysis. With these measures, morbidity is minimized and death from TLS is rare.

Acknowledgments

This work was supported in part by grant CA21765 from the National Institutes of Health and by the American Lebanese Syrian Associated Charities (ALSAC). Dr. Pui is the F.M. Kirby Chair of the American Cancer Society.

References

[1] bu-Alfa AK, Younes A. Tumor lysis syndrome and acute kidney injury: evaluation, prevention, and management. Am J Kidney Dis 2010;55:S1—13.

[2] Cairo MS, Coiffier B, Reiter A, Younes A. Recommendations for the evaluation of risk and prophylaxis of tumour lysis syndrome (TLS) in adults and children with malignant diseases: an expert TLS panel consensus. Br J Haematol 2010;149:578—86.

[3] Gertz MA. Managing tumor lysis syndrome in 2010. Leuk Lymphoma 2010;51:179—80.

[4] Magrath IT, Semawere C, Nkwocha J. Causes of death in patients with Burkitt's lymphoma — the role of supportive care in overall management. East Afr Med J 1974;51:623—32.

[5] Krishnan G, D'Silva K, Al-Janadi A. Cetuximab-related tumor lysis syndrome in metastatic colon carcinoma. J Clin Oncol 2008;26:2406—8.

[6] Noh GY, Choe dH, Kim CH, Lee JC. Fatal tumor lysis syndrome during radiotherapy for non-small-cell lung cancer. J Clin Oncol 2008;26:6005—6.

[7] Godoy H, Kesterson JP, Lele S. Tumor lysis syndrome associated with carboplatin and paclitaxel in a woman with recurrent endometrial cancer. Int J Gynaecol Obstet 2010;109:254.

[8] Joshita S, Yoshizawa K, Sano K, Kobayashi S, Sekiguchi T, Morita S, et al. A patient with advanced hepatocellular carcinoma treated with sorafenib tosylate showed massive tumor lysis with avoidance of tumor lysis syndrome. Intern Med 2010;49:991—4.

[9] Ji J, Mould DR, Blum KA, Ruppert AS, Poi M, Zhao Y, et al. A pharmacokinetic/pharmacodynamic model of tumor lysis syndrome in chronic lymphocytic leukemia patients treated with flavopiridol. Clin Cancer Res 2013;19:1269—80.

[10] Doi M, Okamoto Y, Yamauchi M, Naitou H, Shinozaki K. Bleomycin-induced pulmonary fibrosis after tumor lysis syndrome in a case of advanced yolk sac tumor treated with bleomycin, etoposide and cisplatin (BEP) chemotherapy. Int J Clin Oncol 2012;17:528—31.

[11] Katiman D, Manikam J, Goh KL, Abdullah BJ, Mahadeva S. Tumour lysis syndrome: a rare complication of trans-arterial chemo-embolisation with doxorubicin beads for hepatocellular carcinoma. J Gastrointest Cancer. http://www.ncbi.nlm.nih.gov/pubmed/22692948; 2012 Jun 13 [Epub ahead of print].

[12] Howard SC, Jones DP, Pui CH. The tumor lysis syndrome. N Engl J Med 2011;364:1844—54.

[13] Coiffier B, Altman A, Pui CH, Younes A, Cairo MS. Guidelines for the management of pediatric and adult tumor lysis syndrome: an evidence-based review. J Clin Oncol 2008;26:2767—78.

[14] Cairo MS, Bishop M. Tumour lysis syndrome: new therapeutic strategies and classification. Br J Haematol 2004;127:3—11.

[15] El-Husseini A, Sabucedo A, Lamarche J, Courville C, Peguero A. Acute kidney injury associated with tumor lysis syndrome: a paradigm shift. Am J Emerg Med 2012;30:390—6.

[16] Firwana BM, Hasan R, Hasan N, Alahdab F, Alnahhas I, Hasan S, et al. Tumor lysis syndrome: a systematic review of case series and case reports. Postgrad Med 2012;124:92—101.

[17] Howard SC, Ribeiro RC, Pui C-H. Acute complications. In: Pui C-H, editor. Cambridge: Childhood Leukemias; 2006. p. 709—49.

[18] Feig DI, Kang DH, Johnson RJ. Uric acid and cardiovascular risk. N Engl J Med 2008;359:1811—21.

[19] Shimada M, Johnson RJ, May Jr WS, Lingegowda V, Sood P, Nakagawa T, et al. A novel role for uric acid in acute kidney injury associated with tumour lysis syndrome. Nephrol Dial Transplant 2009;24:2960—4.

[20] Ejaz AA, Mu W, Kang DH, Roncal C, Sautin YY, Henderson G, et al. Could uric acid have a role in acute renal failure? Clin J Am Soc Nephrol 2007;2:16—21.

[21] Hijiya N, Metzger ML, Pounds S, Schmidt JE, Razzouk BI, Rubnitz JE, et al. Severe cardiopulmonary complications consistent with systemic inflammatory response syndrome caused by leukemia cell

lysis in childhood acute myelomonocytic or mono-cytic leukemia. Pediatr Blood Cancer 2005;44:63—9.

[22] Nakamura M, Oda S, Sadahiro T, Hirayama Y, Tateishi Y, Abe R, et al. The role of hypercytokinemia in the pathophysiology of tumor lysis syndrome (TLS) and the treatment with continuous hemodiafiltration using a polymethylmethacrylate membrane hemofil-ter (PMMA-CHDF). Transfus Apher Sci 2009;40:41—7.

[23] Soares M, Feres GA, Salluh JI. Systemic inflammatory response syndrome and multiple organ dysfunction in patients with acute tumor lysis syndrome. Clinics (Sao Paulo) 2009;64:479—81.

[24] LaRosa C, McMullen L, Bakdash S, Ellis D, Krishnamurti L, Wu HY, et al. Acute renal failure from xanthine nephropathy during management of acute leukemia. Pediatr Nephrol 2007;22:132—5.

[25] Greene ML, Fujimoto WY, Seegmiller JE. Urinary xanthine stones — a rare complications of allopurinol therapy. N Engl J Med 1969;280:426—7.

[26] Beshensky AM, Wesson JA, Worcester EM, Sorokina EJ, Snyder CJ, Kleinman JG. Effects of urinary macromolecules on hydroxyapatite crystal formation. J Am Soc Nephrol 2001;12:2108—16.

[27] Wesson JA, Worcester EM, Wiessner JH, Mandel NS, Kleinman JG. Control of calcium oxalate crystal structure and cell adherence by urinary macromole-cules. Kidney Int 1998;53:952—7.

[28] Finlayson B. Physicochemical aspects of urolithiasis. Kidney Int 1978;13:344—60.

[29] Pais Jr VM, Lowe G, Lallas CD, Preminger GM, Assimos DG. Xanthine urolithiasis. Urology 2006;67:1084—11.

[30] Bose P, Qubaiah O. A review of tumour lysis syndrome with targeted therapies and the role of rasburicase. J Clin Pharm Ther 2011;36:299—326.

[31] Dombret H, Hunault M, Faucher C, Dombret MC, Degos L. Acute lysis pneumopathy after chemo-therapy for acute myelomonocytic leukemia with abnormal marrow eosinophils. Cancer 1992;69:1356—61.

[32] Lester WA, Hull DR, Fegan CD, Morris TC. Respira-tory failure during induction chemotherapy for acute myelomonocytic leukaemia (FAB M4Eo) with ara-C and all-trans retinoic acid. Br J Haematol 2000;109:847—50.

[33] Filippatos TD, Milionis HJ, Elisaf MS. Alterations in electrolyte equilibrium in patients with acute leuke-mia. Eur J Haematol 2005;75:449—60.

[34] Stein E, McMahon B, Kwaan H, Altman JK, Frankfurt O, Tallman MS. The coagulopathy of acute promyelocytic leukaemia revisited. Best Pract Res Clin Haematol 2009;22:153—63.

[35] Jeha S. Tumor lysis syndrome. Semin Hematol 2001;38:4—8.

[36] Pui CH, Jeha S, Irwin D, Camitta B. Recombinant urate oxidase (rasburicase) in the prevention and treatment of malignancy-associated hyperuricemia in pediatric and adult patients: results of a compassionate-use trial. Leukemia 2001;15:1505—9.

[37] Howard SC, Pui CH. Pitfalls in predicting tumor lysis syndrome. Leuk Lymphoma 2006;47:782—5.

[38] Michels J, Lassau N, Gross-Goupil M, Massard C, Mejean A, Escudier B. Sunitinib inducing tumor lysis syndrome in a patient treated for renal carcinoma. Invest New Drugs 2010;28:690—3.

[39] Cheson BD. Etiology and management of tumor lysis syndrome in patients with chronic lymphocytic leu-kemia. Clin Adv Hematol Oncol 2009;7:263—71.

[40] Gemici C. Tumor lysis syndrome in solid tumors. J Clin Oncol 2009;27:2738—9.

[41] Huang WS, Yang CH. Sorafenib induced tumor lysis syndrome in an advanced hepatocellular carcinoma patient. World J Gastroenterol 2009;15:4464—6.

[42] Keane C, Henden A, Bird R. Catastrophic tumour lysis syndrome following single dose of imatinib. Eur J Haematol 2009;82:244—5.

[43] Grenader T, Shavit L. Tumor lysis syndrome in a pa-tient with merkel cell carcinoma and provoked path-ologic sequence of acute kidney injury, reduced clearance of carboplatin and fatal pancytopenia. Onkologie 2011;34:626—9.

[44] Rodriguez-Reimundes E, Perazzo F, Vilches AR. Tu-mor lysis syndrome in a patient with a renal carci-noma treated with sunitinib. Medicina (B Aires) 2011;71:158—60.

[45] Cairo MS, Gerrard M, Sposto R, Auperin A, Pinkerton CR, Michon J, et al. Results of a random-ized international study of high-risk central nervous system B non-Hodgkin lymphoma and B acute lymphoblastic leukemia in children and adolescents. Blood 2007;109:2736—43.

[46] Elinoff JM, Salit RB, Ackerman HC. The tumor lysis syndrome. N Engl J Med 2011;365:571—2.

[47] Palevsky PM, Zhang JH, O'Connor TZ, Chertow GM, Crowley ST, Choudhury D, et al. Intensity of renal support in critically ill patients with acute kidney injury. N Engl J Med 2008;359:7—20.

[48] Montesinos P, Lorenzo I, Martin G, Sanz J, Perez-Sirvent ML, Martinez D, et al. Tumor lysis syndrome in patients with acute myeloid leukemia: identifica-tion of risk factors and development of a predictive model. Haematologica 2008;93:67—74.

[49] Mato AR, Riccio BE, Qin L, Heitjan DF, Carroll M, Loren A, et al. A predictive model for the detection of

tumor lysis syndrome during AML induction therapy. Leuk Lymphoma 2006;47:877−83.

[50] Truong TH, Beyene J, Hitzler J, Abla O, Maloney AM, Weitzman S, et al. Features at presentation predict children with acute lymphoblastic leukemia at low risk for tumor lysis syndrome. Cancer 2007;110:1832−9.

[51] Feusner JH, Ritchey AK, Cohn SL, Billett AL. Management of tumor lysis syndrome: need for evidence-based guidelines. J Clin Oncol 2008;26:5657−8.

[52] Agrawal AK, Feusner JH. Management of tumour lysis syndrome in children: what is the evidence for prophylactic rasburicase in non-hyperleucocytic leukaemia? Br J Haematol 2011;153:275−7.

[53] Pui CH, Campana D, Pei D, Bowman WP, Sandlund JT, Kaste SC, et al. Treating childhood acute lymphoblastic leukemia without cranial irradiation. N Engl J Med 2009;360:2730−41.

[54] Conger JD, Falk SA. Intrarenal dynamics in the pathogenesis and prevention of acute urate nephropathy. J Clin Invest 1977;59:786−93.

[55] Pui CH, Mahmoud HH, Wiley JM, Woods GM, Leverger G, Camitta B, et al. Recombinant urate oxidase for the prophylaxis or treatment of hyperuricemia in patients with leukemia or lymphoma. J Clin Oncol 2001;19:697−704.

[56] Goldman SC, Holcenberg JS, Finklestein JZ, Hutchinson R, Kreissman S, Johnson FL, et al. A randomized comparison between rasburicase and allopurinol in children with lymphoma or leukemia at high risk for tumor lysis. Blood 2001;97: 2998−3003.

[57] Tumor lysis syndrome: focus on hyperphosphatemia. http://www cure4kids org/private/lectures/ ppt1468/C4K-1454−0MC-Tumor-Lysis pdf; 2009.

[58] Giraldez M, Puto K. A single, fixed dose of rasburicase (6 mg maximum) for treatment of tumor lysis syndrome in adults. http://www.ncbi.nlm.nih.gov/pubmed? term=Giraldez%20M%5BAuthor%5D&cauthor=true& cauthor_uid=20394650. Eur J Haematol 2010 Aug;85(2): 177−9.

[59] Knoebel RW, Lo M, Crank CW. Evaluation of a low, weight-based dose of rasburicase in adult patients for the treatment or prophylaxis of tumor lysis syndrome. J Oncol Pharm Pract 2011 Sep;17(3):147−54.

[60] Vadhan-Raj S, Fayad LE, Fanale MA, Pro B, Rodriguez A, Hagemeister FB, et al. A randomized trial of a single-dose rasburicase versus five-daily doses in patients at risk for tumor lysis syndrome. Ann Oncol 2012;23:1640−5.

[61] Feng X, Dong K, Pham D, Pence S, Inciardi J, Bhutada NS. Efficacy and cost of single-dose rasburicase in prevention and treatment of adult tumour lysis syndrome: a meta-analysis. J Clin Pharm Ther 2013;38(4):301−8.

[62] Lee AC, Li CH, So KT, Chan R. Treatment of impending tumor lysis with single-dose rasburicase. Ann Pharmacother 2003;37:1614−7.

[63] McDonnell AM, Lenz KL, Frei-Lahr DA, Hayslip J, Hall PD. Single-dose rasburicase 6 mg in the management of tumor lysis syndrome in adults. Pharmacotherapy 2006;26:806−12.

[64] Jeha S, Kantarjian H, Irwin D, Shen V, Shenoy S, Blaney S, et al. Efficacy and safety of rasburicase, a recombinant urate oxidase (Elitek), in the management of malignancy-associated hyperuricemia in pediatric and adult patients: final results of a multicenter compassionate use trial. Leukemia 2005;19:34−8.

[65] Arnold TM, Reuter JP, Delman BS, Shanholtz CB. Use of single-dose rasburicase in an obese female. Ann Pharmacother 2004;38:1428−31.

[66] Trifilio S, Gordon L, Singhal S, Tallman M, Evens A, Rashid K, et al. Reduced-dose rasburicase (recombinant xanthine oxidase) in adult cancer patients with hyperuricemia. Bone Marrow Transplant 2006;37:997−1001.

[67] Hummel M, Reiter S, Adam K, Hehlmann R, Buchheidt D. Effective treatment and prophylaxis of hyperuricemia and impaired renal function in tumor lysis syndrome with low doses of rasburicase. Eur J Haematol 2008;80:331−6.

[68] Coutsouvelis J, Wiseman M, Hui L, Poole S, Dooley M, Patil S, et al. Effectiveness of a single fixed dose of rasburicase 3 mg in the management of tumour lysis syndrome. Br J Clin Pharmacol 2013;75:550−3.

[69] Trifilio SM, Pi J, Zook J, Golf M, Coyle K, Greenberg D, et al. Effectiveness of a single 3-mg rasburicase dose for the management of hyperuricemia in patients with hematological malignancies. Bone Marrow Transplant 2011;46:800−5.

[70] Hobbs DJ, Steinke JM, Chung JY, Barletta GM, Bunchman TE. Rasburicase improves hyperuricemia in infants with acute kidney injury. Pediatr Nephrol 2010;25:305−9.

[71] Hooman N, Otukesh H. Single dose of rasburicase for treatment of hyperuricemia in acute kidney injury: a report of 3 cases. Iran J Kidney Dis 2011;5:130−2.

[72] Jarmolinski T, Zaniew M, Tousty J, Runowski D. Is it the right time to subject children with acute kidney injury to rasburicase trials? Pediatr Nephrol 2012;27:1201−2.

[73] Lin PY, Lin CC, Liu HC, Lee MD, Lee HC, Ho CS, et al. Rasburicase improves hyperuricemia in patients with

acute kidney injury secondary to rhabdomyolysis caused by ecstasy intoxication and exertional heat stroke. Pediatr Crit Care Med 2011;12:e424—7.

[74] Sundy JS, Becker MA, Baraf HS, Barkhuizen A, Moreland LW, Huang W, et al. Reduction of plasma urate levels following treatment with multiple doses of pegloticase (polyethylene glycol-conjugated uricase) in patients with treatment-failure gout: results of a phase II randomized study. Arthritis Rheum 2008;58:2882—91.

[75] Bellinghieri G, Santoro D, Savica V. Emerging drugs for hyperphosphatemia. Expert Opin Emerg Drugs 2007;12:355—65.

[76] Arenas MD, Rebollo P, Malek T, Moledous A, Gil T, varez-Ude F, et al. A comparative study of 2 new phosphate binders (sevelamer and lanthanum carbonate) in routine clinical practice. J Nephrol 2010.

[77] Gutzwiller JP, Schneditz D, Huber AR, Schindler C, Gutzwiller F, Zehnder CE. Estimating phosphate removal in haemodialysis: an additional tool to quantify dialysis dose. Nephrol Dial Transplant 2002;17:1037—44.

[78] Tan HK, Bellomo R, M'Pis DA, Ronco C. Phosphatemic control during acute renal failure: intermittent hemodialysis versus continuous hemodiafiltration. Int J Artif Organs 2001;24:186—91.

[79] Levin A, Warnock DG, Mehta RL, Kellum JA, Shah SV, Molitoris BA, et al. Improving outcomes from acute kidney injury: report of an initiative. Am J Kidney Dis 2007;50:1—4.

[80] Bowman WP, Shuster JJ, Cook B, Griffin T, Behm F, Pullen J, et al. Improved survival for children with B-cell acute lymphoblastic leukemia and stage IV small noncleaved-cell lymphoma: a pediatric oncology group study. J Clin Oncol 1996;14:1252—61.

[81] Cortes J, Moore JO, Maziarz RT, Wetzler M, Craig M, Matous J, et al. Control of plasma uric acid in adults at risk for tumor lysis syndrome: efficacy and safety of rasburicase alone and rasburicase followed by

allopurinol compared with allopurinol alone — results of a multicenter phase III study. J Clin Oncol 2010;28:4207—13.

[82] Patte C, Sakiroglu C, Ansoborlo S, Baruchel A, Plouvier E, Pacquement H, et al. Urate-oxidase in the prevention and treatment of metabolic complications in patients with B-cell lymphoma and leukemia, treated in the Societe Francaise d'Oncologie Pediatrique LMB89 protocol. Ann Oncol 2002;13:789—95.

[83] Coiffier B, Mounier N, Bologna S, Ferme C, Tilly H, Sonet A, et al. Efficacy and safety of rasburicase (recombinant urate oxidase) for the prevention and treatment of hyperuricemia during induction chemotherapy of aggressive non-Hodgkin's lymphoma: results of the GRAAL1 (Groupe d'Etude des Lymphomes de l'Adulte Trial on Rasburicase Activity in Adult Lymphoma) study. J Clin Oncol 2003;21:4402—6.

[84] Bosly A, Sonet A, Pinkerton CR, McCowage G, Bron D, Sanz MA, et al. Rasburicase (recombinant urate oxidase) for the management of hyperuricemia in patients with cancer: report of an international compassionate use study. Cancer 2003;98:1048—54.

[85] Pui CH, Relling MV, Lascombes F, Harrison PL, Struxiano A, Mondesir JM, et al. Urate oxidase in prevention and treatment of hyperuricemia associated with lymphoid malignancies. Leukemia 1997;11:1813—6.

[86] Bouropoulos C, Vagenas N, Klepetsanis PG, Stavropoulos N, Bouropoulos N. Growth of calcium oxalate monohydrate on uric acid crystals at sustained supersaturation. Cryst Res Technol 2004;39:699—704.

[87] Grases F, Sanchis P, Isern B, Perello J, Costa-Bauza A. Uric acid as inducer of calcium oxalate crystal development. Scand J Urol Nephrol 2007;41:26—31.

[88] Howard SC, Jones DP, Pui C-H. The tumor lysis syndrome (letter). N Engl J Med 2011;365:573—4.

Multiple Myeloma and Kidney Disease

Amit Lahoti

MD Anderson Cancer Center, Houston, TX, USA

INTRODUCTION

Multiple myeloma (MM) is characterized by the abnormal proliferation of plasma cells resulting in the excessive secretion of monoclonal proteins into the blood (paraproteins). It is the second most common hematological malignancy behind non-Hodgkin lymphoma with an annual incidence of 4–7 cases per 100,00 in the USA. Median age at diagnosis is 62 years, with less than 2% of patients being younger than 40 years of age. African-Americans are affected more commonly than Caucasians or Asians.

MM is part of a spectrum of plasma cell dyscrasias that can be associated with renal disease. Patients with low levels of serum monoclonal protein (less than 3 gm/dL), low tumor burden (less than 10% plasma cells on bone marrow biopsy) and no evidence of end organ damage are considered to have monoclonal gammopathy of unknown significance (MGUS). This is an asymptomatic pre-malignant phase that requires no specific therapy. However, there is a 1% life-long annual risk of progression to MM or other related conditions. In addition, patients with MGUS may eventually develop renal disease (i.e. light chain deposition disease (LCCD) or light chain (AL) amyloidosis) in the absence of progression to MM. Therefore, periodic observation of patients with MGUS for signs of progressive anemia, hypercalcemia, renal failure, proteinuria, cardiomyopathy and paraproteinemia is essential. Patients with more than 3 gm/dL of serum monoclonal proteins and greater than 10% plasma cells on bone marrow biopsy are diagnosed with MM.

Circulating monoclonal proteins (intact immunoglobulins, light chains, heavy chains, or fragments thereof) may precipitate or deposit within the kidneys and cause injury. At initial presentation, approximately one-half of patients with MM will have renal insufficiency and 10% will require dialysis [1]. Less than 25% of patients that require dialysis will recover renal function [2]. Renal failure is associated with decreased overall survival in patients with MM [3]. Reduction in serum free light chain levels with therapy is associated with renal recovery and increased overall survival [4,5]. Factors associated with renal recovery include lower serum creatinine at presentation, hypercalcemia and proteinuria less than 1 g/day [3]. Not all monoclonal proteins are nephrotoxic and inherent biochemical properties of the

65

proteins determine the specific pattern of renal injury. This is supported by the fact that mice injected with serum from patients with myeloma-related kidney disease will replicate the same pattern of kidney disease as the patient [6]. This chapter will focus on the main patterns of myeloma-related kidney disease: cast nephropathy, AL amyoidosis and LCDD.

CAST NEPHROPATHY

Pathogenesis

Cast nephropathy occurs almost exclusively in the setting of MM, and is the most common manifestation of myeloma-related kidney disease. Cast nephropathy has been described in 32–48% of patients with MM at autopsy. In healthy individuals, the kidneys filter less than 1 gram of polyclonal light chains per day, which are subsequently catabolized by the proximal tubule cells. In MM, the kidneys filter more than 80–90 grams of pathogenic monoclonal light chains (Bence–Jones proteins). Excessive endocytosis of light chains by proximal tubule cells triggers apoptotic, pro-inflammatory, and fibrotic pathways. Light chains are subsequently delivered to the distal tubule and form casts by binding with Tamm–Horsfall protein (THP), which is produced in the thick ascending limb of the loop of Henle. Casts cause intratubular obstruction, interstitial inflammation and fibrosis. In rat models, cast formation is accelerated in the presence of furosemide. Conversely, pretreating rats with colchicine, which decreases urinary levels of THP, inhibits cast formation [7]. Individual light chain affinity for THP predicts the propensity for forming casts. Renal disease is predominantly secondary to intratubular obstruction from cast formation.

Pathology

Casts are strongly eosin positive and have a fractured appearance on light microscopy. Cellular reaction around the casts by monocytes or giant cells leads to basement membrane disruption. This eventually leads to tubular atrophy and interstitial fibrosis in long standing disease. Immunofluorescence reveals monoclonal light chains within the casts with a slight predominance of kappa (60%) versus lambda (40%) light chains. Electron microscopy has limited value in the diagnosis of cast nephropathy.

Clinical Symptoms and Diagnosis

Acute kidney injury is the most common manifestation of cast nephropathy. Proteinuria is generally mild as the glomeruli are free from injury, unless concurrent AL amyloidosis or LCDD is also present. Signs and symptoms related to underlying MM include anemia, hypercalcemia, fatigue, weight loss, bone pain and fractures. Dipstick urinalysis is generally bland with minimal proteinuria or hematuria. In contrast, urine protein electrophoresis (UPEP) may reveal several grams of light chains (Bence–Jones proteins), which are not detectable by standard urinalysis. Over 90% of patients have an M-protein spike on serum protein electrophoresis (SPEP), and serum immunofixation electrophoresis (IFE) demonstrates a monoclonal immunoglobulin. Bone marrow biopsy generally reveals a high tumor burden of plasma cells. Most patients do not require a kidney biopsy, as this does not generally alter clinical management.

Treatment and Prognosis

Advances in treatment of MM have made achieving remission fairly common. Unfortunately, relapses are also common. All treatment is directed at the underlying pathogenic plasma cells. Oral high-dose dexamethasone can be used acutely to suppress the production of light chains by plasma cells. High-dose melphalan with autologous stem cell transplant is the treatment of choice for patients who have a good performance status and are free of multiple comorbidities. Renal failure is not a contraindication for stem cell transplant, although there is higher transplant-related mortality (17–29%) in patients with advanced chronic kidney disease (CKD) [8–10]. Factors associated with renal recovery after stem cell transplant include dialysis duration less than 6 months, greater residual renal function and complete versus partial remission after transplant [2]. Advances in chemotherapy include lenalidomide, which is an immunomodulatory drug with several possible mechanisms: (1) direct cell toxicity, (2) inhibit tumor cell growth factors, (3) anti-angiogenesis, and (4) increase tumor immunity [11]. The kidneys clear the majority of lenalidomide, and dose adjustments are necessary for patients with CKD to prevent drug toxicity (anemia, thrombocytopenia, dehydration, infection) [12]. Bortezomib, which is a reversible proteosome inhibitor, is another novel therapy with high activity against plasma cells. Proteosomes are necessary for the degradation and clearance of proteins including light chains. Bortezomib causes the accumulation of light chains within the plasma cell leading to proteotoxic stress and cell death. No dosing adjustments of bortezomib are necessary for patients with CKD [13]. A significant number of patients have reversal of renal failure with bortezomib-based therapy in the setting of cast nephropathy [14].

Extracorporeal therapy has been studied to increase the clearance of light chains.

Two small older studies demonstrated a benefit of plasma exchange in the setting of myeloma-related kidney disease [15,16]. However, the largest and most recent trial did not show a significant benefit in the composite endpoint of death, dialysis dependence and glomerular filtration rate less than 30 mL/min [17]. All three studies had relatively small sample sizes, did not measure free light chain levels to assess adequacy of treatment and did not use chemotherapy currently available. Nonetheless, current guidelines do not recommend the routine use of plasma exchange in this setting.

Dialysis with a high cut-off filter is more effective in clearing light chains compared to plasma exchange, and is currently being studied in a multicenter randomized European trial for myeloma cast nephropathy [18].

Treatment also includes the avoidance of other nephrotoxic agents such as iodinated contrast and nonsteroidal anti-inflammatory drugs, treatment of hypercalcemia and aggressive hydration to increase urine flow. The value of alkalinization of the urine is unclear as different light chains precipitate and bind to THP at varying pHs depending on the amino acid sequence, and therefore is not routinely recommended.

AL AMYLOIDOSIS

Pathogenesis

Amyloidosis results from the misfolding of pathogenic precursor proteins secondary to mutations, proteolytic events, or local environmental factors. AL amyloidosis occurs when the precursor proteins are monoclonal light chains. AL amyloidosis may develop with or without underlying MM, and approximately 5% of patients with MM have evidence of AL amyloidosis at autopsy [19]. One-third to one-half of patients with AL amyloidosis have renal involvement. Light chains undergo conformational changes and form unstable fragments which self-aggregate and deposit as amyloid fibrils. Fibrils may deposit within the glomerular basement membrane (GBM), mesangium, or vessel walls. Mesangial cells phenotypically behave like macrophages with increased lysozyme production and increased matrix metalloproteinase (MMP) production. This leads to matrix breakdown and amyloid deposition [20].

Pathology

On light microscopy, the mesangium may have an expanded nodular appearance secondary to amyloid deposition. PAS staining is often weak in contrast to LCDD. Congo red staining and apple green birefringence under polarized light are diagnostic of disease. Immunofluorescence staining determines the pathogenic light chain which has a lambda:kappa ratio of 3:1. Electron microscopy may reveal subepithelial spikes along the GBM as well as randomly oriented non-branching 8–12 nanometer fibrils arranged in a beta-pleated sheet configuration within the mesangium.

Clinical Symptoms and Diagnosis

Characteristics of patients with AL amyloidosis and renal involvement are listed in Table 5.1. AL amyloid may deposit within essentially any organ aside from the central nervous system. Nephrotic range proteinuria is common secondary to glomerular basement membrane disease. Renal function may be preserved on initial presentation, but slowly progressive chronic kidney disease generally develops. Rarely, patients with amyloid deposition within the collecting duct may develop nephrogenic diabetes insipidus. Nephrotic range proteinuria

TABLE 5.1 Patient Characteristics and Outcomes of Patients with Renal AL Amyloidosis

	Pinney et al.*	Gertz et al.**	Bergesio et al.***
No. of patients	923	84	237
Age	62	61	65
Gender (male)	57%	62%	56%
Initial SCr (mg/dL)	1.2	1.1	1.2
Initial proteinuria	5.1	7.0	4.9
Kappa:lambda	1:3.4	1:6.5	1:3.5
ESRD progression	24%	42%	26%

* JCO 2011; 29(6): 674–81.
** NDT 2009; 24(10): 3132–7.
*** NDT 2007; 22(6): 1608–18.

may predispose to the development of edema, ascites and effusions. Cardiac deposition commonly leads to restrictive cardiomyopathy and entails a high mortality. Patients may also present with hepatomegaly, gut malabsorption, carpal tunnel syndrome and myopathy secondary to amyloid deposition. In the absence of MM, bone marrow biopsy often reveals only low-grade tumor burden and SPEP may not detect a monoclonal spike. However, serum IFE generally reveals a monoclonal light chain predominance. Diagnosis largely depends on tissue biopsy (e.g. renal, cardiac, abdominal, or rectal fat pad) demonstrating amyloid deposition. Renal biopsy may help to differentiate between AL amyloidosis and LCDD, as both conditions may present with nephrotic range proteinuria and renal failure.

Treatment and Prognosis

Treatment is targeted at decreasing the production of the amyloidogenic light chain. Treatment previously consisted of oral melphalan and prednisone, which increased median survival from 7 months to 12–18 months in two separate trials. High-dose melphalan with autologous stem cell transplant (HDM/SCT) currently offers the best chance for survival [21–23]. In one large retrospective study looking at 497 patients who underwent HDM/SCT over a 14-year period, median survival was 6.3 years. Combination therapy with bortezomib/dexamethasone [24–26] or lenalidomide/dexamethasone [27,28] has also demonstrated promising results. At least one center has used risk-adapted chemotherapy (based on age, renal function and cardiac involvement) followed by consolidative therapy after transplant to maintain durable overall and organ response rates [29]. Patients who achieve a hematologic response have prolonged survival [21], less proteinuria and preserved renal function [30]. Proteinuria generally decreases gradually over years in these patients [31]. Newer therapies directed at serum amyloid P, which is present in all amyloid fibrils regardless of etiology, have demonstrated promising results in animal models [32,33].

LCDD

Pathogenesis

Light chain deposition disease (LCDD) occurs when complete or partial monoclonal immunoglobulins deposit within all compartments within the renal parenchyma as granular deposits. Cationic polypeptides from light chains bind to anionic basement membranes leading to deposition [34]. Mesangial cells phenotypically behave like myofibroblasts with downregulation of matrix metalloproteinase expression. This leads to increased matrix formation and a profibrotic state [20]. Similar to AL amyloidosis, LCDD may develop with or without underlying MM, and 3% of patients with MM have evidence of LCDD at autopsy [19].

Pathology

Light microscopy demonstrates mesangial matrix expansion, often with a nodular appearance. The nodular appearance may be similar to Kimmelstiel–Wilson lesions in diabetes. In contrast to amyloidosis, PAS staining is generally strongly positive and congo red stain is negative. Thickening of the TBM is common secondary to light chain deposits. Immunofluorescence demonstrates a single light chain isotype predominance, with a kappa:lambda ratio of 9:1. Electron microscopy reveals granular powdery deposits as opposed to fibrils within the mesangium, TBM, GBM and blood vessels.

Clinical Symptoms and Diagnosis

Patient characteristics are listed in Table 5.2. Given the glomerular, tubular and vascular

TABLE 5.2 Patient Characteristics and Outcomes of Patients with LCDD

	Lin et al.*	Pozzi et al.**	Nasr et al.***
No. of patients	23	63	51
Age	57	58	55
Gender (male)	52%	64%	65%
Initial SCr (mg/dL)	4.5	3.8	3.8
Initial proteinuria	4.2	2.7	3
+SPEP/UPEP	87%	94%	73%
MM	39%	65%	59%
Kappa:lambda	9:1	7:3	8:2
ESRD progression	48%	57%	39%

* JASN 2001; 12(7): 1482–92.
** AJKD 2003; 42(6): 1154–63.
*** CJASN 2012; 7(2): 231–9.

injury, patients often present with advanced and rapidly progressive acute kidney injury. Nephrotic range proteinuria is common and may lead to edema and effusions. Chronic kidney disease occurs in a majority of patients, and approximately 50% of patients will progress to end stage renal disease within 2 years of diagnosis. Extra-renal disease from light chain deposits is not generally clinically significant. In the absence of underlying MM, it is not unusual for the SPEP and IFE to be negative, and the bone marrow generally has a low percentage of plasma cells. UPEP demonstrates predominantly albuminuria. Kidney biopsy is necessary for a definitive diagnosis.

Treatment and Prognosis

Until recently, patients with LCDD without MM were not treated with systemic therapy, as this was considered primarily a kidney disease. However, practice has shifted towards treating these patients with anti-plasma cell therapy.

High-dose melphalan with autologous stem cell transplant is generally the treatment of choice [35–37]. Unfortunately, patients that present initially with marked acute kidney injury generally progress to ESRD, regardless of treatment.

BISPHOSPHONATES

Bisphosphonates are routinely given during the first 2 years of treatment of MM. They are also used in the setting of hypercalcemia secondary to MM. Caution must be taken as pamidronate has been associated with collapsing focal segmental glomerulosclerosis and zoledronate may cause acute tubular necrosis. Another potential risk of chronic bisphosphonate usage is osteonecrosis of the jaw. In patients with end stage renal disease, bisphosphonates may further worsen adynamic bone disease by further decreasing the rate of bone turnover. A recent Cochrane review of 17 trials determined that the addition of bisphosphonates to the treatment of MM reduces pathological vertebral fractures, skeletal-related events and pain but not mortality [38]. For patients with LCDD or AL amyloidosis in the absence of MM, bisphosphonates are not routinely given except for the treatment of osteoporosis.

RENAL TRANSPLANT

There is a high risk of disease recurrence in the renal allograft if the patient is not in hematologic remission prior to renal transplant. In LCDD, patients with no detectable evidence of a circulating monoclonal immunoglobulin may still have active disease. Rituximab has been successfully used to delay recurrence of light chain deposits in patients with LCDD after renal transplant. Newer treatments such as lenalidomide and bortezomib could also be potentially used after kidney transplant to prevent disease recurrence and increase longevity of the allograft. The optimal time for performing a renal transplant is not entirely clear, and current guidelines are not specific given the lack of evidence.

References

[1] Kyle RA, Gertz MA, Witzig TE, Lust JA, Lacy MQ, Dispenzieri A, et al. Review of 1027 patients with newly diagnosed multiple myeloma. Mayo Clin Proc 2003;78(1):21–33.

[2] Lee CK, Zangari M, Barlogie B, Fassas A, van Rhee F, Thertulien R, et al. Dialysis-dependent renal failure in patients with myeloma can be reversed by high-dose myeloablative therapy and autotransplant. Bone Marrow Transplant 2004;33(8):823–8.

[3] Blade J, Fernandez-Llama P, Bosch F, Montoliu J, Lens XM, Montoto S, et al. Renal failure in multiple myeloma: presenting features and predictors of outcome in 94 patients from a single institution. Arch Intern Med 1998;158(17):1889–93.

[4] Leung N, Gertz MA, Zeldenrust SR, Rajkumar SV, Dispenzieri A, Fervenza FC, et al. Improvement of cast nephropathy with plasma exchange depends on the diagnosis and on reduction of serum free light chains. Kidney Int 2008;73(11):1282–8.

[5] Hutchison CA, Cockwell P, Stringer S, Bradwell A, Cook M, Gertz MA, et al. Early reduction of serum-free light chains associates with renal recovery in myeloma kidney. J Am Soc Nephrol 2011;22(6):1129–36.

[6] Solomon A, Weiss DT, Kattine AA. Nephrotoxic potential of Bence Jones proteins. N Engl J Med 1991;324(26):1845–51.

[7] Sanders PW, Booker BB. Pathobiology of cast nephropathy from human Bence Jones proteins. J Clin Invest 1992;89(2):630–9.

[8] San Miguel JF, Lahuerta JJ, Garcia-Sanz R, Alegre A, Blade J, Martinez R, et al. Are myeloma patients with renal failure candidates for autologous stem cell transplantation? Hematol J 2000;1(1):28–36.

[9] Knudsen LM, Nielsen B, Gimsing P, Geisler C. Autologous stem cell transplantation in multiple myeloma: outcome in patients with renal failure. Eur J Haematol 2005;75(1):27–33.

[10] Badros A, Barlogie B, Siegel E, Roberts J, Langmaid C, Zangari M, et al. Results of autologous stem cell transplant in multiple myeloma patients with renal failure. Br J Haematol 2001;114(4):822–9.

[11] Bartlett JB, Dredge K, Dalgleish AG. The evolution of thalidomide and its IMiD derivatives as anticancer agents. Nat Rev Cancer 2004;4(4):314–22.

[12] Dimopoulos M, Alegre A, Stadtmauer EA, Goldschmidt H, Zonder JA, de Castro CM, et al. The efficacy and safety of lenalidomide plus dexamethasone in relapsed and/or refractory multiple myeloma patients with impaired renal function. Cancer 2010; 116(16):3807−14.

[13] Jagannath S, Barlogie B, Berenson JR, Singhal S, Alexanian R, Srkalovic G, et al. Bortezomib in recurrent and/or refractory multiple myeloma. Initial clinical experience in patients with impared renal function. Cancer 2005;103(6):1195−200.

[14] Dimopoulos MA, Roussou M, Gavriatopoulou M, Zagouri F, Migkou M, Matsouka C, et al. Reversibility of renal impairment in patients with multiple myeloma treated with bortezomib-based regimens: identification of predictive factors. Clin Lymphoma Myeloma 2009;9(4):302−6.

[15] Zucchelli P, Pasquali S, Cagnoli L, Ferrari G. Controlled plasma exchange trial in acute renal failure due to multiple myeloma. Kidney Int 1988;33(6):1175−80.

[16] Johnson WJ, Kyle RA, Pineda AA, O'Brien PC, Holley KE. Treatment of renal failure associated with multiple myeloma. Plasmapheresis, hemodialysis, and chemotherapy. Arch Intern Med 1990;150(4): 863−9.

[17] Clark WF, Stewart AK, Rock GA, Sternbach M, Sutton DM, Barrett BJ, et al. Plasma exchange when myeloma presents as acute renal failure: a randomized, controlled trial. Ann Intern Med 2005;143(11): 777−84.

[18] Hutchison CA, Cook M, Heyne N, Weisel K, Billingham L, Bradwell A, et al. European trial of free light chain removal by extended haemodialysis in cast nephropathy (EuLITE): a randomised control trial. Trials 2008;9:55.

[19] Herrera GA, Joseph L, Gu X, Hough A, Barlogie B. Renal pathologic spectrum in an autopsy series of patients with plasma cell dyscrasia. Arch Pathol Lab Med 2004;128(8):875−9.

[20] Keeling J, Teng J, Herrera GA. AL-amyloidosis and light-chain deposition disease light chains induce divergent phenotypic transformations of human mesangial cells. Lab Invest 2004;84(10):1322−38.

[21] Skinner M, Sanchorawala V, Seldin DC, Dember LM, Falk RH, Berk JL, et al. High-dose melphalan and autologous stem-cell transplantation in patients with AL amyloidosis: an 8-year study. Ann Intern Med 2004;140(2):85−93.

[22] Sanchorawala V, Skinner M, Quillen K, Finn KT, Doros G, Seldin DC. Long-term outcome of patients with AL amyloidosis treated with high-dose melphalan and stem-cell transplantation. Blood 2007;110(10):3561−3.

[23] Gertz MA, Lacy MQ, Dispenzieri A, Hayman SR, Kumar SK, Dingli D, et al. Autologous stem cell transplant for immunoglobulin light chain amyloidosis: a status report. Leuk Lymphoma 2010;51(12): 2181−7.

[24] Wechalekar AD, Lachmann HJ, Offer M, Hawkins PN, Gillmore JD. Efficacy of bortezomib in systemic AL amyloidosis with relapsed/refractory clonal disease. Haematologica 2008;93(2):295−8.

[25] Kastritis E, Wechalekar AD, Dimopoulos MA, Merlini G, Hawkins PN, Perfetti V, et al. Bortezomib with or without dexamethasone in primary systemic (light chain) amyloidosis. J Clin Oncol 2010;28(6): 1031−7.

[26] Reece DE, Sanchorawala V, Hegenbart U, Merlini G, Palladini G, Fermand JP, et al. Weekly and twice-weekly bortezomib in patients with systemic AL amyloidosis: results of a phase 1 dose-escalation study. Blood 2009;114(8):1489−97.

[27] Sanchorawala V, Wright DG, Rosenzweig M, Finn KT, Fennessey S, Zeldis JB, et al. Lenalidomide and dexamethasone in the treatment of AL amyloidosis: results of a phase 2 trial. Blood 2007; 109(2):492−6.

[28] Dispenzieri A, Lacy MQ, Zeldenrust SR, Hayman SR, Kumar SK, Geyer SM, et al. The activity of lenalidomide with or without dexamethasone in patients with primary systemic amyloidosis. Blood 2007;109(2): 465−70.

[29] Cohen AD, Zhou P, Chou J, Teruya-Feldstein J, Reich L, Hassoun H, et al. Risk-adapted autologous stem cell transplantation with adjuvant dexamethasone +/− thalidomide for systemic light-chain amyloidosis: results of a phase II trial. Br J Haematol 2007;139(2):224−33.

[30] Dember LM, Sanchorawala V, Seldin DC, Wright DG, LaValley M, Berk JL, et al. Effect of dose-intensive intravenous melphalan and autologous blood stem-cell transplantation on al amyloidosis-associated renal disease. Ann Intern Med 2001;134(9 Pt 1): 746−53.

[31] Leung N, Dispenzieri A, Fervenza FC, Lacy MQ, Villicana R, Cavalcante JL, et al. Renal response after high-dose melphalan and stem cell transplantation is a favorable marker in patients with primary systemic amyloidosis. Am J Kidney Dis 2005;46(2):270−7.

[32] Bodin K, Ellmerich S, Kahan MC, Tennent GA, Loesch A, Gilbertson JA, et al. Antibodies to human serum amyloid P component eliminate visceral amyloid deposits. Nature 2010;468(7320):93−7.

[33] Pepys MB, Herbert J, Hutchinson WL, Tennent GA, Lachmann HJ, Gallimore JR, et al. Targeted pharmacological depletion of serum amyloid P component

for treatment of human amyloidosis. Nature 2002; 417(6886):254—9.

[34] Kaplan B, Livneh A, Gallo G. Charge differences between in vivo deposits in immunoglobulin light chain amyloidosis and non-amyloid light chain deposition disease. Br J Haematol 2007;136(5):723—8.

[35] Lorenz EC, Gertz MA, Fervenza FC, Dispenzieri A, Lacy MQ, Hayman SR, et al. Long-term outcome of autologous stem cell transplantation in light chain deposition disease. Nephrol Dial Transplant 2008; 23(6):2052—7.

[36] Weichman K, Dember LM, Prokaeva T, Wright DG, Quillen K, Rosenzweig M, et al. Clinical and molecular characteristics of patients with non-amyloid light chain deposition disorders, and outcome following treatment with high-dose melphalan and autologous stem cell transplantation. Bone Marrow Transplant 2006;38(5):339—43.

[37] Royer B, Arnulf B, Martinez F, Roy L, Flageul B, Etienne I, et al. High dose chemotherapy in light chain or light and heavy chain deposition disease. Kidney Int 2004;65(2):642—8.

[38] Mhaskar R, Redzepovic J, Wheatley K, Clark OA, Miladinovic B, Glasmacher A, et al. Bisphosphonates in multiple myeloma. Cochrane Database Syst Rev (3): 2012 May 16;5:CD003188.

6

Kidney Disease in Patients Undergoing Hematopoietic Cell Transplantation

Benjamin L. Laskin[1], Sangeeta R. Hingorani[2]

[1]The Children's Hospital of Philadelphia, Philadelphia, Pennsylvania, USA
[2]Seattle Children's Hospital/University of Washington and
Fred Hutchinson Cancer Research Center, Seattle, Washington, USA

INTRODUCTION

Acute kidney injury (AKI) and chronic kidney disease (CKD) are common complications of hematopoietic cell transplantation (HCT) and their etiology is often multi-factorial (Figure 6.1). Patients undergoing HCT are at risk for kidney injury from pre-existing kidney disease, conditioning chemotherapy, radiation, antimicrobials, infections, sinusoidal obstruction syndrome (SOS, previously known as veno-occlusive disease of the liver), transplantation-associated thrombotic microangiopathy (TA-TMA) and graft-versus-host disease (GVHD) [1,2]. Both AKI and CKD can increase short- and long-term morbidity and mortality [3]. Further complications of HCT, such as fluid imbalances, electrolyte abnormalities, glomerular disease, and hypertension may occur independent of, or concomitant with, reductions in the glomerular filtration rate (GFR).

The expanding indications for HCT include malignancy, immune deficiencies, bone marrow failure syndromes and inherited metabolic diseases [4,5]. The HCT procedure itself has also become more heterogeneous with variables such as myeloablative or reduced intensity conditioning regimens, allogeneic, autologous, related and unrelated donors, bone marrow, peripheral stem cell and cord blood sources, and an ever increasing array of immunomodulatory agents [2,5,6].

Despite improvements in technology and survival, kidney injury remains a significant problem after HCT [4,7−9]. The management of kidney complications requires close collaboration between transplant physicians, oncologists, intensivists and nephrologists [10−12]. Specifically, nephrologists help manage decreased GFR, elevated blood pressure, fluid overload, electrolyte abnormalities, hematuria and nephrotic syndrome. The objective of this chapter is to summarize the most up-to-date literature on the epidemiology, diagnosis and treatment of kidney disease in patients undergoing HCT.

Renal Disease in Cancer Patients
http://dx.doi.org/10.1016/B978-0-12-415948-8.00006-4

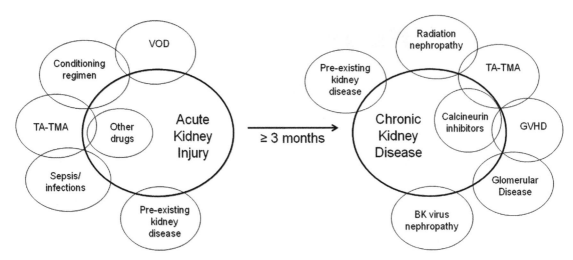

FIGURE 6.1 **Model for the multi-factorial causes of acute kidney injury (AKI) and chronic kidney disease (CKD) in patients receiving hematopoietic stem cell transplantation (HCT).** VOD, veno-occlusive disease of the liver; TA-TMA, transplantation-associated thrombotic microangiopathy; GVHD, graft-versus-host disease. *Adapted from [5].*

CURRENT PRACTICE OF HCT

Source of Infused Hematopoietic Cells

There are various types of HCTs currently being performed, each with varying risks and toxicities (Table 6.1). Autologous HCT involves harvesting a patient's own bone marrow or peripheral blood hematopoietic cells before high-dose myeloablative therapy. To restore hematopoiesis following marrow ablation, the patient's cells are then re-infused. Allogeneic HCT require hematopoietic cells donated from family members (ideally, human leukocyte antigen-

matched siblings), matched unrelated donors, or hematopoietic cells from umbilical cord blood. Syngeneic transplants use cells donated from an identical twin [13].

Conditioning Regimens

In allogeneic HCT, the infusion of donor hematopoietic cells is preceded by either myeloablative therapy (usually a combination of chemotherapy drugs with or without total body irradiation (TBI)) or reduced-intensity (but immunosuppressive) therapy that permits host hematopoietic cells to coexist with donor

TABLE 6.1   Complications Associated with Types of HCT.

Type of conditioning	Donor relationship	Exposure to CNI	Risk for aGVHD	Risk for AKI	Development of SOS	Risk for cGVHD
Myeloablative	Allos	High	High	High	High	High
	Autos	None	+/−	Low	Moderate	None
RIC	Allos	High	Very high	High	Low	High

HCT, hematopoietic cell transplantation; RIC, reduced-intensity conditioning; CNI, calcineurin inhibitor; aGVHD, acute graft-versus-host disease; AKI, acute kidney injury; SOS, sinusoidal obstruction syndrome; cGVHD, chronic graft-versus-host disease; Allos, allogeneic; Autos, autologous.

It is adapted from a review article I wrote for JASN in July of 2006, Vol. 17, No.7, starting on page 1995.

cells (mixed hematopoietic cell chimerism). The distinguishing feature between myeloablative and reduced-intensity allogeneic HCT is the conditioning regimen. The most common myeloablative regimens for allogeneic HCT include cyclophosphamide plus busulfan, fludarabine plus busulfan and cyclophosphamide plus TBI. Myeloablative transplantation involves significant toxicities; the non-myeloablative reduced-intensity regimens are less toxic and therefore can be used in older patients and those with substantial co-morbidities. Reduced-intensity regimens contain lower doses of radiation, for example fludarabine plus 2 to 4 cGy TBI along with intense post-HCT immune suppression. The goal of reduced-intensity regimens is to use immunosuppression which allows for engraftment of the transplanted donor cells, providing a graft-versus-tumor effect against residual malignant cells [13].

Prophylaxis for Complications

Allogeneic graft recipients receive GVHD prophylaxis with immunosuppressive drugs including cyclosporine or tacrolimus plus pulse doses of methotrexate. Mycophenolate mofetil and sirolimus can also be used as GVHD prophylaxis. Prophylactic immunosuppression is typically continued until day +80 (with day zero representing the day of hematopoietic cell infusion) post-HCT transplant after myeloablative conditioning regimens. In patients receiving reduced-intensity conditioning, these medications are often tapered earlier to promote the beneficial graft-versus-tumor effect. Patients who develop acute GVHD (~60% of allograft recipients) are treated initially with high-dose prednisone (1–2 mg/kg/day). Those failing prednisone therapy are treated with more intense immunosuppressive agents including anti-T-cell antibodies (such as anti-thymocyte globulin) and monoclonal antibodies (such as infliximab). Infectious prophylaxis includes acyclovir, trimethoprim/sulfamethoxazole (*Pneumocystic jirovecii*),

fluconazole or voriconazole, and pre-emptive ganciclovir or forscarnet for cytomegalovirus disease in viremic patients. Ursodiol is used to prevent cholestatic liver injury [14–16].

EVALUATION OF KIDNEY DISEASE DURING HCT

The evaluation of suspected kidney disease in a patient undergoing HCT requires careful attention to the medical history, drug exposures (Table 6.2) and the physical examination, combined with targeted laboratory and radiological studies [17].

Kidney Function

Determination of pre-transplant kidney function is important, as those with existing kidney disease may be at higher risk for post-HCT complications due to diminished renal reserve [11,18]. To assist with risk stratification, pre-transplant co-morbidity scales have been validated in adults [19] and children [20]. These scales have defined mild kidney dysfunction as a pre-HCT creatinine of 1.2–2 mg/dL and moderate disease as a creatinine >2 mg/dL, the need for dialysis, or the history of a kidney transplant. However, requiring such severe kidney disease may underestimate the effect of pre-transplant kidney function on later outcome, especially in a high-risk population exposed to multiple prior nephrotoxic medications including chemotherapy, radiation and antimicrobials.

In fact, the influence of pre-transplant kidney function on outcomes remains unclear. Adult leukemia patients with moderately reduced pre-transplant GFR receiving reduced intensity regimens did not have worse survival but did trend towards a higher risk of dialysis in the first year [21]. Similarly, others have reported no change in the later need for dialysis or an increased mortality in those with a pre-HCT

TABLE 6.2   Medications Commonly Associated with Kidney Disease or Hypertension in the HCT Setting [6,18,23,220–222]

Medication	Adverse reactions	Dosing adjust in kidney disease
CONDITIONING THERAPY		
Busulfan	AKI, hypertension, edema, hypomagnesemia, hypokalemia, hypocalcemia, hypophosphatemia	n/a
Cyclophosphamide	Hemorrhagic cystitis, urinary fibrosis	yes
Fludarabine	Edema	yes
Melphalan	–	yes
Alemtuzumab	Hypertension, edema	no
Cisplatin	AKI, CKD	yes
Carboplatin	AKI, hypomagnesemia, hypokalemia, hypocalcemia, hyponatremia	yes
Thiotepa	Hematuria, dysuria, urinary retention	yes
Amifostine	AKI, hypertension, hypomagnesemia, hypocalcemia	n/a
Vincristine	Hyperuricemia, hemolytic uremic syndrome, hypertension, dysuria, polyuria, urinary retention	no
Etoposide	Metabolic acidosis	yes
Carmustine	AKI	yes
Cytarabine	–	yes
Ifosfamide	Metabolic acidosis, hematuria	yes
Radiation	AKI, CKD	consider kidney shielding as appropriate
Dimethyl sulfoxide (stem cell cryopreservative)	Hypertension, kidney injury	n/a
ANTIBACTERIAL AGENTS		
Aminoglycosides	AKI, hypomagnesemia, hypokalemia, hypocalcemia, hyponatremia, proteinuria	yes
Vancomycin	AKI	yes
Sulfamethoxazole/ trimethoprim	AKI, interstitial nephritis, hyperkalemia, proteinuria	yes
ANTIVIRAL AGENTS		
Cidofovir	AKI, proteinuria	yes
Foscarnet	AKI, proteinuria, hypertension, hypomagnesemia, hypokalemia, hypocalcemia, hypophosphatemia, hyperphosphatemia, hyponatremia, proteinuria, dysuria	yes

TABLE 6.2 Medications Commonly Associated with Kidney Disease or Hypertension in the HCT Setting [6,18,23,220−222]—(cont'd)

Medication	Adverse reactions	Dosing adjust in kidney disease
Acyclovir/Ganciclovir	AKI	yes
Immune globulin	AKI, hypertension	yes
ANTIFUNGAL AGENTS		
Amphotericin B	AKI, hypertension, hematuria, hypomagnesemia, hypokalemia, hypocalcemia, hyponatremia	no
Caspofungin	AKI, edema, hypokalemia	yes
Voriconazole	AKI	yes
GVHD PROPHYLAXIS OR TREATMENT		
Calcineurin inhibitors	AKI, hypertension, edema, hypomagnesemia, hypophosphatemia, hyperkalemia, hypokalemia	yes
Rapamycin	Proteinuria, hypertension	no
Methotrexate	AKI, hyperuricemia	yes
Corticosteroids	Hypertension, edema	no

GFR <60 ml/min/1.73 m^2 compared to controls with normal kidney function [22]. Care must be taken in evaluating the effect of baseline kidney function, as those with a higher starting creatinine will have a lower risk of AKI simply because it is harder to double the serum creatinine [17].

Individual centers differ in their assessment of pre- and post-HCT kidney function, which includes creatinine-based estimation and more formal GFR measurement methods [23,24]. The calculation of inulin clearance remains the gold standard for GFR determination, but the procedure is invasive, time consuming and only available at select locations. Newer methods have utilized radioactive isotopes (Tc-DTPA or Cr-EDTA) or iodinated contrast (iothalamate or iohexol) to accurately measure the GFR [11]. However, these techniques are also costly, require repeated blood sampling, and in the case of radioisotopes, necessitate exposure to radiation [25,26].

Therefore, serum creatinine remains the most widely available marker of kidney function in patients undergoing HCT [24]. Creatinine is included in GFR prediction formulas such as the Modification of Diet in Renal Disease (MDRD) equation in adults or the Schwartz formula in children (Table 6.3) [27−29]. Collection of 24-hour urine samples for calculating creatinine clearance may offer improved GFR accuracy over single blood measurements, although adherence with the procedure, especially in children, can be challenging.

Because creatinine is strongly associated with muscle mass, relying on creatinine-based estimates of kidney function has limitations, especially in the HCT population where chronic illness and nutritional deficiencies lead to decreased muscle mass, causing an overestimation of the GFR [4,10,30]. Novel, non-invasive methods using endogenous serum markers such as cystatin C have shown increased performance compared to creatinine in the estimation

TABLE 6.3 Classification of Acute Kidney Injury

Criteria	Risk, injury, failure, loss, end-stage (RIFLE) [55]		Pediatric risk, injury, failure, loss, end stage (pRIFLE) [56]. Higher risk of RRT if persists for >48 hours (No prenal reversal)		Acute kidney injury network (AKIN) [59]		Grade 0–3 Staging [57,58]
	Creatinine	Urine	Creatinine	Urine	Creatinine	Urine	Creatinine
Risk	1.5× ↑creat or >25% ↓GFR*	<0.5 ml/kg/hr × 6 hr	25% ↓GFR†	<0.5 ml/kg/hr× 8hr	1.5× or ≥ 0.3 mg/dL ↑creat	<0.5 ml/kg/h × 6 hr	Grade 0: Decrease in GFR<25% of baseline
Injury	2× ↑creat or >50% ↓GFR*	<0.5 ml/kg/hr × 12hr	50% ↓GFR†	<0.5 ml/kg/hrx 16 hr			Grade 1: Increase in serum creatinine <2 with decrease GFR from 25—<50%
Failure	3× ↑creat, >75% ↓GFR*, or creat >4 mg/dL	<0.3 ml/kg/hr × 24 hr oranuria × 12 hr	>75% ↓GFR† or GFR† <35	<0.3 ml/kg/hr × 24 hr oranuria × 12 hr			Grade 2: Increase in serum creatinine >2 but no dialysis
Loss	Dialysis >4 weeks		Dialysis >4 weeks				Grade 3: Increase in serum creatinine >2 and dialysis
ESRD	Dialysis >3 months		Dialysis >3 months				

*Based on the Modification of Diet in Renal Disease (MDRD) formula: $GFR = [186 \times Creat^{-1.154} \times Age^{-0.203} \times 0.742$ if female $\times 1.210$ if African American] [27].

†Based on the original Schwartz formula [28]: $GFR = [k \times height$ in cm/Creat]; where $k = 0.33$ in premature infants, 0.45 in term infants to 1 year of age, 0.55 in children to 13 years of age, and 0.70 in adolescent males 13–21 years of age. The most recent Schwartz formula uses a $k = 0.413$ in all children [29].

ESRD indicates end stage renal disease; creat, serum creatinine; GFR, glomerular filtration rate (ml/min/1.73 m²); ↑, increased; and ↓, decreased. This research was originally published in Laskin BL, Goebel J, Davies SM, Jodele S. Small vessels, big trouble in the kidneys and beyond: hematopoietic stem cell transplantation-associated thrombotic microangiopathy. Blood 2011;118(6):1452–62. © The American Society of Hematology. Adapted from [10].

of GFR in other high-risk populations such as pediatric and adult solid organ transplant recipients [31,32]. Preliminary data support that cystatin C predicts GFR in the HCT population [33−37], although cystatin C concentrations may be affected by corticosteroid use, thyroid function and inflammation [38,39].

Further Evaluation of Kidney Disease after HCT

When taking the initial medical history, focus should be on the time course of symptoms in reference to baseline/pre-HCT findings, changing laboratory values and non-renal co-morbidities. Key questions to ask include an assessment of thirst and fluid intake, urinary symptoms such as frequency, pain, or hematuria, and the presence of facial or lower extremity swelling.

A careful review of current and past medications is critical for both identifying agents with the potential to cause kidney toxicity (chemotherapy, antimicrobials and calcineurin inhibitors) or hypertension (corticosteroids and calcineurin inhibitors) and to ensure other medications are accurately dosed based on GFR [17]. As hypertension is a common complication of HCT, close attention to a patient's sodium intake from enteral, medication and parenteral nutrition sources is important.

Accurate measurement of patient weight is critical in the evaluation of kidney disease after HCT, especially given that excessive fluid gains have been associated with worse survival [17,18,40,41]. All patients should have at least daily weights, including using bed scales for those unable to ambulate. Meticulous attention to intake and urine and other losses is also vital. Key points in the physical examination include evaluation of the pulse, a properly measured blood pressure in an upper extremity and an assessment of pain as a cause of hypertension, especially during periods of mucositis. Fluid status should be determined with a careful inspection for edema and evaluation of the cardiovascular and respiratory condition [17].

Obtaining a baseline urinalysis prior to transplant allows for future comparison, particularly in patients with pre-existing kidney disease, hypertension, or diabetes mellitus [11,18,24]. Evaluation of a fresh urine sample can aid greatly in the diagnosis of several diseases after HCT. A low urine specific gravity may indicate a concentrating defect as with interstitial nephritis, although careful interpretation is required in those receiving large amounts of intravenous fluids. The presence of glucose and/or protein in the urine may indicate proximal tubular dysfunction. Hematuria, defined as more than five red blood cells per high powered field, can be lower urinary tract as in the case of hemorrhagic cystitis, or upper tract secondary to glomerular injury. Urine microscopy aids in determining the bleeding source, as dysmorphic red cells or red cell casts are diagnostic for glomerulonephritis [17].

A positive urine dipstick for blood without red blood cells raises the suspicion for pigment nephropathy from myoglobinuria/rhabdomyolysis. Albuminuria, as discussed later, is an important finding after HCT with potential prognostic and therapeutic significance [42]. Proteinuria may be secondary to AKI, CKD, urinary infection, or nephrotic syndrome. First morning void spot urine protein to creatinine ratios can assist in the quantification of proteinuria, especially when 24-hour collections are not feasible. After 2 years of age, a spot urine protein to creatinine ratio of >0.2 mg/mg is abnormal and a ratio >2.0 mg/mg indicates nephrotic range proteinuria [43].

The urine electrolyte composition provides diagnostic information in those with electrolyte abnormalities. Urinary potassium is important to measure in those with unexplained hyper- or hypokalemia, urine sodium and osmolarity will aid in the diagnosis of sodium imbalances, and the fractional excretion of sodium can sometimes help in the classification of AKI into prerenal and intrinsic renal disease. However, these values should be interpreted carefully in reference to intravenous fluid intake and the use of diuretic therapy, both of which are common after HCT.

In terms of imaging, renal ultrasound provides useful information regarding obstructive uropathy and the assessment of unexplained significant hypertension [23,44]. A pre-transplant ultrasound is warranted in patients at high risk for congenital genitourinary malformations, such as those with Fanconi anemia [45].

Finally, in certain situations, a kidney biopsy may be necessary in the diagnosis and management of kidney disease after HCT [11,23, 24,44,46]. Indications for kidney biopsy are not absolute but typically include severe unexplained kidney dysfunction, nephrotic syndrome (edema, hypoalbuminemia and proteinuria), prolonged, isolated nephrotic range proteinuria, glomerulonephritis, or to assess for cyclosporine toxicity [47−49]. Biopsy specimens are evaluated using light microscopy, immunofluorescence and electron microscopy. These techniques evaluate for the presence of viral inclusions (BK or adenovirus nephropathy), immune deposition (C4d staining or IgA nephropathy), vascular changes (TA-TMA), or tubular and interstitial inflammation/atrophy (GVHD) [46,50−52].

The HCT population is at high risk of bleeding, so the potential benefits of kidney biopsy should be weighed against the risks [5,53]. Coagulation parameters, hemoglobin and the platelet count should be optimized, the patient should remain in bed for at least 12 hours after the procedure, with limited to no physical activity over the ensuing 2−3 days. Careful monitoring of post-procedure vital signs, blood counts and a very low threshold for serial renal ultrasounds are mandatory if there are any concerns for bleeding. While no studies have specifically addressed the complications of kidney biopsy after HCT, it is important to understand that the procedure, while typically well tolerated, is not without risks even in healthier populations. With ultrasound guidance prospective studies have identified a 1.2% significant complication rate (defined as the need for a blood transfusion or surgical embolization to stop bleeding) in adults undergoing kidney biopsy [54]. The authors identified that the risk for any bleeding, significant or not, was higher in women, younger patients and those with a higher, pre-procedure partial thromboplastin time.

ACUTE KIDNEY INJURY

AKI is defined as a reduction in the GFR resulting in an elevated creatinine, decreased urine output, or both. Several criteria have been published to characterize the timing and severity of kidney injury (Table 6.3). The Risk, Injury, Failure, Loss and End-Stage (RIFLE) are perhaps the most widely utilized criteria in the critical care setting [55]. The GFR estimation relies on the MDRD formula, the creatinine-based method for evaluating kidney function in adults [27]. In pediatric patients, a similar pRIFLE [56] system has been developed, where GFR is estimated with the creatinine-based original Schwartz formula [28]. Others have categorized AKI on a four-point scale from Grade 0 (<25% decrease in estimated GFR) to Grade 3 (more than two times risk in serum creatinine and needing dialysis) [57,58]. Finally, the Acute Kidney Injury Network (AKIN) criteria define AKI as a 1.5 times elevation in baseline creatinine, a creatinine elevation of at least 0.3 mg/dL, or a reduction in urine output to <0.5 ml/kg/hr over a 6-hour period [59].

While most of these equations have been developed for use in a wide range of populations at risk for kidney injury, many have been specifically studied in subjects undergoing HCT. AKIN has assessed AKI in pediatric [45] and adult [37] HCT recipients and the RIFLE criteria have been utilized in adult allogeneic patients [60,61]. A study by Ando et al. [10]

compared the three most commonly cited AKI staging systems shown in Table 6.2 (AKIN, RIFLE and the four-point grading system proposed by Parikh et al. [57,58]) in a heterogeneous adult HCT population including myeloablative, reduced intensity and autologous HCT recipients. They concluded that while all three criteria predicted mortality, the AKIN system had less sensitivity for detecting lower AKI stages. Therefore, they recommended using the RIFLE criteria in the HCT population.

There is wide variation in the reported percentage of patients with AKI after HCT. This is likely due to differences in study designs, patient populations, the definitions of kidney injury and conditioning regimens. Overall, when AKI is defined as at least a doubling of serum creatinine or a 50% reduction in estimated GFR (RIFLE "I") anytime during the first 100 days after stem cell infusion, the reported prevalence ranges from 15 to 73%, but likely occurs in about one-third of recipients [1,2,33,42,58,62–72]. In the largest study to date in allogeneic recipients, up to a third of all patients (children and adults) doubled their serum creatinine in the first 100 days, 10% tripled their creatinine and 5% required acute dialysis [8].

There are multiple causes for AKI after HCT (Figure 6.1). Sepsis is a risk factor for kidney injury, leading to decreased renal blood flow as well as cytokine and complement-induced inflammation [18]. Furthermore, antimicrobials used to treat sepsis, most notably vancomycin and the aminoglycosides, can further decrease kidney function. SOS has been identified as an independent risk factor for AKI and is typically associated with poor outcomes. SOS is likely on the spectrum of hepatorenal syndromes, as damage to liver endothelial cells results in edema and decreased urinary sodium concentration [73]. Other causes of AKI include calcineurin inhibitor use, which acutely leads to renal arteriolar vasoconstriction and has also been associated with the development of TA-TMA [11]. GVHD has been associated with AKI, even independent of calcineurin inhibitor exposure. GVHD likely causes tissue and endothelial damage via T-cell and cytokine mediated injury [2,5].

Myeloablative Conditioning

In patients receiving myeloablative conditioning for allogeneic HCT, Parikh et al. conducted a meta-analysis of studies reporting AKI in the first 100 days after HCT [74]. AKI, defined as a doubling of serum creatinine, was reported in six adult studies through 2003. Patients with AKI had a 2–3 times risk of death compared to those without AKI and recipients needing dialysis had a mortality >80%. More recent studies have supported these findings in both adult and pediatric patient populations. In a prospective evaluation of 61 children after allogeneic myeloablative HCT, patients developing AKI had an increased risk of death [45]. AKI, defined as at least a 1.5 times increase in the baseline serum creatinine, was independently associated with SOS and amphotericin use. Conversely, other prospective evaluations of AKI in small studies of children and adults after myeloablative allogeneic HCT have been unable to find an association between AKI and underlying diagnosis, patient age, sepsis, SOS, acute GVHD, TA-TMA, or vancomycin use during the first 100 days after HCT [33,63].

In larger, retrospective analyses, reported risk factors for the development of AKI have varied. Kersting et al. studied 363 adults who received myeloablative HCT with fractionated total body irradiation (TBI) and partial kidney shielding [62]. AKI was identified in 50% of their cohort and multivariate associations with AKI included pre-HCT hypertension and admission to the intensive care unit. Interestingly, AKI was not associated with mortality after correction for co-morbid conditions such as high-grade acute GVHD, TA-TMA and SOS. Serum creatinine levels at 12 months post-HCT levels were no different between those who did and did not develop AKI. Hingorani et al. conducted a nested case–control study in pediatric and adult allogeneic recipients receiving conditioning with cyclophosphamide and TBI that was fractionated but given without renal shielding [1]. There was no difference in AKI risk between children and adults. In their multivariate model, AKI was associated with amphotericin use, SOS and a lower baseline serum creatinine. Other reported independent risk factors for AKI after myeloablative conditioning included vancomycin, increased bilirubin and acute GVHD [60,64].

Reduced Intensity Conditioning

Reduced intensity protocols are increasingly used in patients with non-malignant HCT indications and those with older age and greater co-morbidities at the time of transplant. Liu et al. prospectively studied 26 adults receiving non-myeloablative conditioning for chronic myelogenous leukemia. Including lower grades of AKI (less than two times baseline creatinine) their reported risk for AKI was 19% in the first 100 days [69]. In 188 adults undergoing allogeneic reduced intensity conditioning with busulfan/fludarabine, cyclophosphamide/melphalan, or low dose TBI, the prevalence of AKI (defined as a less than two-fold increase in creatinine during the first year) was 52% [75]. Eighty-one percent of these AKI episodes occurred in the first 100 days. AKI was associated with higher non-relapse mortality at both 100 days and 1 year. Independent risk factors for AKI included methotrexate use, more than three prior chemotherapy courses before HCT and a history of diabetes.

When stricter AKI criteria (doubling of serum creatinine in the first 100 days) have been used in those receiving reduced intensity conditioning, the prevalence of AKI has been reported to be slightly lower at 33% [68]. In this study, risk factors for AKI were the absence of

cardiovascular disease and lower baseline creatinine and patients with higher grade AKI and concomitant acute GVHD had worse survival. Similarly, Parikh et al. studied 253 adults receiving reduced intensity conditioning that included TBI and found that 40.4% had at least a doubling of serum creatinine in the first 3 months [58]. The need for mechanical ventilation was independently associated with AKI and survival was worse as the grade of AKI increased. Finally, another study by the same author found that AKI developed in 56% of 358 patients receiving reduced intensity conditioning and TBI. At a median follow-up of 3 years, overall mortality (but not non-relapse mortality) and chronic GVHD were associated with AKI [70]. The authors speculated that AKI is associated with higher mortality because improper drug dosing may lead to chronic GVHD or graft loss.

When comparing the risk of AKI between myeloablative and reduced intensity regimens, most studies report that the risk is higher after myeloablative conditioning, despite the fact that recipients of non-myeloablative regimens are often older. Accordingly, the prevalence of AKI during the first 100 days was 47% in adult reduced intensity recipients who were 10 years older and far more likely to have GFR of <90 ml/min/1.73 m^2 at baseline compared to myeloablative recipients, in whom 73% developed AKI over this time period [71]. The authors hypothesized that myeloablative preparatory regimens may have a greater risk of AKI because kidney stem cells are destroyed, limiting the ability of the kidney to repair itself after HCT.

Additional studies have compared the risk of AKI between myeloablative and reduced intensity regimens in the same study population. In children [66] and adults [76] some have reported that both myeloablative and reduced intensity recipients have a similar risk for AKI. However, while myeloablative conditioning may be associated with a higher risk of AKI and death from kidney injury [2,10,65], others have found that reduced intensity regimens carry a greater risk of kidney injury [67].

Autologous HCT

Only a few recent studies have assessed the risk of AKI in patients receiving autologous HCT. Lopes et al. compared percentage of patients with a doubling of serum creatinine in the first 100 days between autologous and allogeneic recipients [72]. The overall risk of AKI was 21.5%, and trended towards being higher in the allogeneic (27%) compared to the autologous 12% recipients ($p = 0.07$). Similarly, Ando et al. studied 249 adults in an observational cohort and found a risk for AKI in autologous recipients of 10–19%, depending on the staging system used [10]. In comparison, the risk for AKI in the MA group was 62–66%. Finally, Beyzadeoglu et al. compared two conditioning regimens in autologous HCT recipients [77]. Forty-seven patients received ifosfamide, carboplatin, etoposide and the remaining 21 received TBI and cyclophosphamide. Although the study population was small, the risk of AKI was four times higher in the ifosfamide group (23.4%) than the TBI group (4.8%, $p = 0.06$).

Acute Dialysis

The reported risk of needing acute dialysis after HCT-associated AKI varies widely in the literature. The most recent literature cites a risk of dialysis ranging from 0 to 30% [33,40,58,62,66,70,72], but is likely closer to about 5% and probably higher in myeloablative compared to reduced intensity recipients [71]. However, there is less uncertainty concerning the outcome of patients requiring acute renal replacement therapy as almost all report that acute dialysis in this population is associated with an extremely high mortality rate, often approaching 80–100% [2,10,58,62,66,70,72,77].

The indications for initiating renal replacement therapy after HCT are identical to the non-transplant population and include refractory acidosis, electrolyte abnormalities (hyperkalemia), iatrogenic ingestions (vancomycin toxicity), fluid overload and uremia. However, there is increasing evidence from the critical care literature that earlier initiation of renal replacement therapy may provide clinical benefits, although results are conflicting [78]. In the HCT population, Michael et al. retrospectively reviewed the outcome of 272 pediatric recipients. By univariate analysis, survival was worse in those requiring ventilation, having more severe illness, and in those with >10% fluid overload [40]. In support of the importance of fluid overload as a predictor of mortality, Sutherland et al. in a multi-center, prospective observational study of 297 children (one-third of whom had a history of malignancy or HCT) receiving intensive care found that mortality increased by 3% for every 1% increase in fluid overload. In those children with ≥20% fluid overload, mortality was eight times higher compared to those with <20% fluid overload [41].

Aggressive fluid control with careful attention to fluid balance relative to the admission weight is important. Once fluid overload reaches 5%, some suggest starting furosemide infusions and limiting further intake unless a patient shows firm signs of volume depletion [12,40]. However, diuretics must be used cautiously in the intensive care setting, as they may have unproven benefit and can even result in harm [79]. At 10% fluid overload, some support the initiation of renal replacement therapy [40,80].

In terms of dialysis modality, continuous therapies may be more desirable in the intensive care setting, allowing for fluid removal in hemodynamically unstable patients. Furthermore, continuous hemofiltration, given at a replacement rate of 35 ml/kg/hr (2000 ml/1.73 m^2/hr) offers convective removal of larger inflammatory molecules which cannot be cleared using the diffusive properties of continuous hemodialysis [12,80]. Whether removal of these larger molecules provides clinical benefit in this population remains uncertain. Flores et al. reviewed 51 children receiving continuous renal replacement therapy after HCT [81]. At dialysis initiation, each patient's mean percent fluid overload was 12.4% and half were receiving diuretic therapy. Overall, 45% survived to discharge from the intensive care unit, and mortality was higher in those requiring ventilatory support with higher mean airway pressures. Patients receiving convective clearance with continuous hemofiltration had improved survival (59%) compared to those prescribed only diffusive clearance with continuous hemodialysis (27% survival).

CHRONIC KIDNEY DISEASE

CKD is defined as kidney disease or a GFR of <60 ml/min/1.73 m^2 for ≥3 months [27]. The five stages of CKD (Table 6.4) range from mild (Stage I) to the need for chronic renal replacement therapy (Stage V). This classification system is important for following the progression of CKD over time, standardizing patient definitions for research studies and optimizing

TABLE 6.4 Staging of Chronic Kidney Disease: Renal Damage or a Glomerular Filtration Rate less than 60 ml/min/1.73 m^2 for at Least 3 Months

Stage	Description	GFR (ml/min/1.73 m^2)
I	Kidney disease with normal GFR	90
II	Mild	60−89
III	Moderate	30−59
IV	Severe	15−29
V	End stage renal disease	<15 or on renal replacement therapy

This research was originally published in Laskin BL, Goebel J, Davies SM, Jodele S. Small vessels, big trouble in the kidneys and beyond: hematopoietic stem cell transplantation-associated thrombotic microangiopathy. Blood 2011;118(6):1452−62. © The American Society of Hematology.
Adapted from [27].

management strategies which may vary based on the degree of kidney dysfunction.

As with AKI, there is wide variation in the proportion of patients developing CKD after HCT due to different study designs, lengths of follow-up, definitions of CKD and conditioning regimens. Nevertheless, the prevalence of CKD after HCT, when defined as an estimated GFR <60 ml/min/1.73 m^2 for ≥3 months [27], is reported as 5−49% but is likely about 20−30% [9,52,61,76,82−88]. These studies may underestimate the impact of kidney disease in this population, as the exclusive reliance on creatinine-based methods of GFR estimation may have limitations in those with reduced muscle mass, as mentioned above.

CKD before HCT

While kidney injury after HCT remains a significant complication, there are increasing numbers of patients entering the transplant process with pre-existing kidney disease (reviewed in Heher et al. [6]). Most of these patients have a history of multiple myeloma or sickle cell disease. HCT for these diseases can treat both the underlying hematological process and possibly slow the progression of CKD. Other conditions that carry a high risk of pre-HCT CKD include renal cell carcinoma, Wilms tumor, neuroblastoma, Fanconi anemia and aplastic anemia [6].

Parikh et al. retrospectively analyzed 46 adults with a history of multiple myeloma and a pre-HCT serum creatinine of >2 mg/dL [89]. In fact, 20% of patients were on chronic dialysis at the time of transplant. Patients received autologous HCT with high-dose melphalan. After a median follow-up of 34 months, two-thirds of patients were alive and 39% were progression free. Thirty percent of patients (who did not have pre-HCT end stage kidney disease) had improvement in kidney function after HCT. Similarly, a recent case report of a patient with amyloidosis and nephrotic syndrome treated with autologous HCT had a decrease in proteinuria 3 years post-transplant [90].

Current indications for reduced intensity HCT in sickle cell patients >16 years of age include an elevated creatinine (1.5 times normal) or biopsy proven disease [91]. Fludarabine conditioning has been reported in a patient with sickle cell disease receiving hemodialysis prior to HCT [92]. Using pharmacokinetic studies in combination with daily dialysis (6 hours of dialysis given 12 hours after fludarabine dosing), the authors advised that reducing the fludarabine dose by 20% was effective and produced fludarabine exposures similar to those with normal kidney function. Patients with diabetic nephropathy receiving chronic dialysis prior to HCT have also been successfully treated by using daily dialysis during the conditioning regimen [93].

Longer-term reports of follow-up in patients with pre-existing chronic kidney disease receiving reduced intensity conditioning have also been encouraging. In 141 adult patients with leukemia and pre-transplant kidney dysfunction, non-myeloablative conditioning with fludarabine and melphalan was fairly well tolerated [21]. At 1 year, these patients did not have worse survival than those with normal kidney function; however, there was a trend towards the need for more dialysis. This lack of decreased survival in those with baseline CKD has also been reported in a smaller group of patients followed until almost 3 years post-HCT [22].

Finally, there have even been reports of patients receiving an HCT after a previous kidney transplant (reviewed in [6]). These transplants are often quite challenging and have been reported to have a high risk of kidney rejection, even in those who had received an HLA identical kidney.

CKD after HCT

As in the AKI literature, studies reporting the risk of CKD after HCT are difficult to compare because the definitions of CKD are not consistent, the populations are often heterogeneous and follow-up times vary [4]. While several disease processes such as TA-TMA, radiation nephritis, nephrotic syndrome, chronic GVHD and BK virus nephropathy have been associated with CKD after HCT, much of the long-term kidney injury in this population remains unexplained (Figure 6.1) [5]. GVHD may lead to CKD via direct T-cell damage, cytokine-induced inflammation, or may be associated with CKD due to concomitant calcineurin therapy [85].

Chronic radiation-induced kidney injury may be caused by tissue fibrosis, vessel damage and overactivation of the renin–angiotensin system and is typically apparent by about 9 months after HCT [47]. Glezerman et al. retrospectively assessed the risk of TBI (fractionated without kidney shielding) on CKD in adult HCT recipients receiving T-cell-depleted grafts [52]. At 2 years follow-up, CKD (GFR <60 ml/min/ 1.73 m^2) was 29% in the non-TBI group and 48.8% in the TBI group. While some studies have supported that TBI is a risk factor for CKD [83,94], others have failed to show an association between radiation and the development of CKD, possibly due to different radiation doses, use of fractionation and kidney shielding [9,61,85,95].

Ellis et al. conducted a meta-analysis to review the literature on CKD after HCT through 2006 [4]. Patients in the included studies had to survive past 100 days and only 18% of the identified studies were prospective. Kidney function was assessed with creatinine-based, radioisotope, or inulin GFR. The overall prevalence of CKD was 16.6% (range of 3.6–89%) and was similar in those receiving autologous and allogeneic transplants, although the allogeneic patients had a greater decrement in kidney function. The risk of CKD was noted to be higher in adults than in children. At 2 years post-HCT, overall estimated GFR decreased from about 102 ml/min/ 1.73 m^2 pre-transplant to 77 ml/min/1.73 m^2 (25% decrease). Risk factors for CKD reported by more than two studies included a history of AKI, chronic GVHD, long-term cyclosporine use and TBI. Study heterogeneity precluded an accurate assessment of the significance of these risk factors across cohorts. Compared to the community population, GFR decreased more rapidly in the HCT recipients (0.75 ml/min/1.73 m^2 per year versus 12−25 ml/min/1.73 m^2 per year after HCT) and the risk of CKD after HCT was almost double that reported in the age-matched Framingham cohort (9.4% versus 16.6%).

More recent reports have supported these findings on both the burden of CKD after HCT and its associated risk factors. At 1 year post-HCT, children have a 10% risk of CKD following allogeneic HCT [45], a percentage increasing to 27% at 10 years [94]. Cohorts including both children and adults note a CKD prevalence of 19% at 1 year [42] and 7% at least 2 years after HCT with a mean estimated GFR of 46 ml/min/1.73 m^2 [83].

In studies including only adult myeloablative allogeneic recipients, the prevalence of CKD varies from 17 to 40% [61,82,84,96]. Risk factors for the development of CKD in this population include longer survival after HCT, AKI, hypertension, age >45 years, acute GVHD and a baseline GFR <90 ml/min/1.73 m^2 [61,82,94].

In recipients receiving reduced intensity conditioning, the reported prevalence of CKD has ranged from 7−30% up to 3 years after HCT [76,83,85]. While one study found reduced intensity conditioning to be a risk factor for CKD [85], another did not [76]. Other independent risk factors for CKD in these studies have included acute and chronic GVHD, older patient age, prolonged cyclosporine use (>6 months) and AKI [76,83,85].

Looking directly at populations only receiving non-myeloablative conditioning, risk factors for CKD have included baseline kidney function, AKI, prior autologous HCT, chronic GVHD and prolonged calcineurin use [87,88]. The prevalence of CKD up to 4 years after HCT is about 20% [87,88]. Only one recent study

included a larger percentage of autologous recipients (47%) and found after a median of 7 years follow-up, the prevalence of CKD was 5% and was higher in those who were older, had calcineurin inhibitor exposure, or a diagnosis of multiple myeloma [9].

Complications of CKD after HCT and their Management

Proteinuria, hypertension and anemia are common complications of CKD in the non-transplant population and are also amenable to treatment.

Proteinuria

Proteinuria can be tubular (low-molecular weight, such as beta-2 microglobulin) or glomerular (albumin) in origin. In a large prospective cohort, Hingorani et al. assessed the impact of microalbuminuria (morning albumin to creatinine ratio (ACR) of ≥30 mg/g creatinine) and overt proteinuria (≥300 mg/g creatinine) on outcomes after HCT [42]. Microalbuminuria at day 100 was associated with a four times greater risk of CKD and overt proteinuria at 100 days was associated with a seven times greater risk of non-relapse mortality. Others have found microalbuminuria without overt proteinuria in children followed 18 years after transplant [36]. Conversely, a retrospective analysis in 158 adults receiving myeloablative allogeneic HCT identified a prevalence of proteinuria (defined as a dipstick of 1+ or greater) of 23% at 3 years post-transplant and this level of proteinuria was not associated with the development of CKD [82]. In pediatric autologous recipients, urinary albumin excretion was reported as normal at 2 years post-HCT [97].

Recent consensus guidelines recommend screening urinalyses for ACR as part of the day +80 post-HCT evaluation and then yearly screening after HCT [23,36]. Routine urinalyses can be used to test for hematuria and proteinuria. Patients with proteinuria should have a urine protein to creatinine evaluation performed. Similarly, microalbuminuria testing should be done at day +80 and then yearly, with more frequent monitoring every 3—6 months if elevated [23]. Anti-proteinuric therapy with angiotensin converting enzyme inhibitors (ACE-I) and/or angiotensin receptor blockers (ARB) have not been studied in controlled trials in HCT recipients with proteinuria, although it seems reasonable to speculate they would have benefit [11,42]. Patients with overt proteinuria of >300 mg/g on one check or persistent microalbuminuria >30 mg/g may benefit from treatment [23]. However, a randomized trial of 50 patients on the use of short-term ACE-I therapy to prevent radiation nephropathy after TBI and allogeneic HCT did not find any statistical impact on survival or the development of CKD [98,99].

Low-molecular weight or tubular proteinuria occurs in those receiving an HCT and serves as a marker of tubular damage. This proteinuria may be transient, returning to pre-transplant values after the first 30 days [33], or may persist in association with other markers of tubular dysfunction such as hyperphosphaturia [36,83,97].

Hypertension

The definition and accurate classification of hypertension (Table 6.5) is important, as elevations in blood pressure are a common complication of HCT. In adults (>18 years of age), the Seventh Report of the Joint National Committee on Prevention, Detection, Evaluation and Treatment of High Blood Pressure defines hypertension as a blood pressure ≥140/90 on at least two separate occasions when properly obtained (i.e. correct cuff size) with seated measurements in the office setting [100]. In children, the Fourth Report on the Diagnosis, Evaluation and Treatment of High Blood Pressure in Children and Adolescents defines hypertension as a systolic or diastolic blood pressure >95th percentile based on gender, age and height [101]. Because there are no guidelines for the classification of

TABLE 6.5 Definition and Classification of Hypertension in Adults and Children (Systolic and/or Diastolic) [100,101]

	Adults (>18 years of age)	Children and adolescents*
Normal	<120/80	<90th percentile
Pre-hypertension	120—139/80—89	90th to <95th percentile or if >120/80
Stage 1 hypertension	140—159/90—99	95th—99th percentile plus 5 mm Hg
Stage 2 hypertension	≥160/100	>99th percentile plus 5 mm Hg

Percentile values based on gender, age and height.

hypertension in the inpatient setting, the above outpatient criteria are often used for those admitted to hospital.

In pediatric and adult HCT recipients, Majhail et al. reported on a hypertension prevalence of 70% during the first 2 years with a median time to onset of 1 month post-transplant [102]. Almost 90% of these patients were receiving drug therapy. Cyclosporine use was an independent risk factor for hypertension. Other studies have reported a hypertension prevalence of 15—72%, depending on the length of follow-up [36,84,88,96,103].

In a retrospective analysis of children and adults over a median of 16 years, the prevalence of hypertension was 17% [104]. Antihypertensive therapy was prescribed for 65% of patients with hypertension. Independent predictors of hypertension include AKI, TBI, autologous transplant (mostly neuroblastoma), obesity and diabetes. Hypertension has also been closely associated with the development of TA-TMA [30,52].

Effective treatment of hypertension is important to decrease cardiovascular risk and slow the progression of CKD [84,105]. Blood pressure screening should be performed at all follow-up visits, and at least once a year [23,36,44]. ACE-I or ARB therapy should be considered first line chronic therapy, given their anti-proteinuria and renoprotective properties [11,47]. However, caution must be exercised in those with hyperkalemia, AKI and females of reproductive age. Additional therapeutic options should include sodium restriction and lifestyle medication [104].

Anemia

Only a few studies have examined the prevalence of anemia in HCT recipients developing CKD. One reported lower levels of mean hemoglobin compared to patients without CKD at mean follow-up of 5 years [84]. Another study noted lower erythropoietin levels in children developing TA-TMA and those treated with recombinant erythropoietin therapy had a decrease in transfusion requirements [106]. While some have supported the use of erythrocyte stimulating therapy in those with HCT renal injury nephropathy [47], caution should be used in those with a history of malignancy [107].

End Stage Kidney Disease and Kidney Transplant after HCT

There are limited data on the risk of end stage renal disease after HCT. The reported prevalence ranges from 0.4 to 4.4% (the latter when followed for a mean of 10 years after HCT) [4,61,82,96,104]. Relative to the non-transplant population, the rate of end stage kidney disease after HCT is reported to be 900 times higher than an age-matched Japanese population [82]. Furthermore, Cohen et al. calculated that by 20 years post-HCT, transplant recipients had a risk of end stage kidney disease 16 times higher than the general population [108]. As a comparison, the rate of *de novo* solid tumors occurring after HCT, a commonly cited long-term complication, was only 2.7 higher than the general population.

There are several reports of successful kidney transplantation in both children and adults developing end stage kidney disease after HCT [5,10,47,104,109]. Some of these patients have successfully received a kidney transplant from the original stem cell donor, allowing for a reduction or even cessation of immunosuppression [47,110,111].

The search for methods to enhance tolerance after solid organ transplant has in part been guided by these successful reports of HCT recipients receiving a kidney transplant from the same donor. The concept of mixed chimerism, whereby a recipient is able to stop immunosuppression after "combined" HCT-kidney transplantation, has become an active area of research. The original reports of these "combined" transplants were in patients with multiple myeloma [6]. Although the patient numbers are small, 5/7 of the original recipients have survived 4–11 years after transplant, with 3/5 remaining off immunosuppression.

These reports have prompted expansion of this procedure to patients with primary kidney disease, utilizing a reduced intensity HCT to achieve microchimerism and long-term solid organ tolerance. Mixed chimerism, as opposed to complete donor chimerism, may offer the benefits of transplant tolerance with lower risks of GVHD [112]. In one protocol, lymphoid radiation and 5 days of thymoglobulin have allowed immunosuppression to be weaned off over 6 months post-transplant [112]. At a mean follow-up of 25 months, 8/12 patients have remained off immunosuppression [113]. A second protocol has utilized conditioning with cyclophosphamide, anti-CD2 antibody, thymic radiation and rituximab (in an effort to decrease the risk of antibody mediated rejection) [114]. The patients demonstrated only transient chimerism, did not develop GVHD and had increased FOXP3$^+$ cells, indicative of peripheral tolerance. In the five patients undergoing this procedure, successful withdrawal of immunosuppression occurred at about 1 year in 4/5 recipients and they remain well 2–5 years post-transplant.

These exciting interactions between the fields of solid organ and stem cell transplantation may greatly enhance our understanding of transplant immunology, perhaps allowing for dramatic improvements in the clinical care of high-risk patients [115]. As mentioned, case reports have demonstrated that HCT is possible in those with pre-existing end stage kidney disease, kidney transplant can be successful after HCT and a combined HCT–kidney transplant may allow for the achievement of long-term tolerance (Figure 6.2).

SPECIFIC KIDNEY DISEASES AFTER HCT

TA-TMA

TA-TMA is a pathologically defined entity characterized as endothelial damage leading to thickened glomerular and arteriolar vessels, the presence of fragmented red blood cells, thrombosis and endothelial cell swelling [11,116]. TA-TMA can lead to subclinical disease, AKI, or CKD after HCT [5,30,118]. Given the challenges of obtaining kidney tissue in the HCT population, two consensus guidelines have been published outlining clinical criteria for the diagnosis of TA-TMA [119,120]. Both guidelines require the presence of schistocytes on peripheral smear and an elevated lactate dehydrogenase. The BMT Clinical Trials Network also includes AKI (doubling of serum creatinine), unexplained CNS dysfunction and a negative Coombs test [119]. The International Guidelines from the European Group for Blood and Marrow Transplantation include thrombocytopenia, anemia and a decreased haptoglobin [120]. Diagnosing TA-TMA remains challenging and often requires a high index of suspicion, as

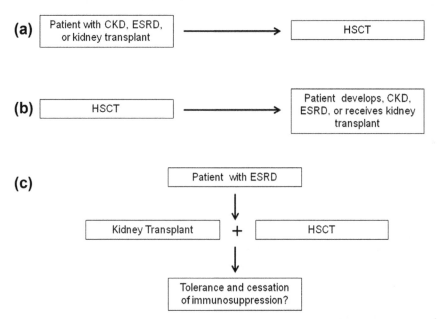

FIGURE 6.2 **Interactions between chronic kidney disease (CKD), kidney transplantation and hematopoietic stem cell transplantation (HCT) [6].** (a) Patients with pre-existing CKD, end stage renal disease (ESRD), or kidney transplants have successfully received later HCT. (b) Patients with HCT commonly develop later CKD, which can progress to ESRD/kidney transplantation. (c) Patients receiving combined kidney and HCT may develop tolerance and no longer require lifelong immunosuppression.

supported by validation studies [121] and autopsy studies where clinical criteria often do not correlate with histological findings [53,117,122].

Whether TA-TMA is a distinct disease after HCT, or merely a manifestation of other post-HCT complications such as GVHD or infections, is a matter of ongoing debate [53,103,123,124]. However, the distinct histological findings support the importance of endothelial cell damage, primarily in the renal vasculature, in the pathogenesis of TA-TMA. While several risk factors have been associated with the development of TA-TMA, it is more likely that the disease is caused by different processes in different patients.

Specifically, factors associated with TA-TMA include infections, especially viral infections (CMV, adenovirus, parvovirus B19, HHV-6 and BK virus) [48,116,125,126], GVHD prophylaxis including calcineurin inhibitors (tacrolimus and cyclosporine) and mammalian target of rapamycin inhibitors (rapamycin) [127–131], and GVHD [53,128,132–137]. TA-TMA is likely more common after allogeneic compared to autologous HCT [30,116], and is reported after both myeloablative and RIC conditioning [128,138]. Specific agents associated with TA-TMA include busulfan, fludarabine, cisplatin and radiation [106,124,128,138,139].

The exact pathogenesis and mechanisms of endothelial injury for TA-TMA remain unknown. Although histologically similar, TA-TMA appears to be distinct from TTP, in that TA-TMA patients do not have markedly low levels of ADAMTS13 [116,124]. Current theories on the pathogenesis of renal endothelial injury include hypotheses based on abnormalities of the coagulation cascade and the complement system [50,51,140–142]. A recent case report has identified the potential role of NK cell dysregulation in the pathogenesis of TA-TMA [143].

TA-TMA in the kidney may reflect direct injury to endothelial cells of the kidney by GVHD. More recent clinical and pathologic studies of TA-TMA after HCT have supported both acute and chronic GVHD as potential risk factors for its development. The risk of TA-TMA diagnosed on renal pathology at autopsy was increased four-fold in patients with acute GVHD after transplant [53]. Endothelial injury in the kidney may be secondary to circulating inflammatory cytokines related to GVHD elsewhere in the body or may reflect direct injury to endothelial cells of the kidney by GVHD [53]. Endothelial injury has been described in patients with chronic GVHD, and it is thought that endothelial cells are direct targets of cytotoxic donor T-lymphocytes [144]. Plasma markers of endothelial injury and coagulation activation are elevated in patients with acute GVHD after HCT suggesting an association between endothelial injury, acute GVHD and the subsequent development of TA-TMA [145,146]. Newer evidence suggests a role for vascular endothelial growth factor (VEGF) in the development of TA-TMA as well as GVHD [147,148]. Loss of function of VEGF or inhibition of VEGF leads to development of proteinuria and glomerular endothelial injury consistent with TA-TMA [147], and lower levels of VEGF have been associated with more severe forms of acute GVHD [148]. Perhaps GVHD leads to endothelial injury in the kidney through a reduction in serum VEGF levels and therefore loss of the protective effects of VEGF on the glomerular filtration barrier. The increased risk of TA-TMA in recipient/donor gender mismatch pairs further supports the theory that acute GVHD may play a role in the pathogenesis of TA-TMA after HCT [53]. Acute GVHD is increased in gender mismatch pairs, possibly due to the presence of sex-specific antigens [53,149].

Treatment for TA-TMA remains challenging and current studies have been limited by retrospective study designs and the inclusion of heterogeneous patient populations. Current options include adjustment of GVHD prophylaxis (especially either stopping or reducing calcineurin inhibitor dosing), the use of therapeutic plasma exchange (TPE), rituximab and defibrotide [119,121,130,150,151]. The most recent response rates for TPE are reported at 27–80% in uncontrolled studies [126,128,137, 139,152–154], but the procedure is not without risks, including requiring separate large vessel central access [155,156]. Worel et al. reported a 64% response rate in a prospective study of patients with TA-TMA treated with both TPE and cyclosporine withdrawal [139]. Rituximab, which may work by reducing inciting antibodies (complement mediated or otherwise), has been shown to have benefit in case reports [142,150,157–161].

BK Virus

BK virus is a double-stranded DNA virus in the polyomavirus family. Infection with the virus is almost ubiquitous by early adulthood as seroprevalence rates of 80% have been reported in healthy blood donors [162]. The virus then remains dormant in the urothelial cells without clinical effects in immunocompetent individuals. In the immunosuppressed population, BK virus has most commonly been associated with nephropathy after kidney transplant and hemorrhagic cystitis (>1 week after stem cell infusion) after HCT [163]. In transplant recipients, primary BK virus infection may be acquired from the environment, blood transfusions, or donor [164].

Current treatment options for hemorrhagic cystitis have not been assessed in controlled trials and include pain control, bladder irrigation and urological intervention for clot removal or obstruction. Pharmacological interventions include cidofovir, leflunomide and fluoroquinolones [165–167]. Ciprofloxacin has been reported to decrease BK urinary viral loads, but not the risk of hemorrhagic cystitis, when given as prophylaxis during the first 2 months after HCT [168]. CMX100, an oral formulation of cidofovir with activity against double-stranded DNA viruses, may have less kidney toxicity and clinical trials are currently ongoing [169]. As decreases in cell-mediated immunity have been associated with worse BK virus disease, novel therapeutic approaches include the development of exogenous BK-specific T-cells and manipulation of immunosuppression to maximize a patient's own immune response [170–172]. Given the nephrotoxicity of cidofovir, its use should be restricted to those with biopsy evidence of BK nephropathy.

After HCT, BK virus-associated hemorrhagic cystitis occurs in 10–25% of patients and leads to prolonged hospitalization, surgical interventions and even death [163,173,174]. Cesaro et al. prospectively studied BK virus in pediatric patients undergoing allogeneic HCT and reported a 22% prevalance of hemorrhagic cystitis when including grade I (isolated microscopic hematuria) along with higher grades of bladder bleeding [173]. Hemorraghic cystitis developed at a median of 35 days post HCT and was associated with worse survival. Giraud et al. prospectively studied 175 adults and children and found a 15% prevalence of hemorrhagic cystitis (85% of whom were BK positive) [175]. Patients receiving unrelated donor transplants were more likely to develop BK, and hemorrhagic cystitis was associated with BK infection and myeloablative conditioning. Other reported risk factors for BK viruria include higher pre-HCT BK IgG levels, while GVHD and higher levels of BK viruria have been associated with the development of hemorrhagic cystitis [176].

In patients with hemorrhagic cystitis, BK virus can lead to AKI if significant obstruction of the bladder or ureters occurs [177]. While the association between nephropathy and BK virus is established in the kidney transplantation literature, less evidence is available supporting the virus's ability to directly cause kidney damage after HCT. As increased levels of immunosuppression are hypothesized to lead to BK virus reactivation and subsequent pathology after kidney transplant, it seems reasonable to assume that a similar process could occur after HCT [166,178]. Several case reports have identified HCT recipients with biopsy proven BK nephropathy [179–182]. Adenovirus infection after HCT has also been reported to cause nephropathy [183].

Although the reported BK viremia prevalence is 10–30% after HCT, less is known about the relationship between BK viremia and nephropathy in this population [164,174,184]. BK viremia has been associated with concomitant CMV infection and an underlying diagnosis of leukemia or lymphoma [184]. O'Donnell et al. followed 124 adult allogeneic HCT recipients for BK infection and reported that 65% developed viruria and 17% viremia after a median follow-up of 454 days [164]. Only 2/21 patients had persistent viremia and biopsy proven nephropathy, while the remaining 19 cases of viremia were mild and transient. Nevertheless, BK viremia was independently associated with an increase in post-HCT creatinine. In kidney transplant recipients, BK viremia >10,000 copies/ml has high positive predictive value for biopsy proven nephropathy [185]. After HCT, a blood BK level of >10,000 has been associated with the development of hemorrhagic cystitis [186]. Similarly, Haines et al. reported that children with a peak plasma BK viral load of >10,000 copies/ml during the first year after HCT, regardless of urine viral load, had worse renal and urological disease compared to those with viremia of <10,000 copies/ml [187]. Specifically, subjects with a high peak viremia level were more likely to undergo surgical intervention for obstructive uropathy, had a higher peak serum creatinine relative to baseline and were more likely to require dialysis compared to those with lower viremia. This preliminary evidence, combined with the fact that plasma levels of BK virus (viremia) correlate with the development of nephropathy in kidney transplant recipients, supports the monitoring of plasma BK PCR levels after HCT. BK viruria, while helpful in the diagnosis of hemorrhagic cystitis, likely has poor predictive value for the development of nephropathy. Nevertheless, definitive diagnosis of BK nephropathy requires a kidney biopsy, especially in patients with persistent elevations in serum creatinine.

GVHD-related CKD

Many HCT survivors developing CKD will not present with nephrotic syndrome, meet criteria for a diagnosis of TA-TMA, or have a documented viral infection. These patients are typically labeled as idiopathic CKD (Figure 6.1). Recent data may support a more appropriate label of acute or chronic GVHD-related CKD, especially in patients receiving non-TBI-based conditioning regimens [85,88]. In a large retrospective study of 1635 HCT recipients, neither TBI nor cyclosporine use were associated with the development of CKD (defined as a GFR <60 ml/min/1.73 m^2) at 1 year post-transplant. A sub-group analysis of all patients receiving cyclosporine further supported the theory that GVHD, independent of calcineurin inhibitor therapy, increased the risk of CKD [85].

The renal manifestations of GVHD may be mediated by two different mechanisms. First, the kidney could be a direct target of T-cell-mediated renal damage. Second, the chronic systemic inflammatory state of GVHD could lead to cytokine-mediated tissue damage. These mechanisms are likely not mutually exclusive, as T-cell-mediated injury in GVHD occurs concomitant with cytokine effects and the effects of cyclosporine can be potentiated by a chronic inflammatory state [85].

In reference to cell-mediated damage, an autopsy study of 26 autologous and allogeneic HCT recipients found evidence of renal tubulitis identical to that seen in renal allograft rejection in 67% of patients [122]. Furthermore, in a report of minimal change nephrotic syndrome that developed after HCT, a large number of CD8$^+$ donor T-cells were found infiltrating the interstitium and peri-glomerular areas of the kidney

[188]. Finally, in a mouse model of kidney GVHD, progressive venulitis, endothelialitis and tubulitis were noted within 2 weeks of transplant. These mechanisms of tissue injury are distinct from the histological findings typically seen in other organs affected by acute GVHD [189].

The cytokine cascade activated by GVHD can also lead to kidney damage independent of the direct T-cell-mediated injury implicated in the pathogenesis of GVHD involving the skin, gastrointestinal tract, or liver [190,191]. Increased plasma cytokine levels have correlated with post-transplant complications and organ dysfunction in the HCT population [135,192]. In animal models, tissue damage from acute GVHD does not require alloantigen expression on target epithelial cells; injury can be mediated solely by inflammatory cytokines [193].

As with acute GVHD, chronic GVHD also involves the activation of B-cells and the production of cytokines such as transforming growth factor-beta 1 (TGF-β1) [194]. TGF-β1 is important for collagen synthesis, involved with matrix deposition in the kidney [195,196], and also appears to be important in the development of cyclosporine-induced kidney fibrosis [197]. The damaging effects of cyclosporine can be potentiated by increased production of TGF-β1 [198]. It is possible that a percentage of CKD currently classified as idiopathic is not secondary to TBI or cyclosporine use, but rather is caused by a combination of factors including GVHD and the accompanying chronic inflammatory state. Careful examination of kidney tissue may increase our understanding of the pathophysiology of idiopathic CKD and the potential role of GVHD and chronic inflammation in its development and progression. Therapy can then be tailored accordingly.

Glomerular Disease

Given the risks of performing kidney biopsies in HCT recipients, only a few studies have been able to report histological findings after transplant. As mentioned previously, indications for biopsy are typically proteinuria, nephrotic syndrome and/or unexplained kidney dysfunction [48,199]. The largest published biopsy cohorts have included a maximum of 20 patients. Supporting that kidney biopsy is a rare procedure after HCT, one study reported that over a period of 8 years and 2208 transplants, only 11 biopsies were performed [46]. In decreasing order of frequency, the most commonly reported pathologies in these biopsy studies have included membranous nephropathy, acute tubular necrosis, TA-TMA, focal segmental glomerular sclerosis (FSGS), BK nephropathy, IgA nephropathy, minimal change disease, hypertensive vasculopathy, amyloidosis and cyclosporine toxicity [46,48,199]. Autopsy studies have also noted a high proportion of TA-TMA in HCT recipients [117,122].

While nephrotic syndrome and glomerular disease are not common complications of HCT, membranous nephropathy, characterized by sub-epithelial deposits on electron microscopy and IgG deposition on immunofluoresence, seems to be the most common finding in this subset of patients [11]. In a review of 95 subjects, the overall prevalence of glomerular disease was 1—6% higher than the general population [200]. Membranous nephropathy was the common finding (64%), followed by minimal change disease (19%). Glomerular disease was more frequently identified in peripheral blood compared to bone marrow recipients and occurred at about 15 months after transplant. Usually, but not always, disease was noted while patients were not receiving immunosuppression. At median follow-up of 1 year, those diagnosed with glomerular disease had an 87% survival rate and 70% were in remission (no or decreased proteinuria).

Others have also reported a cumulative risk of nephrotic syndrome of 3.5—6% at a median of 3—5 years after transplant [201,202]. The increasing number of case reports in the literature points to the fact that glomerular disease after HCT may not be such a rare occurrence. Specifically, both pediatric and adult HCT recipients with a wide range of underlying diagnoses have been reported to develop membranous nephropathy [203–211], minimal change disease [210,212], FSGS [213,214], type I membranoproliferative glomerulonephritis [215], IgA nephropathy [216,217] and secondary amyloidosis [218].

The pathophysiology of post-HCT glomerular disease remains poorly understood, but likely is an immune-mediated process. Support for this hypothesis includes the association with chronic GVHD in patients developing nephrotic syndrome after transplant [49]. However, although the majority of reported cases of post-HCT glomerular disease occur in patients with GVHD [203,206,210,211,213–215,218], this is not a universal finding [200,205,207,212,216].

There are a wide range of potential pathophysiological mechanisms leading to glomerular disease including increased cytokine expression [210], kidney deposition of antibody/antigen complexes in patients with GVHD [11], decreased numbers of regulatory T-cells [201], antibody production by recipient B-cells that have survived reduced intensity regimens [202], immune-mediated podocyte damage [49] and overactive recipient T-cells, as has been shown in patients with both graft loss and nephrotic syndrome [212].

As in patients with GVHD-related kidney damage, there is histological evidence for an immune-mediated process in post-transplant glomerular disease. Similar to findings of both cellular and antibody-mediated allograft rejection in kidney transplant recipients, studies in HCT recipients have shown staining with the complement degradation product C4d [46,50,51] and evidence of tubulitis [122,219].

The treatment of post-HCT glomerular injury also supports an immunological mechanism of injury, as many patients have responded to increases in immunosuppression including steroids, calcineurin inhibitors, cyclophosphamide, azathioprine and rituximab [201,203–205,208,210–216]. However, there are reports of positive responses with the use of only ACE-I and ARB, either alone [209] or in combination with increased immunosupression [211,213,214,216]. As no controls exist, these results must be interpreted with caution and the optimal treatment regimen for post-HCT glomerular disease remains unknown. In fact, careful attention to the particular pathological findings is extremely important, as some diseases, such as TA-TMA, may in fact respond to a reduction in immunosuppression [136].

CONCLUSION

Advances in technology and care have decreased morbidity and mortality after HCT, but kidney disease remains a significant complication. AKI and CKD affect at least 20–30% of HCT recipients and lead to hypertension, anemia and proteinuria. Other diagnoses to consider are glomerular disease (nephrotic syndrome), electrolyte abnormalities and BK virus nephropathy. The etiologies of these complications are often multi-factorial with risks including conditioning chemotherapy, radiation, nephrotoxic antimicrobials, infections, sinusoidal obstruction syndrome of the liver, transplantation-associated thrombotic microangiopathy and graft-versus-host disease (GVHD) (Figure 6.1). Continued prospective evaluations are needed to gain knowledge on the most relevant, modifiable factors associated with post-HCT kidney disease. The association between kidney injury and GVHD after HCT mirrors allograft dysfunction and rejection after kidney transplant and supports immune-mediated mechanisms of tissue damage. Increasing our understanding of the mechanisms involving cellular, antibody-mediated and complement-directed pathways of kidney disease will pave the way for therapeutic trials to hopefully improve outcomes in this high-risk population.

References

[1] Hingorani SR, Guthrie K, Batchelder A, Schoch G, Aboulhosn N, Manchion J, et al. Acute renal failure after myeloablative hematopoietic cell transplant: incidence and risk factors. Kidney Int 2005;67(1):272–7.

[2] Parikh CR, Coca SG. Acute renal failure in hematopoietic cell transplantation. Kidney Int 2006;69(3):430–5.

[3] Go AS, Chertow GM, Fan D, McCulloch CE, Hsu CY. Chronic kidney disease and the risks of death, cardiovascular events, and hospitalization. N Engl J Med 2004;351(13):1296–305.

[4] Ellis MJ, Parikh CR, Inrig JK, Kanbay M, Patel UD. Chronic kidney disease after hematopoietic cell transplantation: a systematic review. Am J Transplant 2008;8(11):2378–90.

[5] Hingorani S. Chronic kidney disease in long-term survivors of hematopoietic cell transplantation: epidemiology, pathogenesis, and treatment. J Am Soc Nephrol 2006;17(7):1995–2005.

[6] Heher EC, Spitzer TR. Hematopoietic stem cell transplantation in patients with chronic kidney disease. Semin Nephrol 2010;30(6):602–14.

[7] Oeffinger KC, Mertens AC, Sklar CA, Kawashima T, Hudson MM, Meadows AT, et al. Chronic health conditions in adult survivors of childhood cancer. N Engl J Med 2006;355(15):1572–82.

[8] Gooley TA, Chien JW, Pergam SA, Hingorani S, Sorror ML, Boeckh M, et al. Reduced mortality after allogeneic hematopoietic-cell transplantation. N Engl J Med 2010;363(22):2091–101.

[9] Choi M, Sun CL, Kurian S, Carter A, Francisco L, Forman SJ, et al. Incidence and predictors of delayed chronic kidney disease in long-term survivors of hematopoietic cell transplantation. Cancer 2008;113(7):1580–7.

[10] Ando M, Mori J, Ohashi K, Akiyama H, Morito T, Tsuchiya K, et al. A comparative assessment of the RIFLE, AKIN and conventional criteria for acute kidney injury after hematopoietic SCT. Bone Marrow Transplant 2010;45(9):1427–34.

[11] Hingorani S. Chronic kidney disease after liver, cardiac, lung, heart-lung, and hematopoietic stem cell transplant. Pediatr Nephrol 2008;23(6):879–88.

[12] DiCarlo J, Alexander SR. Acute kidney injury in pediatric stem cell transplant recipients. Semin Nephrol 2008;28(5):481–7.

[13] Chao NJ. Pharmacology and use of immunosuppressive agents after hematopoietic cell transplantation. In: Thomas ED, Blume KG, Forman SJ, editors. Hematopoietic cell transplantation. 2nd ed. Malden: Blackwell Science; 1999. p. 176–85.

[14] Ito J. Herpes simplex virus infections. In: Appelbaum FR, Blume KG, Forman SJ, editors. Thomas' hematopoietic cell transplant. 4th ed. Malden: Wiley-Blackwell; 2009. p. 1382–7.

[15] Leather HL, Wingard JR. Bacterial infections. In: Appelbaum FR, Blume KG, Forman SJ, editors. Thomas' hematopoietic cell transplant. 4th ed. Malden: Wiley-Blackwell; 2009. p. 1325–45.

[16] Zaia JA. Cytomegalovirus infections. In: Appelbaum FR, Blume KG, Forman SJ, editors. Thomas' hematopoietic cell transplant. 4th ed. Malden: Wiley-Blackwell; 2009. p. 1367–81.

[17] Zappitelli M. Epidemiology and diagnosis of acute kidney injury. Semin Nephrol 2008;28(5):436–46.

[18] Kogon A, Hingorani S. Acute kidney injury in hematopoietic cell transplantation. Semin Nephrol 2010;30(6):615–26.

[19] Sorror ML, Maris MB, Storb R, Baron F, Sandmaier BM, Maloney DG, et al. Hematopoietic cell transplantation (HCT)-specific comorbidity index: a new tool for risk assessment before allogeneic HCT. Blood 2005;106(8):2912–9.

[20] Smith AR, Majhail NS, MacMillan ML, DeFor TE, Jodele S, Lehmann LE, et al. Hematopoietic cell transplantation comorbidity index predicts transplantation outcomes in pediatric patients. Blood 2011;117(9):2728–34.

[21] de Souza JA, Saliba RM, Patah P, Rondon G, Ribeiro R, de Padua Silva L, et al. Moderate renal function impairment does not affect outcomes of reduced-intensity conditioning with fludarabine and melphalan for allogeneic hematopoietic stem cell transplantation. Biol Blood Marrow Transplant 2009;15(9):1094–9.

[22] Kersting S, Verdonck LF. Successful outcome after nonmyeloablative allogeneic hematopoietic stem cell transplantation in patients with renal dysfunction. Biol Blood Marrow Transplant 2008;14(11):1312–6.

[23] Pulsipher MA, Skinner R, McDonald GB, Hingorani S, Armenian SH, Cooke KR, et al. National Cancer Institute, National Heart, Lung and Blood Institute/Pediatric Blood and Marrow Transplantation Consortium First International Consensus Conference on late effects after pediatric hematopoietic cell transplantation: the need for pediatric-specific long-term follow-up guidelines. Biol Blood Marrow Transplant 2012;18(3):334–47.

[24] Tichelli A, Rovo A, Gratwohl A. Late pulmonary, cardiovascular, and renal complications after hematopoietic stem cell transplantation and recommended screening practices. Hematology Am Soc Hematol Educ Program 2008:125–33.

[25] Andersen TB, Eskild-Jensen A, Frokiaer J, Brochner-Mortensen J. Measuring glomerular filtration rate in children; can cystatin C replace established methods? A review. Pediatr Nephrol 2009;24(5): 929–41.

[26] Kletzel M, Pirich L, Haut P, Cohn RA. Comparison of Tc-99 measurement of glomerular filtration rate vs. calculated creatinine clearance to assess renal function pretransplant in pediatric patients undergoing hematopoietic stem cell transplantation. Pediatr Transplant 2005;9(5):584–8.

[27] Levey AS, Coresh J, Balk E, Kausz AT, Levin A, Steffes MW, et al. National Kidney Foundation practice guidelines for chronic kidney disease: evaluation, classification, and stratification. Ann Intern Med 2003;139(2):137–47.

[28] Schwartz GJ, Brion LP, Spitzer A. The use of plasma creatinine concentration for estimating glomerular filtration rate in infants, children, and adolescents. Pediatr Clin North Am 1987;34(3):571–90.

[29] Schwartz GJ, Munoz A, Schneider MF, Mak RH, Kaskel F, Warady BA, et al. New equations to estimate GFR in children with CKD. J Am Soc Nephrol 2009;20(3):629–37.

[30] Laskin BL, Goebel J, Davies SM, Khoury JC, Bleesing JJ, Mehta PA, et al. Early clinical indicators of transplant-associated thrombotic micro-angiopathy in pediatric neuroblastoma patients undergoing auto-SCT. Bone Marrow Transplant 2011; 46(5):682–9.

[31] Boudville N, Salama M, Jeffrey GP, Ferrari P. The inaccuracy of cystatin C and creatinine-based equations in predicting GFR in orthotopic liver transplant recipients. Nephrol Dial Transplant 2009;24(9): 2926–30.

[32] White C, Akbari A, Hussain N, Dinh L, Filler G, Lepage N, et al. Estimating glomerular filtration rate in kidney transplantation: a comparison between serum creatinine and cystatin C-based methods. J Am Soc Nephrol 2005;16(12):3763–70.

[33] Hazar V, Gungor O, Guven AG, Aydin F, Akbas H, Gungor F, et al. Renal function after hematopoietic stem cell transplantation in children. Pediatr Blood Cancer 2009;53(2):197–202.

[34] Bacchetta J, Cochat P, Rognant N, Ranchin B, Hadj-Aissa A, Dubourg L. Which creatinine and cystatin C equations can be reliably used in children? Clin J Am Soc Nephrol 2011;6(3):552–60.

[35] Aydin F, Tezcan G, Gungor O, Cengiz AK, Hazar V, Akman S, et al. Can serum cystatin C reflect the glomerular filtration rate accurately in pediatric patients under chemotherapeutic treatment? A comparative study with Tc-99m DTPA two-plasma sample method. Nucl Med Commun 2010;31(4): 301–6.

[36] Frisk P, Arvidson J, Neveus T. Glomerular and tubular function in young adults treated with stem-cell transplantation in childhood. Pediatr Nephrol 2010;25(7):1337–42.

[37] Muto H, Ohashi K, Ando M, Akiyama H, Sakamaki H. Cystatin C level as a marker of renal function in allogeneic hematopoietic stem cell transplantation. Int J Hematol 2010;91(3):471–7.

[38] Poge U, Gerhardt T, Stoffel-Wagner B, Palmedo H, Klehr HU, Sauerbruch T, et al. Cystatin C-based calculation of glomerular filtration rate in kidney transplant recipients. Kidney Int 2006;70(1):204–10.

[39] Stevens LA, Schmid CH, Greene T, Li L, Beck GJ, Joffe MM, et al. Factors other than glomerular filtration rate affect serum cystatin C levels. Kidney Int 2009;75(6):652–60.

[40] Michael M, Kuehnle I, Goldstein SL. Fluid overload and acute renal failure in pediatric stem cell transplant patients. Pediatr Nephrol 2004;19(1):91–5.

[41] Sutherland SM, Zappitelli M, Alexander SR, Chua AN, Brophy PD, Bunchman TE, et al. Fluid overload and mortality in children receiving continuous renal replacement therapy: the prospective pediatric continuous renal replacement therapy registry. Am J Kidney Dis 2010;55(2):316–25.

[42] Hingorani SR, Seidel K, Lindner A, Aneja T, Schoch G, McDonald G. Albuminuria in hematopoietic cell transplantation patients: prevalence, clinical associations, and impact on survival. Biol Blood Marrow Transplant 2008;14(12):1365–72.

[43] Langlois V. Laboratory evaluation at different ages. In: Geary DF, Schaefer F, editors. Comprehensive Pediatric Nephrology. Philadelphia: Mosby Elsevier; 2008. p. 39–54.

[44] Majhail NS, Rizzo JD, Lee SJ, Aljurf M, Atsuta Y, Bonfim C, et al. Recommended screening and preventive practices for long-term survivors after hematopoietic cell transplantation. Biol Blood Marrow Transplant 2012;18(3):348–71.

[45] Ileri T, Ertem M, Ozcakar ZB, Ince EU, Biyikli Z, Uysal Z, et al. Prospective evaluation of acute and chronic renal function in children following matched related donor hematopoietic stem cell transplantation. Pediatr Transplant 2010;14(1):138–44.

[46] Troxell ML, Pilapil M, Miklos DB, Higgins JP, Kambham N. Renal pathology in hematopoietic cell transplantation recipients. Mod Pathol 2008;21(4): 396–406.

[47] Cohen EP, Pais P, Moulder JE. Chronic kidney disease after hematopoietic stem cell transplantation. Semin Nephrol 2010;30(6):627–34.

[48] Chang A, Hingorani S, Kowalewska J, Flowers ME, Aneja T, Smith KD, et al. Spectrum of renal pathology in hematopoietic cell transplantation: a series of 20 patients and review of the literature. Clin J Am Soc Nephrol 2007;2(5):1014−23.

[49] Terrier B, Delmas Y, Hummel A, Presne C, Glowacki F, Knebelmann B, et al. Post-allogeneic haematopoietic stem cell transplantation membranous nephropathy: clinical presentation, outcome and pathogenic aspects. Nephrol Dial Transplant 2007;22(5):1369−76.

[50] Mii A, Shimizu A, Kaneko T, Fujita E, Fukui M, Fujino T, et al. Renal thrombotic microangiopathy associated with chronic graft-versus-host disease after allogeneic hematopoietic stem cell transplantation. Pathol Int 2011;61(9):518−27.

[51] Mii A, Shimizu A, Masuda Y, Fujino T, Kaneko T, Utsumi K, et al. Renal thrombotic microangiopathy associated with chronic humoral graft versus host disease after hematopoietic stem cell transplantation. Pathol Int 2011;61(1):34−41.

[52] Glezerman IG, Jhaveri KD, Watson TH, Edwards AM, Papadopoulos EB, Young JW, et al. Chronic kidney disease, thrombotic microangiopathy, and hypertension following T cell-depleted hematopoietic stem cell transplantation. Biol Blood Marrow Transplant 2010;16(7):976−84.

[53] Changsirikulchai S, Myerson D, Guthrie KA, McDonald GB, Alpers CE, Hingorani SR. Renal thrombotic microangiopathy after hematopoietic cell transplant: role of GVHD in pathogenesis. Clin J Am Soc Nephrol 2009;4(2):345−53.

[54] Manno C, Strippoli GF, Arnesano L, Bonifati C, Campobasso N, Gesualdo L, et al. Predictors of bleeding complications in percutaneous ultrasound-guided renal biopsy. Kidney Int 2004;66(4):1570−7.

[55] Bellomo R, Ronco C, Kellum JA, Mehta RL, Palevsky P. Acute renal failure − definition, outcome measures, animal models, fluid therapy and information technology needs: the Second International Consensus Conference of the Acute Dialysis Quality Initiative (ADQI) Group. Crit Care 2004;8(4): R204−12.

[56] Akcan-Arikan A, Zappitelli M, Loftis LL, Washburn KK, Jefferson LS, Goldstein SL. Modified RIFLE criteria in critically ill children with acute kidney injury. Kidney Int 2007;71(10):1028−35.

[57] Parikh CR, McSweeney PA, Korular D, Ecder T, Merouani A, Taylor J, et al. Renal dysfunction in allogeneic hematopoietic cell transplantation. Kidney Int 2002;62(2):566−73.

[58] Parikh CR, Sandmaier BM, Storb RF, Blume KG, Sahebi F, Maloney DG, et al. Acute renal failure after nonmyeloablative hematopoietic cell transplantation. J Am Soc Nephrol 2004;15(7):1868−76.

[59] Mehta RL, Kellum JA, Shah SV, Molitoris BA, Ronco C, Warnock DG, et al. Acute Kidney Injury Network: report of an initiative to improve outcomes in acute kidney injury. Crit Care 2007;11(2):R31.

[60] Bao YS, Xie RJ, Wang M, Feng SZ, Han MZ. An evaluation of the RIFLE criteria for acute kidney injury after myeloablative allogeneic haematopoietic stem cell transplantation. Swiss Med Wkly 2011;141: w13225.

[61] Touzot M, Elie C, van Massenhove J, Maillard N, Buzyn A, Fakhouri F. Long-term renal function after allogenic haematopoietic stem cell transplantation in adult patients: a single-centre study. Nephrol Dial Transplant 2010;25(2):624−7.

[62] Kersting S, Koomans HA, Hene RJ, Verdonck LF. Acute renal failure after allogeneic myeloablative stem cell transplantation: retrospective analysis of incidence, risk factors and survival. Bone Marrow Transplant 2007;39(6):359−65.

[63] Tokgoz B, Kocyigit I, Polat G, Eser B, Unal A, Kaynar L, et al. Acute renal failure after myeloablative allogeneic hematopoietic stem cell transplantation: incidence, risk factors, and relationship with the quantity of transplanted cells. Ren Fail 2010;32(5):547−54.

[64] Mae H, Ooi J, Takahashi S, Tomonari A, Tsukada N, Konuma T, et al. Early renal injury after myeloablative cord blood transplantation in adults. Leuk Lymphoma 2008;49(3):538−42.

[65] Yu ZP, Ding JH, Chen BA, Liu BC, Liu H, Li YF, et al. Risk factors for acute kidney injury in patients undergoing allogeneic hematopoietic stem cell transplantation. Chin J Cancer 2010;29(11):946−51.

[66] Satwani P, Bavishi S, Jin Z, Jacobson JS, Baker C, Duffy D, et al. Risk factors associated with kidney injury and the impact of kidney injury on overall survival in pediatric recipients following allogeneic stem cell transplant. Biol Blood Marrow Transplant 2011;17(10):1472−80.

[67] Kagoya Y, Kataoka K, Nannya Y, Kurokawa M. Pretransplant predictors and posttransplant sequels of acute kidney injury after allogeneic stem cell transplantation. Biol Blood Marrow Transplant 2011; 17:394−400.

[68] Kersting S, Dorp SV, Theobald M, Verdonck LF. Acute renal failure after nonmyeloablative stem cell transplantation in adults. Biol Blood Marrow Transplant 2008;14(1):125−31.

[69] Liu H, Ding JH, Liu BC, Zhao G, Chen BA. Early renal injury after nonmyeloablative allogeneic peripheral blood stem cell transplantation in patients

with chronic myelocytic leukemia. Am J Nephrol 2007;27(4):336—41.

[70] Parikh CR, Yarlagadda SG, Storer B, Sorror M, Storb R, Sandmaier B. Impact of acute kidney injury on long-term mortality after nonmyeloablative hematopoietic cell transplantation. Biol Blood Marrow Transplant 2008;14(3):309—15.

[71] Parikh CR, Schrier RW, Storer B, Diaconescu R, Sorror ML, Maris MB, et al. Comparison of ARF after myeloablative and nonmyeloablative hematopoietic cell transplantation. Am J Kidney Dis 2005; 45(3):502—9.

[72] Lopes JA, Jorge S, Silva S, de Almeida E, Abreu F, Martins C, et al. Acute renal failure following myeloablative autologous and allogeneic hematopoietic cell transplantation. Bone Marrow Transplant 2006;38(10):707.

[73] Coppell JA, Richardson PG, Soiffer R, Martin PL, Kernan NA, Chen A, et al. Hepatic veno-occlusive disease following stem cell transplantation: incidence, clinical course, and outcome. Biol Blood Marrow Transplant 2010;16(2):157—68.

[74] Parikh CR, McSweeney P, Schrier RW. Acute renal failure independently predicts mortality after myeloablative allogeneic hematopoietic cell transplant. Kidney Int 2005;67(5):1999—2005.

[75] Pinana JL, Valcarcel D, Martino R, Barba P, Moreno E, Sureda A, et al. Study of kidney function impairment after reduced-intensity conditioning allogeneic hematopoietic stem cell transplantation. A single-center experience. Biol Blood Marrow Transplant 2009;15(1):21—9.

[76] Al-Hazzouri A, Cao Q, Burns LJ, Weisdorf DJ, Majhail NS. Similar risks for chronic kidney disease in long-term survivors of myeloablative and reduced-intensity allogeneic hematopoietic cell transplantation. Biol Blood Marrow Transplant 2008;14(6):658—63.

[77] Beyzadeoglu M, Arpaci F, Surenkok S, Ozyigit G, Oysul K, Caglar K, et al. Acute renal toxicity of 2 conditioning regimens in patients undergoing autologous peripheral blood stem-cell transplantation. Total body irradiation-cyclophosphamide versus ifosfamide, carboplatin, etoposide. Saudi Med J 2008;29(6):832—6.

[78] Karvellas CJ, Farhat MR, Sajjad I, Mogensen SS, Leung AA, Wald R, et al. A comparison of early versus late initiation of renal replacement therapy in critically ill patients with acute kidney injury: a systematic review and meta-analysis. Crit Care 2011;15(1):R72.

[79] Bagshaw SM, Bellomo R, Kellum JA. Oliguria, volume overload, and loop diuretics. Crit Care Med 2008;36(Suppl. 4):S172—8.

[80] DiCarlo JV, Alexander SR, Agarwal R, Schiffman JD. Continuous veno-venous hemofiltration may improve survival from acute respiratory distress syndrome after bone marrow transplantation or chemotherapy. J Pediatr Hematol Oncol 2003;25(10): 801—5.

[81] Flores FX, Brophy PD, Symons JM, Fortenberry JD, Chua AN, Alexander SR, et al. Continuous renal replacement therapy (CRRT) after stem cell transplantation. A report from the prospective pediatric CRRT Registry Group. Pediatr Nephrol 2008;23(4): 625—30.

[82] Ando M, Ohashi K, Akiyama H, Sakamaki H, Morito T, Tsuchiya K, et al. Chronic kidney disease in long-term survivors of myeloablative allogeneic haematopoietic cell transplantation: prevalence and risk factors. Nephrol Dial Transplant 2010;25(1): 278—82.

[83] Abboud I, Porcher R, Robin M, de Latour RP, Glotz D, Socie G, et al. Chronic kidney dysfunction in patients alive without relapse 2 years after allogeneic hematopoietic stem cell transplantation. Biol Blood Marrow Transplant 2009;15(10):1251—7.

[84] Kersting S, Hene RJ, Koomans HA, Verdonck LF. Chronic kidney disease after myeloablative allogeneic hematopoietic stem cell transplantation. Biol Blood Marrow Transplant 2007;13(10):1169—75.

[85] Hingorani S, Guthrie KA, Schoch G, Weiss NS, McDonald GB. Chronic kidney disease in long-term survivors of hematopoietic cell transplant. Bone Marrow Transplant 2007;39(4):223—9.

[86] Hingorani S. Chronic kidney disease after pediatric hematopoietic cell transplant. Biol Blood Marrow Transplant 2008;14(1 Suppl. 1):84—7.

[87] Kersting S, Verdonck LF. Chronic kidney disease after nonmyeloablative stem cell transplantation in adults. Biol Blood Marrow Transplant 2008;14(4): 403—8.

[88] Weiss AS, Sandmaier BM, Storer B, Storb R, McSweeney PA, Parikh CR. Chronic kidney disease following non-myeloablative hematopoietic cell transplantation. Am J Transplant 2006;6(1):89—94.

[89] Parikh GC, Amjad AI, Saliba RM, Kazmi SM, Khan ZU, Lahoti A, et al. Autologous hematopoietic stem cell transplantation may reverse renal failure in patients with multiple myeloma. Biol Blood Marrow Transplant 2009;15(7):812—6.

[90] Akay OM, Sahin G, Kabukcuoglu S, Yalcin AU, Gulbas Z. Successful treatment of nephrotic syndrome due to systemic AL amyloidosis after autologous stem cell transplantation: renal response is an important therapeutic end point. Clin Nephrol 2008;69(4):294—7.

[91] Hsieh MM, Fitzhugh CD, Tisdale JF. Allogeneic hematopoietic stem cell transplantation for sickle cell disease: the time is now. Blood 2011;118(5):1197—207.

[92] Horwitz ME, Spasojevic I, Morris A, Telen M, Essell J, Gasparetto C, et al. Fludarabine-based nonmyeloablative stem cell transplantation for sickle cell disease with and without renal failure: clinical outcome and pharmacokinetics. Biol Blood Marrow Transplant 2007;13(12):1422—6.

[93] Choi HS, Kim SY, Lee JH, Yoon SY, Cho YH, Lee HG. Successful allogeneic stem-cell transplantation in a patient with myelodysplastic syndrome with hemodialysis-dependent end-stage renal disease. Transplantation 2011;92(6):e28—9.

[94] Leung W, Ahn H, Rose SR, Phipps S, Smith T, Gan K, et al. A prospective cohort study of late sequelae of pediatric allogeneic hematopoietic stem cell transplantation. Medicine (Baltimore) 2007;86(4):215—24.

[95] Kal HB, van Kempen-Harteveld ML. Chronic kidney disease after myeloablative allogeneic hematopoietic stem cell transplantation. Biol Blood Marrow Transplant 2007;13(12):1525.

[96] Munakata W, Sawada T, Kobayashi T, Kakihana K, Yamashita T, Ohashi K, et al. Mortality and medical morbidity beyond 2 years after allogeneic hematopoietic stem cell transplantation: experience at a single institution. Int J Hematol 2011;93(4):517—22.

[97] Patzer L, Ringelmann F, Kentouche K, Fuchs D, Zintl F, Brandis M, et al. Renal function in long-term survivors of stem cell transplantation in childhood. A prospective trial. Bone Marrow Transplant 2001;27(3):319—27.

[98] Cohen EP, Irving AA, Drobyski WR, Klein JP, Passweg J, Talano JA, et al. Captopril to mitigate chronic renal failure after hematopoietic stem cell transplantation: a randomized controlled trial. Int J Radiat Oncol Biol Phys 2008;70(5):1546—51.

[99] Cohen EP, Bedi M, Irving AA, Jacobs E, Tomic R, Klein J, et al. Mitigation of late renal and pulmonary injury after hematopoietic stem cell transplantation. Int J Radiat Oncol Biol Phys 2012;83(1):292—6.

[100] Chobanian AV, Bakris GL, Black HR, Cushman WC, Green LA, Izzo Jr JL, et al. Seventh report of the Joint National Committee on Prevention, Detection, Evaluation, and Treatment of High Blood Pressure. Hypertension 2003;42(6):1206—52.

[101] The fourth report on the diagnosis, evaluation, and treatment of high blood pressure in children and adolescents. Pediatrics 2004;114(2 Suppl. 4th Report): 555—76.

[102] Majhail NS, Challa TR, Mulrooney DA, Baker KS, Burns LJ. Hypertension and diabetes mellitus in adult and pediatric survivors of allogeneic hematopoietic cell transplantation. Biol Blood Marrow Transplant 2009;15(9):1100—7.

[103] Tichelli A, Passweg J, Wojcik D, Rovo A, Harousseau JL, Masszi T, et al. Late cardiovascular events after allogeneic hematopoietic stem cell transplantation: a retrospective multicenter study of the Late Effects Working Party of the European Group for Blood and Marrow Transplantation. Haematologica 2008;93(8):1203—10.

[104] Hoffmeister PA, Hingorani SR, Storer BE, Baker KS, Sanders JE. Hypertension in long-term survivors of pediatric hematopoietic cell transplantation. Biol Blood Marrow Transplant 2010;16(4):515—24.

[105] Wuhl E, Trivelli A, Picca S, Litwin M, Peco-Antic A, Zurowska A, et al. Strict blood-pressure control and progression of renal failure in children. N Engl J Med 2009;361(17):1639—50.

[106] Hale GA, Bowman LC, Rochester RJ, Benaim E, Heslop HE, Krance RA, et al. Hemolytic uremic syndrome after bone marrow transplantation: clinical characteristics and outcome in children. Biol Blood Marrow Transplant 2005;11(11):912—20.

[107] Bohlius J, Schmidlin K, Brillant C, Schwarzer G, Trelle S, Seidenfeld J, et al. Recombinant human erythropoiesis-stimulating agents and mortality in patients with cancer: a meta-analysis of randomised trials. Lancet 2009;373(9674):1532—42.

[108] Cohen EP, Drobyski WR, Moulder JE. Significant increase in end-stage renal disease after hematopoietic stem cell transplantation. Bone Marrow Transplant 2007;39(9):571—2.

[109] Bunin N, Guzikowski V, Rand ER, Goldfarb S, Baluarte J, Meyers K, et al. Solid organ transplants following hematopoietic stem cell transplant in children. Pediatr Transplant 2010;14(8):1030—5.

[110] Tanaka T, Ishida H, Shirakawa H, Amano H, Nishida H, Tanabe K. Renal transplantation after myeloablative and non-myeloablative hematopoietic cell transplantation from the same donor. Int J Urol 2007;14(11):1044—5.

[111] Fangmann J, Kathrin Al-Ali H, Sack U, Kamprad M, Tautenhahn HM, Faber S, et al. Kidney transplant from the same donor without maintenance immunosuppression after previous hematopoietic stem cell transplant. Am J Transplant 2011;11(1): 156—62.

[112] Scandling JD, Busque S, Dejbakhsh-Jones S, Benike C, Millan MT, Shizuru JA, et al. Tolerance and chimerism after renal and hematopoietic-cell transplantation. N Engl J Med 2008;358(4):362—8.

[113] Scandling JD, Busque S, Shizuru JA, Engleman EG, Strober S. Induced immune tolerance for kidney transplantation. N Engl J Med 2011;365(14):1359—60.

[114] Kawai T, Cosimi AB, Spitzer TR, Tolkoff-Rubin N, Suthanthiran M, Saidman SL, et al. HLA-mismatched renal transplantation without maintenance immunosuppression. N Engl J Med 2008; 358(4):353–61.

[115] Starzl TE. Immunosuppressive therapy and tolerance of organ allografts. N Engl J Med 2008;358(4): 407–11.

[116] Batts ED, Lazarus HM. Diagnosis and treatment of transplantation-associated thrombotic microangiopathy: real progress or are we still waiting? Bone Marrow Transplant 2007;40(8):709–19.

[117] Siami K, Kojouri K, Swisher KK, Selby GB, George JN, Laszik ZG. Thrombotic microangiopathy after allogeneic hematopoietic stem cell transplantation: an autopsy study. Transplantation 2008;85(1):22–8.

[118] Laskin BL, Goebel J, Davies SM, Jodele S. Small vessels, big trouble in the kidneys and beyond: hematopoietic stem cell transplantation-associated thrombotic microangiopathy. Blood 2011;118(6): 1452–62.

[119] Ho VT, Cutler C, Carter S, Martin P, Adams R, Horowitz M, et al. Blood and marrow transplant clinical trials network toxicity committee consensus summary: thrombotic microangiopathy after hematopoietic stem cell transplantation. Biol Blood Marrow Transplant 2005;11(8):571–5.

[120] Ruutu T, Barosi G, Benjamin RJ, Clark RE, George JN, Gratwohl A, et al. Diagnostic criteria for hematopoietic stem cell transplant-associated microangiopathy: results of a consensus process by an International Working Group. Haematologica 2007;92(1):95–100.

[121] Cho BS, Yahng SA, Lee SE, Eom KS, Kim YJ, Kim HJ, et al. Validation of recently proposed consensus criteria for thrombotic microangiopathy after allogeneic hematopoietic stem-cell transplantation. Transplantation 2010;90(8):918–26.

[122] El-Seisi S, Gupta R, Clase CM, Forrest DL, Milandinovic M, Couban S. Renal pathology at autopsy in patients who died after hematopoietic stem cell transplantation. Biol Blood Marrow Transplant 2003;9(11):683–8.

[123] George JN. Hematopoietic stem cell transplantation-associated thrombotic microangiopathy: defining a disorder. Bone Marrow Transplant 2008;41(11): 917–8.

[124] Kojouri K, George JN. Thrombotic microangiopathy following allogeneic hematopoietic stem cell transplantation. Curr Opin Oncol 2007;19(2):148–54.

[125] Lopes da Silva R, Ferreira I, Teixeira G, Cordeiro D, Mafra M, Costa I, et al. BK virus encephalitis with thrombotic microangiopathy in an allogeneic hematopoietic stem cell transplant recipient. Transpl Infect Dis. Prepublished on November 5, 2010 as DOI 10.1111/j.1399–3062.2010.00581.x.

[126] Uderzo C, Bonanomi S, Busca A, Renoldi M, Ferrari P, Iacobelli M, et al. Risk factors and severe outcome in thrombotic microangiopathy after allogeneic hematopoietic stem cell transplantation. Transplantation 2006;82(5):638–44.

[127] Rosenthal J, Pawlowska A, Bolotin E, Cervantes C, Maroongroge S, Thomas SH, et al. Transplant-associated thrombotic microangiopathy in pediatric patients treated with sirolimus and tacrolimus. Pediatr Blood Cancer. Prepublished on November 23, 2010 as DOI 10.1002/pbc.22861.

[128] Willems E, Baron F, Seidel L, Frere P, Fillet G, Beguin Y. Comparison of thrombotic microangiopathy after allogeneic hematopoietic cell transplantation with high-dose or nonmyeloablative conditioning. Bone Marrow Transplant 2010;45(4): 689–93.

[129] Rodriguez R, Nakamura R, Palmer JM, Parker P, Shayani S, Nademanee A, et al. A phase II pilot study of tacrolimus/sirolimus GVHD prophylaxis for sibling donor hematopoietic stem cell transplantation using 3 conditioning regimens. Blood 2010;115(5):1098–105.

[130] Cutler C, Henry NL, Magee C, Li S, Kim HT, Alyea E, et al. Sirolimus and thrombotic microangiopathy after allogeneic hematopoietic stem cell transplantation. Biol Blood Marrow Transplant 2005; 11(7):551–7.

[131] Platzbecker U, von Bonin M, Goekkurt E, Radke J, Binder M, Kiani A, et al. Graft-versus-host disease prophylaxis with everolimus and tacrolimus is associated with a high incidence of sinusoidal obstruction syndrome and microangiopathy: results of the EVTAC trial. Biol Blood Marrow Transplant 2009;15(1):101–8.

[132] Tichelli A, Gratwohl A. Vascular endothelium as "novel" target of graft-versus-host disease. Best Pract Res Clin Haematol 2008;21(2):139–48.

[133] Cooke KR, Jannin A, Ho V. The contribution of endothelial activation and injury to end-organ toxicity following allogeneic hematopoietic stem cell transplantation. Biol Blood Marrow Transplant 2008;14(1 Suppl. 1):23–32.

[134] Biedermann BC. Vascular endothelium and graft-versus-host disease. Best Pract Res Clin Haematol 2008;21(2):129–38.

[135] Takatsuka H, Takemoto Y, Yamada S, Wada H, Tamura S, Fujimori Y, et al. Complications after bone marrow transplantation are manifestations of

systemic inflammatory response syndrome. Bone Marrow Transplant 2000;26(4):419—26.

[136] Nakamura Y, Yujiri T, Ando T, Hisano S, Tanizawa Y. Nephrotic syndrome associated with thrombotic microangiopathy following allogeneic stem-cell transplantation for myelodysplastic syndrome. Br J Haematol 2007;136(6):857—9; author reply 9—60.

[137] Cho BS, Min CK, Eom KS, Kim YJ, Kim HJ, Lee S, et al. Clinical impact of thrombotic microangiopathy on the outcome of patients with acute graft-versus-host disease after allogeneic hematopoietic stem cell transplantation. Bone Marrow Transplant 2008; 41(9):813—20.

[138] Nakamae H, Yamane T, Hasegawa T, Nakamae M, Terada Y, Hagihara K, et al. Risk factor analysis for thrombotic microangiopathy after reduced-intensity or myeloablative allogeneic hematopoietic stem cell transplantation. Am J Hematol 2006;81(7):525—31.

[139] Worel N, Greinix HT, Leitner G, Mitterbauer M, Rabitsch W, Rosenmayr A, et al. ABO-incompatible allogeneic hematopoietic stem cell transplantation following reduced-intensity conditioning: close association with transplant-associated micro-angiopathy. Transfus Apher Sci 2007;36(3):297—304.

[140] Takatsuka H, Nakajima T, Nomura K, Okikawa Y, Wakae T, Toda A, et al. Changes of clotting factors (7,9 and 10) and hepatocyte growth factor in patients with thrombotic microangiopathy after bone marrow transplantation. Clin Transplant 2006;20(5):640—3.

[141] Takatsuka H, Nakajima T, Nomura K, Wakae T, Toda A, Itoi H, et al. Heparin cofactor II as a pre-dictor of thrombotic microangiopathy after bone marrow transplantation. Hematology 2006;11(2): 101—3.

[142] Jodele S, Bleesing J, Mehta PA, Filipovich AH, Laskin BL, Goebel J, et al. Successful early intervention for hyperacute transplant-associated thrombotic micro-angiopathy following pediatric hematopoietic stem cell transplantation. Pediatr Transplant. Prepub-lished on November 5, 2010 as DOI 10.1111/ j.1399—3046.2010.01408.x.

[143] Ansari M, Vukicevic M, Rougemont AL, Moll S, Parvex P, Gumy-Pause F, et al. Do NK cells contribute to the pathophysiology of transplant-associated thrombotic microangiopathy? Am J Transplant 2011;11(8):1748—52.

[144] Biedermann BC, Sahner S, Gregor M, Tsakiris DA, Jeanneret C, Pober JS, et al. Endothelial injury mediated by cytotoxic T lymphocytes and loss of microvessels in chronic graft versus host disease. Lancet 2002;359(9323):2078—83.

[145] Kanamori H, Maruta A, Sasaki S, Yamazaki E, Ueda S, Katoh K, et al. Diagnostic value of

hemostatic parameters in bone marrow transplant-associated thrombotic microangiopathy. Bone Marrow Transplant 1998;21(7):705—9.

[146] Matsuda Y, Hara J, Osugi Y, Tokimasa S, Fujisaki H, Takai K, et al. Serum levels of soluble adhesion molecules in stem cell transplantation-related com-plications. Bone Marrow Transplant 2001;27(9): 977—82.

[147] Eremina V, Jefferson JA, Kowalewska J, Hochster H, Haas M, Weisstuch J, et al. VEGF inhibition and renal thrombotic microangiopathy. N Engl J Med 2008;358(11):1129—36.

[148] Min CK, Kim SY, Lee MJ, Eom KS, Kim YJ, Kim HJ, et al. Vascular endothelial growth factor (VEGF) is associated with reduced severity of acute graft-versus-host disease and nonrelapse mortality after allogeneic stem cell transplantation. Bone Marrow Transplant 2006;38(2):149—56.

[149] Randolph SS, Gooley TA, Warren EH, Appelbaum FR, Riddell SR. Female donors contribute to a selective graft-versus-leukemia effect in male recipients of HLA-matched, related he-matopoietic stem cell transplants. Blood 2004;103(1): 347—52.

[150] Choi CM, Schmaier AH, Snell MR, Lazarus HM. Thrombotic microangiopathy in haematopoietic stem cell transplantation: diagnosis and treatment. Drugs 2009;69(2):183—98.

[151] Kennedy GA, Kearey N, Bleakley S, Butler J, Mudie K, Durrant S. Transplantation-associated thrombotic microangiopathy: effect of concomitant GVHD on efficacy of therapeutic plasma exchange. Bone Marrow Transplant 2010;45(4):699—704.

[152] Hahn T, Alam AR, Lawrence D, Ford L, Baer MR, Bambach B, et al. Thrombotic microangiopathy after allogeneic blood and marrow transplantation is associated with dose-intensive myeloablative condi-tioning regimens, unrelated donor, and methyl-prednisolone T-cell depletion. Transplantation 2004;78(10):1515—22.

[153] Erdbruegger U, Woywodt A, Kirsch T, Haller H, Haubitz M. Circulating endothelial cells as a prog-nostic marker in thrombotic microangiopathy. Am J Kidney Dis 2006;48(4):564—70.

[154] Oran B, Donato M, Aleman A, Hosing C, Korbling M, Detry MA, et al. Transplant-associated microangiopathy in patients receiving tacrolimus following allogeneic stem cell transplantation: risk factors and response to treatment. Biol Blood Marrow Transplant 2007;13(4):469—77.

[155] Nguyen L, Terrell DR, Duvall D, Vesely SK, George JN. Complications of plasma exchange in patients treated for thrombotic thrombocytopenic

purpura. IV. An additional study of 43 consecutive patients, 2005 to 2008. Transfusion 2009;49(2):392—4.

[156] Shemin D, Briggs D, Greenan M. Complications of therapeutic plasma exchange: a prospective study of 1,727 procedures. J Clin Apher 2007;22(5):270—6.

[157] Marr H, McDonald EJ, Merriman E, Smith M, Mangos H, Stoddart C, et al. Successful treatment of transplant-associated microangiopathy with rituximab. N Z Med J 2009;122(1292):72—4.

[158] Naina HV, Gertz MA, Elliott MA. Thrombotic microangiopathy during peripheral blood stem cell mobilization. J Clin Apher 2009;24(6):259—61.

[159] Carella AM, D'Arena G, Greco MM, Nobile M, Cascavilla N. Rituximab for allo-SCT-associated thrombotic thrombocytopenic purpura. Bone Marrow Transplant 2008;41(12):1063—5.

[160] Au WY, Ma ES, Lee TL, Ha SY, Fung AT, Lie AK, et al. Successful treatment of thrombotic microangiopathy after haematopoietic stem cell transplantation with rituximab. Br J Haematol 2007; 137(5):475—8.

[161] Sakai M, Ikezoe T, Bandobashi K, Togitani K, Yokoyama A. Successful treatment of transplantation-associated thrombotic microangiopathy with recombinant human soluble thrombomodulin. Bone Marrow Transplant 2010;45(4):803—5.

[162] Egli A, Infanti L, Dumoulin A, Buser A, Samaridis J, Stebler C, et al. Prevalence of polyomavirus BK and JC infection and replication in 400 healthy blood donors. J Infect Dis 2009;199(6):837—46.

[163] Dropulic LK, Jones RJ. Polyomavirus BK infection in blood and marrow transplant recipients. Bone Marrow Transplant 2008;41(1):11—8.

[164] O'Donnell PH, Swanson K, Josephson MA, Artz AS, Parsad SD, Ramaprasad C, et al. BK virus infection is associated with hematuria and renal impairment in recipients of allogeneic hematopoetic stem cell transplants. Biol Blood Marrow Transplant 2009;15(9):1038—48 e1.

[165] Egli A, Binggeli S, Bodaghi S, Dumoulin A, Funk GA, Khanna N, et al. Cytomegalovirus and polyomavirus BK posttransplant. Nephrol Dial Transplant 2007;22(Suppl. 8):viii72—82.

[166] Ramos E, Drachenberg CB, Wali R, Hirsch HH. The decade of polyomavirus BK-associated nephropathy: state of affairs. Transplantation 2009;87(5):621—30.

[167] Hirsch HH. BK virus: opportunity makes a pathogen. Clin Infect Dis 2005;41(3):354—60.

[168] Leung AY, Chan MT, Yuen KY, Cheng VC, Chan KH, Wong CL, et al. Ciprofloxacin decreased polyoma BK virus load in patients who underwent allogeneic hematopoietic stem cell transplantation. Clin Infect Dis 2005;40(4):528—37.

[169] Dropulic LK, Cohen JI. Update on new antivirals under development for the treatment of double-stranded DNA virus infections. Clin Pharmacol Ther 2010;88(5):610—9.

[170] Blyth E, Clancy L, Simms R, Gaundar S, O'Connell P, Micklethwaite K, et al. BK virus-specific T cells for use in cellular therapy show specificity to multiple antigens and polyfunctional cytokine responses. Transplantation 2011;92(10):1077—84.

[171] Schachtner T, Muller K, Stein M, Diezemann C, Sefrin A, Babel N, et al. BK virus-specific immunity kinetics: a predictor of recovery from polyomavirus BK-associated nephropathy. Am J Transplant 2011; 11(11):2443—52.

[172] Schneidawind D, Schmitt A, Wiesneth M, Mertens T, Bunjes D, Freund M, et al. Polyomavirus BK-specific $CD8^+$ T cell responses in patients after allogeneic stem cell transplant. Leuk Lymphoma 2010; 51(6):1055—62.

[173] Cesaro S, Facchin C, Tridello G, Messina C, Calore E, Biasolo MA, et al. A prospective study of BK-virus-associated haemorrhagic cystitis in paediatric patients undergoing allogeneic haematopoietic stem cell transplantation. Bone Marrow Transplant 2008; 41(4):363—70.

[174] Gorczynska E, Turkiewicz D, Rybka K, Toporski J, Kalwak K, Dyla A, et al. Incidence, clinical outcome, and management of virus-induced hemorrhagic cystitis in children and adolescents after allogeneic hematopoietic cell transplantation. Biol Blood Marrow Transplant 2005;11(10):797—804.

[175] Giraud G, Priftakis P, Bogdanovic G, Remberger M, Dubrulle M, Hau A, et al. BK-viruria and haemorrhagic cystitis are more frequent in allogeneic haematopoietic stem cell transplant patients receiving full conditioning and unrelated-HLA-mismatched grafts. Bone Marrow Transplant 2008;41(8):737—42.

[176] Wong AS, Chan KH, Cheng VC, Yuen KY, Kwong YL, Leung AY. Relationship of pre-transplantation polyoma BK virus serologic findings and BK viral reactivation after hematopoietic stem cell transplantation. Clin Infect Dis 2007;44(6):830—7.

[177] Khan H, Oberoi S, Mahvash A, Sharma M, Rondon G, Alousi A, et al. Reversible ureteral obstruction due to polyomavirus infection after percutaneous nephrostomy catheter placement. Biol Blood Marrow Transplant 2011;17(10):1551—5.

[178] Dharnidharka VR, Abdulnour HA, Araya CE. The BK virus in renal transplant recipients-review of pathogenesis, diagnosis, and treatment. Pediatr Nephrol 2011;26(10):1763—74.

[179] Lekakis LJ, Macrinici V, Baraboutis IG, Mitchell B, Howard DS. BK virus nephropathy after allogeneic

stem cell transplantation: a case report and literature review. Am J Hematol 2009;84(4):243–6.

[180] Limaye AP, Smith KD, Cook L, Groom DA, Hunt NC, Jerome KR, et al. Polyomavirus nephropathy in native kidneys of non-renal transplant recipients. Am J Transplant 2005;5(3):614–20.

[181] Sanchez-Pinto LN, Laskin BL, Jodele S, Hummel TR, Yin HJ, Goebel J. BK virus nephropathy in a pediatric autologous stem-cell transplant recipient. Pediatr Blood Cancer 2011;56(3):495–7.

[182] Verghese PS, Finn LS, Englund JA, Sanders JE, Hingorani SR. BK nephropathy in pediatric hematopoietic stem cell transplant recipients. Pediatr Transplant 2009;13(7):913–8.

[183] Bruno B, Zager RA, Boeckh MJ, Gooley TA, Myerson DH, Huang ML, et al. Adenovirus nephritis in hematopoietic stem-cell transplantation. Transplantation 2004;77(7):1049–57.

[184] Erard V, Storer B, Corey L, Nollkamper J, Huang ML, Limaye A, et al. BK virus infection in hematopoietic stem cell transplant recipients: frequency, risk factors, and association with postengraftment hemorrhagic cystitis. Clin Infect Dis 2004;39(12):1861–5.

[185] Hirsch HH, Knowles W, Dickenmann M, Passweg J, Klimkait T, Mihatsch MJ, et al. Prospective study of polyomavirus type BK replication and nephropathy in renal-transplant recipients. N Engl J Med 2002;347(7):488–96.

[186] Erard V, Kim HW, Corey L, Limaye A, Huang ML, Myerson D, et al. BK DNA viral load in plasma: evidence for an association with hemorrhagic cystitis in allogeneic hematopoietic cell transplant recipients. Blood 2005;106(3):1130–2.

[187] Haines HL, Laskin BL, Goebel J, Davies SM, Yin HJ, Lawrence J, et al. Blood, and not urine, BK viral load predicts renal outcome in children with hemorrhagic cystitis following hematopoietic stem cell transplantation. Biol Blood Marrow Transplant. Prepublished on March 7, 2011 as DOI 10.1016/j.bbmt. 2011.02.012.

[188] Romagnani P, Lazzeri E, Mazzinghi B, Lasagni L, Guidi S, Bosi A, et al. Nephrotic syndrome and renal failure after allogeneic stem cell transplantation: novel molecular diagnostic tools for a challenging differential diagnosis. Am J Kidney Dis 2005;46(3):550–6.

[189] Niculescu F, Niculescu T, Nguyen P, Puliaev R, Papadimitriou JC, Gaspari A, et al. Both apoptosis and complement membrane attack complex deposition are major features of murine acute graft-vs.-host disease. Exp Mol Pathol 2005;79(2):136–45.

[190] Krenger W, Hill GR, Ferrara JL. Cytokine cascades in acute graft-versus-host disease. Transplantation 1997;64(4):553–8.

[191] Couriel D, Caldera H, Champlin R, Komanduri K. Acute graft-versus-host disease: pathophysiology, clinical manifestations, and management. Cancer 2004;101(9):1936–46.

[192] Seconi J, Watt V, Ritchie DS. Nephrotic syndrome following allogeneic stem cell transplantation associated with increased production of TNF-alpha and interferon-gamma by donor T cells. Bone Marrow Transplant 2003;32(4):447–50.

[193] Teshima T, Ordemann R, Reddy P, Gagin S, Liu C, Cooke KR, et al. Acute graft-versus-host disease does not require alloantigen expression on host epithelium. Nat Med 2002;8(6):575–81.

[194] Kansu E. The pathophysiology of chronic graft-versus-host disease. Int J Hematol 2004;79(3):209–15.

[195] Kitamura M, Suto TS. TGF-beta and glomerulonephritis: anti-inflammatory versus prosclerotic actions. Nephrol Dial Transplant 1997;12(4):669–79.

[196] Negri AL. Prevention of progressive fibrosis in chronic renal diseases: antifibrotic agents. J Nephrol 2004;17(4):496–503.

[197] Langham RG, Egan MK, Dowling JP, Gilbert RE, Thomson NM. Transforming growth factor-beta1 and tumor growth factor-beta-inducible gene-H3 in nonrenal transplant cyclosporine nephropathy. Transplantation 2001;72(11):1826–9.

[198] Disel U, Paydas S, Dogan A, Gulfiliz G, Yavuz S. Effect of colchicine on cyclosporine nephrotoxicity, reduction of TGF-beta overexpression, apoptosis, and oxidative damage: an experimental animal study. Transplant Proc 2004;36(5):1372–6.

[199] Chan GS, Lam MF, Au WY, Chim S, Tse KC, Lo SH, et al. Clinicopathologic analysis of renal biopsies after haematopoietic stem cell transplantation. Nephrology (Carlton) 2008;13(4):322–30.

[200] Hu SL. The role of graft-versus-host disease in haematopoietic cell transplantation-associated glomerular disease. Nephrol Dial Transplant 2011; 26(6):2025–31.

[201] Luo XD, Liu QF, Zhang Y, Sun J, Wang GB, Fan ZP, et al. Nephrotic syndrome after allogeneic hematopoietic stem cell transplantation: etiology and pathogenesis. Blood Cells Mol Dis 2011;46(2):182–7.

[202] Srinivasan R, Balow JE, Sabnis S, Lundqvist A, Igarashi T, Takahashi Y, et al. Nephrotic syndrome: an under-recognised immune-mediated complication of non-myeloablative allogeneic haematopoietic cell transplantation. Br J Haematol 2005;131(1):74–9.

[203] Lam MF, Au WY, Tse KC, Chan TM, Chan GS, Chan KW, et al. Late onset membranous nephropathy complicating donor lymphocyte infusion for leukaemia relapse after allogeneic stem cell transplantation. Am J Hematol 2007;82(4):327–8.

[204] Kalayoglu-Besisik S, Yurci A, Yazici H, Yonal I, Sargin D. Long-term outcome of nephrotic syndrome in an allogeneic hematopoietic stem cell recipient without typical features of graft versus host disease. Transplantation 2007;83(10):1407−8.

[205] Ferrannini M, Vischini G, Di Daniele N. Rituximab in membranous nephropathy after haematopoietic stem cell transplantation. Nephrol Dial Transplant 2008;23(8):2700−1; author reply 1.

[206] Motoyama O, Uchino Y, Tokuyama M, Iitaka K, Ohara A. A boy with membranous nephropathy after allogeneic bone marrow transplantation. Clin Exp Nephrol 2009;13(5):508−11.

[207] Sugimoto T, Tanaka Y, Sakaguchi M, Osawa N, Uzu T, Kashiwagi A. A case of post-allogeneic haematopoietic stem cell transplantation membranous nephropathy. Nephrol Dial Transplant 2007;22(11): 3362−3.

[208] Vischini G, Cudillo L, Ferrannini M, Di Daniele N, Cerretti R, Arcese W. Rituximab in post allogeneic hematopoietic stem cell transplantation membranous nephropathy: a case report. J Nephrol 2009;22(1):160−3.

[209] Gupta A, Lal C, Bhowmik D. De novo membranous nephropathy after hematopoietic stem cell transplantation. Saudi J Kidney Dis Transpl 2011;22(5): 1035−6.

[210] Kaminska D, Bernat B, Vakulenko O, Kuzniar J, Tyran B, Suchnicki K, et al. Glomerular lesion and increased cytokine gene expression in renal tissue in patients with decompensated nephrotic syndrome due to chronic GvHD. Ren Fail 2010;32(4):510−4.

[211] Mattei D, Sorasio R, Guarnieri A, Marazzi F, Formica M, Fortunato M, et al. Long-term results of rituximab treatment for membranous nephropathy after allogeneic hematopoietic SCT: a case report. Bone Marrow Transplant 2010;45(6):1111−2.

[212] Petropoulou AD, Robin M, Rocha V, Ribaud P, Xhaard A, Abboud I, et al. Nephrotic syndrome associated with graft rejection after unrelated double cord blood transplantation. Transplantation 2010;90(7):801−2.

[213] Lopes JA, Martins C, Jorge S, Melo MJ, Resina C, Moreno R, et al. Focal segmental glomerulosclerosis: a very unusual complication of allogeneic hematopoietic cell transplantation (HCT). Bone Marrow Transplant 2011;46(7):1019−20.

[214] Fofi C, Barberi S, Stoppacciaro A, Punzo G, Mene P. Focal segmental glomerulosclerosis as a complication of graft-versus-host disease. Nat Rev Nephrol 2009;5(4):236−40.

[215] Kim JY, Lee MY, Kim B, Park CW, Chang YS, Chung S. Membranoproliferative glomerulonephritis following allogeneic hematopoietic stem cell transplantation. Clin Exp Nephrol 2010;14(6): 630−2.

[216] Hu SL, Colvin GA, Rifai A, Suzuki H, Novak J, Esparza A, et al. Glomerulonephritis after hematopoietic cell transplantation: IgA nephropathy with increased excretion of galactose-deficient IgA1. Nephrol Dial Transplant 2010;25(5):1708−13.

[217] Navaneethan SD, Taylor J, Goldman B, Bose A. Anti-neutrophil cytoplasmic antibody associated crescentic IgA nephropathy in hematopoietic stem cell transplantation. Clin Nephrol 2009;71(1):59−62.

[218] Ben-Dov IZ, Pizov G, Ben-Chetrit E, Rubinger D, Or R. Fatal nephrotic syndrome complicating allogeneic stem cell transplantation: a case report. Nephrol Dial Transplant 2009;24(9):2946−9.

[219] Kusumi E, Kami M, Hara S, Hoshino J, Yamaguchi Y, Murashige N, et al. Postmortem examination of the kidney in allogeneic hematopoietic stem cell transplantation recipients: possible involvement of graft-versus-host disease. Int J Hematol 2008;87(2): 225−30.

[220] Saleh AJ, Al Mohareb F, Al Rabiah F, Chaudhri N, Al Sharif F, Al Zahrani H, et al. High efficacy and low toxicity of short-course oral valganciclovir as preemptive therapy for hematopoietic stem cell transplant cytomegalovirus infection. Hematol Oncol Stem Cell Ther 2010;3(3):116−20.

[221] Hayakawa J, Joyal EG, Gildner JF, Washington KN, Phang OA, Uchida N, et al. 5% dimethyl sulfoxide (DMSO) and pentastarch improves cryopreservation of cord blood cells over 10% DMSO. Transfusion 2010;50(10):2158−66.

[222] Lexicomp Online. Lexi-Comp I, http://www.crlonline.com; 2012 [accessed 02.04.2012].

Radiation-associated Kidney Injury

Amber S. Podoll, Mark J. Amsbaugh

The University of Texas Medical School at Houston, Houston, Texas, USA

INTRODUCTION

Ionizing radiation was first used to treat breast cancer in 1896, a year after the discovery of X-rays. Since that time, it has become an increasingly utilized modality in the treatment of malignant and benign conditions alike. For almost as long, it is known that irradiation of normal tissue can produce toxic effects. Modern-day radiation therapy seeks to balance the curative potential of ionizing radiation with the potentially serious side-effect profile on normal tissue.

Previously, the kidneys were believed to be very radiation resistant organs and the true renal sensitivity to ionizing radiation was not fully appreciated [1]. Today, however, the kidney is often the dose-limiting organ for total body irradiation, many gynecologic cancers, gastrointestinal cancers, sarcomas and lymphomas.

Radiation-associated kidney injury, or previously termed radiation nephritis or radiation nephropathy, as its name suggests stems from ionizing radiation's effects, both acute and chronic on the kidney. The entity was first observed in 1906 and more fully described by Hall and Whipple in 1919 but was quickly

dismissed. Later, irradiation of the abdomen leading to renal insufficiency was again described in humans in 1950 [1–3]. Pathologists at the Children's Hospital of Michigan and the Children's Hospital of Detroit reported three cases of death occurring 5–7 months following irradiation. Each of the children who died exhibited clinical manifestations of renal failure combined with hematuria, albuminuria, azotemia and anemia. On post-mortem exam, the authors described "complete scarring glomerular obstruction of long standing, recent degenerative changes and acute necrosis... [involving] primarily the endothelium and basement membrane" [3]. It is now accepted that exposure to ionizing radiation can produce both acute and chronic effects on the kidneys.

PATHOGENESIS

The pathogenesis of radiation-associated kidney injury is poorly understood in humans. Much of the published research focuses on long-term clinical outcomes of patients with renal insufficiency who have received radiation in the past. Few studies focus on the actual mechanism of injury to the kidney, and those that do have primarily been completed in animals. Radiation appears to harm both the endocrine as well as mechanical filtration function of the human kidney.

Radiation causes cellular damage through direct and indirect mechanisms. One-third of cellular radiation damage is caused by direct ionization of DNA leading to double strand breaks. Two-thirds of damage is indirectly due to a combination of free electrons released when ionizing radiation strikes an intracellular molecule and intracellular free radicals interacting with DNA. The result of both direct and indirect damage is aberrations in cellular DNA. Normal cells can repair small amounts of damage. Irradiation of humans, as a treatment for cancer, was validated when it was discovered many tumor cells have difficulty repairing this damage leading to cellular dysfunction and apoptosis [4].

It was originally postulated that radiation-induced tubular cell damage was the primary mechanism of renal dysfunction; later the glomerular and juxtaglomerular cells were believed also to be injured [5,6]. It appears that the actual pattern of injury is a combination of both tubular and glomerular lesions [5,7,8]. The pattern of damage varies between species studied, but all species develop reactive changes in the tubule with atrophy and mesangiolysis/thrombosis with accompanying glomerulosclerosis [7]. Radiation-damaged glomeruli exhibit basement membrane duplication and vascular changes including capillary loop thickening with subendothelial expansion [7]. The glomerulosclerosis tends to increase in severity from the cortex to the medulla and is accelerated with increased dose [7].

In addition to the early changes, characteristic late findings include loss of renal mass and volume, sclerosed intralobular and arcuate arteries and associated interstitial fibrosis. Late endothelial damage in the small blood vessels will encourage fibrin deposition leading to platelet aggregation and red blood cell injury [9]. Animal studies suggest that these changes begin to cause functional changes within several weeks of exposure to radiation [10]. The initial response is probably one of compensatory increased kidney blood flow and an associated increase in glomerular filtration rate (GFR). Following this short initial period, renal blood flow and corresponding GFR decrease within 6−8 weeks of radiation exposure [7,11].

Prospective studies following patients who received radiation with urinalysis and blood urea nitrogen (BUN) levels did not note any abnormalities within the first year they were followed, although there is some evidence in animal studies that increased permeability of albumin can occur shortly after treatment on a sub-clinical level [7,12]. This highlights the insidious nature of radiation-associated kidney injury. Many of the changes are subtle at first and become more pronounced over time. The long lag time before these changes become clinically evident can contribute to the misdiagnosis of radiation nephropathy because the clinical changes are often attributed to other medical factors.

Due in part to the observation that angiotensin converting enzyme (ACE) inhibitors and angiotensin-II receptor blockers (ARB) help to mitigate the effects of radiation damage on the kidney it was long believed that activation of the renin−angiotensin−aldosterone system (RAAS) was at the root of the clinical signs and symptoms of radiation-induced kidney injury [7,13]. This was supported by studies that showed no benefit from anti-hypertensive agents that did not inhibit the RAAS [14]. Although some evidence for this has been observed in select animal models, most studies now point towards a different mechanism. Interestingly, the protective effect of ACE inhibitors is still evident at drastically reduced doses. This indicates that it might be an unknown effect independent of systemic blood pressure control [15].

As the effects of ionizing radiation on the body become increasingly known, it has been proposed that chronic renal failure after radiation might be associated with chronic oxidative stress [13]. Current evidence suggests that while this effect may be a contributing factor, more research is needed to determine whether this factor plays a significant role in the pathogenesis of kidney injury [16].

EPIDEMIOLOGY

Cases of radiation-associated kidney injury are likely underreported due to the variable time it can take for the effect of radiation to become clinically evident [17]. Incidence can be further confounded by the multiple medical co-morbidities that are present in many cancer patients and the variety of systemic therapies used in conjunction with radiation therapy. The differences between typical treatment fields and dosage schedules based on diseases and treatment centers make it difficult to predict whether a patient is at risk for kidney injury.

Bilateral Kidney Irradiation

Radiation-associated kidney injury is uncommon even in patients receiving large doses of radiation to one or both kidneys. In a large British series a cohort of patients who received over 25 gray (Gy) to both kidneys reported that only 20% of the subjects developed renal side-effects [18]. Other series report a wide range of kidney injury depending on patient and treatment-related factors [12,18—23]. Rates of kidney injury can be as high as 71—76% in ovarian cancer patients receiving abdominal radiation and cisplatin [23]. Rates can be significantly lower for patients receiving no chemotherapy and/or a low dose of radiation [20,22]. Cassady reviewed the data on bilateral whole kidney irradiation in several studies and

concluded that the threshold dose for renal damage was 15 Gy over a 3—5-week period. Furthermore, Cassady concluded that the 5-year risk for injury was 5% at 18 Gy and 50% at 28 Gy, respectively [5].

Unilateral Kidney Irradiation

Radiation-associated injury can also occur after unilateral or partial kidney irradiation, although somewhat less often than when both kidneys are in the radiation field [22,24—34]. Kunkler et al., in a 1952 series of 60 patients undergoing radiation for seminoma, described no patients developing elevated blood pressure and albuminuria when the dose to 33% of the volume of the kidneys was kept under 18 Gy [22]. Thompson et al., however, described a clear dose—response relationship with higher doses resulting in increasing kidney atrophy. All patients had 50% of their total kidney volume receive 15—35 Gy of radiation. Overall, 46% of the study subjects who received radiation for peptic ulcer disease developed some degree of kidney atrophy [32]. It is currently accepted that the 5-year risk for injury was 5% at 30 Gy and 50% at 40 Gy for radiation exposure to two-thirds of the total kidney volume, although these are based largely on speculation [35].

Total Body Irradiation and Transplantation

Total body irradiation (TBI) has been used to prepare both pediatric and adult patients for bone marrow transplantation (BMT). Radiation-associated injury can occur at a much lower dose during total body irradiation versus bilateral whole kidney radiation [36—45]. This is commonly attributed to the fact that radiation for BMT is given in higher dose per fraction which does not allow the normal tissue to undergo appropriate DNA injury repair. Published cases series report rates of renal toxicity to be anywhere from 0 to 46.7% in children and adults depending on dose and dose rate [36–38,40–43,45–47]. Cheng et al. conducted a meta-analysis of 12 studies involving adults and children receiving total body irradiation. Dose was found to be the only significant factor in adults. When studies with patients of all ages were included, dose rate, dose and use of fludarabine chemotherapy were significant factors in the incidence of renal side-effects [48].

Several authors describe radiation nephropathy following irradiation for BMT as a separate and distinct clinical syndrome called BMT nephropathy [39]. This syndrome tends to occur in a more acute time course than chronic forms of radiation-associated kidney injury and can occur at much lower doses of radiation. Severe cases can mimic the presentation of hemolytic uremic syndrome (HUS), and hypertension is more consistently present than radiation nephropathy from other causes [36,39,49].

MODERN RADIATION AND THE KIDNEYS

Modern radiation therapy continues to evolve; today's treatment techniques are much different than those employed when many of the clinical studies observing radiation's long-term effects on the kidney were reported. Recent advances in the field of therapeutic radiation oncology, including 3D CT-based simulation, better planning software and intensity modulated radiation therapy, mean that not only can normal tissues now be increasingly protected, but physicians can calculate the appropriate dose to any part of an organ before the dose is administered. The increasing utilization of proton therapy for pediatric malignancies promises to reduce the incidence of radiation-related toxicities, including renal toxicity. A recent study reports that mean kidney doses alone in childhood abdominal cancers can be reduced by

40–60% [50]. It remains to be seen if these reductions in dose result in clinical significance.

As knowledge of radiation toxicity in both the short- and the long-term increases, greater care is taken to avoid damaging nearby structures. Physicians delivering radiation make an effort to stay under acceptable dose constraints to the kidneys. Individual cases may require a physician to exceed dose constraints in order to deliver an acceptable minimum dose to the clinical target volume. In these cases, the patient can be closely followed for signs of toxicity and the radiation oncologist can collaborate with a nephrologist to ensure the patient is adequately treated if signs of renal injury do manifest.

Dose Constraints

The acceptable dose to the kidney for both bilateral and partial kidney irradiation is unknown. Many of the currently published studies do not have enough follow-up and are not designed to test for long-term complications of irradiation of the kidneys. Currently accepted dose–volume constraints for TBI and non-TBI bilateral kidney irradiation are <10 Gy mean dose and <18 Gy mean dose, respectively [5,17,48]. Dose constraints for partial kidney irradiation are more complicated and less well accepted. Jansen et al. recommend keeping the volume of bilateral kidney receiving 20 Gy under 30%, while Welz et al. recommend keeping the volume receiving 12 Gy under 55% [27,33]. It is important to keep in mind, however, that dosing schedule, radiosensitizing chemotherapy, nephrotoxic drugs and interactions of clinical factors may all contribute to radiation damage.

Radiation-associated Secondary Malignancies

The incidence of radiation-associated secondary malignancies originating in the kidney is somewhat unknown but believed to be low.

High levels of radiation can cause renal cell carcinoma in experimental animal models [51]. Low levels of radiation rarely result in renal tumor formation, although recent data from the Life Span Study of Japanese atomic bomb survivors did find a positive association between both renal cell carcinoma and cancers of the renal pelvis/ureter and radiation [52].

CLINICAL PRESENTATION

Luxton and Kunkler first characterized the four clinical syndromes (Table 7.1) produced by radiation damage to the kidneys in the 1950s while studying the effects of abdominal radiation for seminomas [18,22,53]. Further clinical reporting has reinforced this characterization but also shown that these groups can significantly overlap and are often progressive [5,25,31,32,34]. Late toxicity to the kidneys is currently graded by the joint RTOG/EORTC Late Radiation Morbidity Scoring Scheme [54].

History

A previous exposure to ionizing radiation is essential when radiation-associated kidney injury is suspected but often the patient may not have the specific information about the dose and areas of exposure. It is important to note that as radiation therapy becomes a larger part of cancer care, radiation will not cause all renal dysfunction in previously irradiated patients. In fact, as modern radiation therapy

TABLE 7.1 Clinical Syndromes in Radiation-associated Kidney Injury

Acute Radiation Nephropathy.

Chronic radiation nephropathy

Proteinuria

Malignant hypertension

develops more conformal delivery modalities and better targeting technology, the diagnosis of radiation nephropathy will become less likely. Today's radiation oncologists are aware of the potential side-effects of irradiating normal kidney tissue and usually attempt to minimize the radiation to the kidney providing the dose to the underlying cancer is not compromised.

Radiation-associated kidney injury has a long latency period. With the exception of BMT-nephropathy, there is not an acute form that presents during or shortly after radiation therapy. Patients do not experience signs of kidney dysfunction until 6 months following radiation, and for many patients it may take several years to progress to overt renal dysfunction [5,17,55].

Patients will often not present with an obvious prodrome of symptoms or with a rapid onset of renal failure [55]. Common symptoms of radiation-associated kidney injury include swelling, fluid retention, increased weight and malaise. Additionally, symptoms can overlap with those of other renal diseases such as malignant hypertension (headaches, vomiting and blurry vision) and other end organ damage (dyspnea, confusion and coma). It is important to recognize that these symptoms in themselves do not differentiate radiation nephropathy from many other causes of renal failure.

Laboratory Findings

The complete blood count may reveal a microangiopathic hemolytic anemia with schistocytes on the peripheral smear. Thrombocytopenia will also be present [5,17,32,55]. These findings are similar to what is seen in patients with malignant hypertension or HUS.

Urinalysis typically demonstrates proteinuria, granular casts and microscopic hematuria. Although present, proteinuria usually does not reach nephrotic range levels. These finding are not typically present until 6 months or more after irradiation and may increase in severity as time progresses and symptoms begin to become more clinically evident [5,12,55].

There are no specific findings for radiation-associated kidney injury for most modalities of diagnostic imaging. CT and MR imaging will reveal progressive kidney atrophy beginning 6 months to 1 year after radiation with the possibility of asymmetric contrast uptake if only one kidney was in the target field. 99mTechnetium diethylene triamine penta-acetic acid renography will reveal decreased glomerular function and 99mTechnetium dimercaptosuccinyl acid renography shows decreased tubular function. 131Iodine radio hippurate scintigraphy will likely show a perfusion defect [17].

DIAGNOSIS

The diagnosis of radiation nephropathy is made by comparing a clinical picture of progressive renal dysfunction in a cancer patient who received radiation to the total body, spine, abdomen, or pelvis. A thorough history and physical exam should be performed and the clinician should have a strong index of suspicion for patients with a past history of radiation therapy. It is important to contact the radiation oncologist who delivered the radiation to determine what dose of radiation the kidneys received. A kidney biopsy does not necessarily need to be performed. Many of the histopathologic findings in radiation nephropathy are non-specific and common to a large host of other causes of renal failure. Renal biopsy may demonstrate the finding of thrombotic microangiopathy. Unless the biopsy needs to be performed for another reason the added diagnostic information is often not worth the cost and potential harm to the patient.

TREATMENT

The best way to manage radiation-associated kidney disease is prevention. Due to the uncertainty of factors that contribute to radiation

nephropathy in some patients the avoidance of as much healthy renal tissue as possible is the best way to achieve this end. Modern targeting systems make this increasingly possible.

Of historical interest, aspirin and other prostaglandin inhibitors were originally shown in animal models to prevent radiation-associated kidney injury [56]. They are not currently used since it was found that ACE inhibitors can act as a protective agent in humans.

Patients who receive drugs inhibiting the RAAS after exposure to radiation have a lower incidence of radiation-associated kidney injury [14,57]. This protective effect was first shown with the ACE inhibitor captopril but has now been shown with other ACE inhibitors and ARBs [14,15,57−63]. One randomized trial suggested that the protective effect in bone marrow transplant patients was significant (15% incidence for placebo vs. 3.7% for captopril) [57].

Blockade of the RAAS is also useful once radiation-induced injury has developed. Various studies have shown that angiotensin-1 (AT1) receptor blockers and ACE inhibitors have similar beneficial effects on the course of the disease. As opposed to treatment prior to the development of clinical disease, the use of ARBs does not appear to be effective [63]. It is unclear why this discrepancy exists although it may be related to the degree of blood pressure control [63].

PROGNOSIS

The prognosis for patients who develop radiation-associated kidney injury is generally poor. Once kidney injury caused by radiation therapy becomes clinically evident it will continue to progress and renal function will eventually decline. The time course of progression is somewhat variable and many patients can remain stable for years while others rapidly decompensate. A case−control study conducted by Cohen and his colleagues in patients who developed chronic end stage kidney disease after irradiation for BMT showed that they had poorer survival than other controls with no history of irradiation [64]. This highlights the need for preventive measures and early diagnosis of radiation-induced kidney injury so that management can begin early in the course of the disease.

Like other patients with chronic kidney disease, patients diagnosed with radiation nephropathy should make every effort to avoid nephrotoxic medications and maintain acceptable blood pressure control. These steps will help to slow the eventual further decline in renal function.

SUMMARY

Radiation-associated kidney injury, also known as radiation nephropathy, can occur in both the acute and chronic phase, but most commonly occurs 6−12 months after exposure. It is difficult to predict who is at risk for radiation nephropathy because of the varying doses, dosing fractionation and other systemic treatments cancer patients receive. Patients typically present with hypertension, edema and proteinuria consistent with an acute kidney injury but can also be accompanied by microangiopathic hemolytic anemia with schistocytes and thrombocytopenia. Renal biopsy findings are not specific to radiation injury and are more typical of HUS. Progression to chronic renal failure and ultimately to dialysis dependence is common. ACE inhibitors and ARBs are increasingly being used as successful treatment. The development of end stage renal disease is a poor prognostic event in these patients and survival on chronic dialysis is poor compared to that of age-matched non-diabetic and diabetic patients.

References

[1] McQuarrie I, Whipple GH. A study of renal function in Roentgen ray intoxication: resistance of renal epithelium to direct radiation. J Exp Med 1922;35(2):225−42.

[2] Edsall D. The attitude of the clinician with regard to exposing the patient to the x-ray. JAMA 1906;47(18):1425−9.

[3] Zuelzer WW, Palmer HD, Newton WA. Unusual glomerulonephritis in young children probably radiation nephritis. Am J Pathol 1950;26(6):1019−39.

[4] Hall EJ, Giaccia A. Radiobiology for the Radiologist. 7th ed. Lippincott Williams & Wilkins; 2011.

[5] Cassady JR. Clinical radiation nephropathy. Int J Radiat Oncol Biol Phys 1995;31(5):1249−56.

[6] Glatstein E, Fajardo LF, Brown JM. Radiation injury in the mouse kidney − I. Sequential light microscopic study. Int J Radiat Oncol Biol Phys 1977;2(9−10):933−43.

[7] Cohen EP, Robbins ME. Radiation nephropathy. Semin Nephrol 2003;23(5):486−99.

[8] Robbins ME, Bonsib SM. Radiation nephropathy: a review. Scanning Microsc 1995;9(2):535−60.

[9] White DC. The histopathologic basis for functional decrements in late radiation injury in diverse organs. Cancer 1976;37(Suppl. 2):1126−43.

[10] Hoopes PJ, Gillette EL, Benjamin SA. The pathogenesis of radiation nephropathy in the dog. Radiat Res 1985;104(3):406−19.

[11] Robbins ME, Hopewell JW, Gunn Y. Effects of single doses of X-rays on renal function in unilaterally irradiated pigs. Radiother Oncol 1985;4(2):143−51.

[12] Avioli LV, Lazor MZ, Cotlove E, Brace KC, Andrews JR. Early effects of radiation on renal function in man. Am J Med 1963;34:329−37.

[13] Robbins ME, Zhao W, Davis CS, Toyokuni S, Bonsib SM. Radiation-induced kidney injury: a role for chronic oxidative stress? Micron 2002;33(2):133−41.

[14] Cohen EP, Moulder JE, Fish BL, Hill P. Prophylaxis of experimental bone marrow transplant nephropathy. J Lab Clin Med 1994;124(3):371−80.

[15] Moulder JE, Fish BL, Cohen EP. Radiation nephropathy is treatable with an angiotensin converting enzyme inhibitor or an angiotensin II type-1 (AT1) receptor antagonist. Radiother Oncol 1998;46(3):307−15.

[16] Lenarczyk M, Cohen EP, Fish BL, Irving AA, Sharma M, Driscoll CD, et al. Chronic oxidative stress as a mechanism for radiation nephropathy. Radiat Res 2009;171(2):164−72.

[17] Dawson LA, Kavanagh BD, Paulino AC, Das SK, Miften M, Li XA, et al. Radiation-associated kidney injury. Int J Radiat Oncol Biol Phys 2010;76(Suppl. 3):S108−15.

[18] Luxton RW. Radiation nephritis. A long-term study of 54 patients. Lancet 1961;2(7214):1221−4.

[19] Churchill DN, Hong K, Gault MH. Radiation nephritis following combined abdominal radiation and chemotherapy (bleomycin-vinblastine). Cancer 1978;41(6):2162–4.

[20] Irwin C, Fyles A, Wong CS, Cheung CM, Zhu Y. Late renal function following whole abdominal irradiation. Radiother Oncol 1996;38(3):257–61.

[21] Keane WF, Crosson JT, Staley NA, Anderson WR, Shapiro FL. Radiation-induced renal disease. A clinicopathologic study. Am J Med 1976;60(1):127–37.

[22] Kunkler PB, Farr RF, Luxton RW. The limit of renal tolerance to x-rays; an investigation into renal damage occurring following the treatment of tumours of the testis by abdominal baths. Br J Radiol 1952;25(292): 192–201.

[23] Schneider DP, Marti HP, Von Briel C, Frey FJ, Greiner RH. Long-term evolution of renal function in patients with ovarian cancer after whole abdominal irradiation with or without preceding cisplatin. Ann Oncol 1999;10(6):677–83.

[24] Birkhead BM, Dobbs CE, Beard MF, Tyson JW, Fuller EA. Assessment of renal function following irradiation of the intact spleen for Hodgkin disease. Radiology 1979;130(2):473–5.

[25] Dewit L, Verheij M, Valdes Olmos RA, Arisz L. Compensatory renal response after unilateral partial and whole volume high-dose irradiation of the human kidney. Eur J Cancer 1993;29A(16):2239–43.

[26] Flentje M, Hensley F, Gademann G, Menke M, Wannenmacher M. Renal tolerance to non-homogenous irradiation: comparison of observed effects to predictions of normal tissue complication probability from different biophysical models. Int J Radiat Oncol Biol Phys 1993;27(1):25–30.

[27] Jansen EPM, Saunders MP, Boot H, Oppedijk V, Dubbelman R, Porritt B, et al. Prospective study on late renal toxicity following postoperative chemoradiotherapy in gastric cancer. Int J Radiat Oncol Biol Phys 2007;67(3):781–5.

[28] Kim TH, Freeman CR, Webster JH. The significance of unilateral radiation nephropathy. Int J Radiat Oncol Biol Phys 1980;6(11):1567–71.

[29] Kim TH, Somerville PJ, Freeman CR. Unilateral radiation nephropathy – the long-term significance. Int J Radiat Oncol Biol Phys 1984;10(11):2053–9.

[30] Köst S, Dörr W, Keinert K, Glaser F-H, Endert G, Herrmann T. Effect of dose and dose-distribution in damage to the kidney following abdominal radiotherapy. Int J Radiat Biol 2002;78(8):695–702.

[31] Le Bourgeois JP, Meignan M, Parmentier C, Tubiana M. Renal consequences of irradiation of the spleen in lymphoma patients. Br J Radiol 1979;52(613): 56–60.

[32] Thompson PL, Mackay IR, Robson GS, Wall AJ. Late radiation nephritis after gastric x-irradiation for peptic ulcer. Q J Med 1971;40(157):145–57.

[33] Welz S, Hehr T, Kollmannsberger C, Bokemeyer C, Belka C, Budach W. Renal toxicity of adjuvant chemoradiotherapy with cisplatin in gastric cancer. Int J Radiat Oncol Biol Phys 2007;69(5):1429–35.

[34] Willett CG, Tepper JE, Orlow EL, Shipley WU. Renal complications secondary to radiation treatment of upper abdominal malignancies. Int J Radiat Oncol Biol Phys 1986;12(9):1601–4.

[35] Emami B, Lyman J, Brown A, Coia L, Goitein M, Munzenrider JE, et al. Tolerance of normal tissue to therapeutic irradiation. Int J Radiat Oncol Biol Phys 1991;21(1):109–22.

[36] Borg M, Hughes T, Horvath N, Rice M, Thomas AC. Renal toxicity after total body irradiation. Int J Radiat Oncol Biol Phys 2002;54(4):1165–73.

[37] Bradley J, Reft C, Goldman S, Rubin C, Nachman J, Larson R, et al. High-energy total body irradiation as preparation for bone marrow transplantation in leukemia patients: treatment technique and related complications. Int J Radiat Oncol Biol Phys 1998;40(2): 391–6.

[38] Chou RH, Wong GB, Kramer JH, Wara DW, Matthay KK, Crittenden MR, et al. Toxicities of total-body irradiation for pediatric bone marrow transplantation. Int J Radiat Oncol Biol Phys 1996;34(4): 843–51.

[39] Cohen EP. Radiation nephropathy after bone marrow transplantation. Kidney Int 2000;58(2):903–18.

[40] Frisk P, Bratteby LE, Carlson K, Lonnerholm G. Renal function after autologous bone marrow transplantation in children: a long-term prospective study. Bone Marrow Transplant 2002;29(2):129–36.

[41] Miralbell R, Bieri S, Mermillod B, Helg C, Sancho G, Pastoors B, et al. Renal toxicity after allogeneic bone marrow transplantation: the combined effects of total-body irradiation and graft-versus-host disease. J Clin Oncol 1996;14(2):579–85.

[42] Rabinowe SN, Soiffer RJ, Tarbell NJ, Neuberg D, Freedman AS, Seifter J, et al. Hemolytic-uremic syndrome following bone marrow transplantation in adults for hematologic malignancies. Blood 1991; 77(8):1837–44.

[43] Tarbell NJ, Guinan EC, Chin L, Mauch P, Weinstein HJ. Renal insufficiency after total body irradiation for pediatric bone marrow transplantation. Radiother Oncol 1990;18(Suppl. 1):139–42.

[44] Tarbell NJ, Guinan EC, Niemeyer C, Mauch P, Sallan SE, Weinstein HJ. Late onset of renal dysfunction in survivors of bone marrow transplantation. Int J Radiat Oncol Biol Phys 1988;15(1):99–104.

[45] Van Why SK, Friedman AL, Wei LJ, Hong R. Renal insufficiency after bone marrow transplantation in children. Bone Marrow Transplant 1991;7(5):383—8.

[46] Delgado J, Cooper N, Thomson K, Duarte R, Jarmulowicz M, Cassoni A, et al. The importance of age, fludarabine, and total body irradiation in the incidence and severity of chronic renal failure after allogeneic hematopoietic cell transplantation. Biol Blood Marrow Transplant 2006;12(1):75—83.

[47] Lawton CA, Cohen EP, Murray KJ, Derus SW, Casper JT, Drobyski WR, et al. Long-term results of selective renal shielding in patients undergoing total body irradiation in preparation for bone marrow transplantation. Bone Marrow Transplant 1997;20(12): 1069—74.

[48] Cheng JC, Schultheiss TE, Wong JYC. Impact of drug therapy, radiation dose, and dose rate on renal toxicity following bone marrow transplantation. Int J Radiat Oncol Biol Phys 2008;71(5):1436—43.

[49] Igaki H, Karasawa K, Sakamaki H, Saito H, Nakagawa K, Ohtomo K, et al. Renal dysfunction after total-body irradiation. Significance of selective renal shielding blocks. Strahlenther Onkol 2005;181(11): 704—8.

[50] Hillbrand M, Georg D, Gadner H, Potter R, Dieckmann K. Abdominal cancer during early childhood: a dosimetric comparison of proton beams to standard and advanced photon radiotherapy. Radiother Oncol 2008;89(2):141—9.

[51] Maldague P. Comparative study of experimentally induced cancer of the kidney in mice and rats with X-rays. Radiation-Induced Cancer Vienna International Atomic Energy Agency 1969. Athens, Greece: 439—58.

[52] Richardson DB, Hamra G. Ionizing radiation and kidney cancer among Japanese atomic bomb survivors. Radiat Res 2010;173(6):837—42.

[53] Luxton RW, Kunkler PB. Radiation nephritis. Acta Radiol 1964;2:169—78.

[54] Cox JD, Stetz J, Pajak TF. Toxicity criteria of the Radiation Therapy Oncology Group (RTOG) and the European Organization for Research and Treatment of Cancer (EORTC). Int J Radiat Oncol Biol Phys 1995;31(5):1341—6.

[55] Krochak RJ, Baker DG. Radiation nephritis. Clinical manifestations and pathophysiologic mechanisms. Urology 1986;27(5):389—93.

[56] Verheij M, Stewart FA, Oussoren Y, Weening JJ, Dewit L. Amelioration of radiation nephropathy by acetylsalicylic acid. Int J Radiat Biol 1995;67(5):587—96.

[57] Cohen EP, Irving AA, Drobyski WR, Klein JP, Passweg J, Talano JA, et al. Captopril to mitigate chronic renal failure after hematopoietic stem cell transplantation: a randomized controlled trial. Int J Radiat Oncol Biol Phys 2008;70(5):1546—51.

[58] Cohen EP, Fish BL, Sharma M, Li XA, Moulder JE. Role of the angiotensin II type-2 receptor in radiation nephropathy. Transl Res 2007;150(2):106—15.

[59] Cohen EP, Hussain S, Moulder JE. Successful treatment of radiation nephropathy with angiotensin II blockade. Int J Radiat Oncol Biol Phys 2003;55(1): 190—3.

[60] Moulder JE, Cohen EP, Fish BL. Captopril and losartan for mitigation of renal injury caused by single-dose total-body irradiation. Radiat Res 2011;175(1): 29—36.

[61] Moulder JE, Fish BL, Cohen EP. Treatment of radiation nephropathy with ACE inhibitors. Int J Radiat Oncol Biol Phys 1993;27(1):93—9.

[62] Moulder JE, Fish BL, Cohen EP. Noncontinuous use of angiotensin converting enzyme inhibitors in the treatment of experimental bone marrow transplant nephropathy. Bone Marrow Transplant 1997;19(7): 729—35.

[63] Moulder JE, Fish BL, Cohen EP. Treatment of radiation nephropathy with ACE inhibitors and AII type-1 and type-2 receptor antagonists. Curr Pharm Des 2007;13(13):1317—25.

[64] Cohen EP, Piering WF, Kabler-Babbitt C, Moulder JE. End-stage renal disease (ESRD) after bone marrow transplantation: poor survival compared to other causes of ESRD. Nephron 1998;79(4):408—12.

Molecular-targeted Therapy for Renal Cell Carcinoma

Robert J. Amato[1], Mika Stepankiw[2], Nwabugwu S. Ochuwa[3]

[1]University of Texas Health Science Center at Houston (Medical School), University of Texas Memorial Hermann Cancer Center, Houston, TX, USA

[2]University of Texas Health Science Center at Houston, Houston, TX, USA

[3]University of Texas Memorial Hermann Cancer Center, Houston, TX, USA

INTRODUCTION

The incidence of kidney cancer is highest in Europe, North American and Australia and lowest in India, Japan, Africa and China. Renal cell carcinoma (RCC) accounts for approximately 5% (40,250) of all new cancer cases in men and approximately 3% (24,520) of all new cancer cases for women in 2012 in the United States [1]. It is the 10th most common cancer in Europe [2]. Well-established risk factors for RCC include cigarette smoking, excess body weight and hypertension [3]. Patients who smoke have an increased risk of developing RCC in comparison to patients who do not smoke by 50% in men and 20% in women [4]. Worldwide prospective studies found that patients who were overweight or obese at baseline had an increased risk for RCC by 24% in men and 34% in women for every $5\,kg/m^2$ increase in BMI [5–9]. Long-term hypertension

can lead to conditions that may predispose patients to the development of RCC, including chronic kidney disease, worsening renal function and enhancing progression to end stage renal disease [3,10,11]. Additional suspected risk factors include diabetes mellitus, end stage renal disease, parity in women, trichloroethylene exposure and genetic predisposition. There is also a suspected inverse association between RCC and alcohol consumption or regular exercise.

Diagnostic testing to determine if a renal cell tumor is present includes complete blood and urine laboratory tests, cross-sectional CT scans of the abdomen, an MRI, an ultrasound and an intravenous pyelogram. After a patient receives a differential diagnosis, staging is done to determine if the cancer has spread within the kidney or to other parts of the body. In stage I, the tumor is 7 centimeters or smaller and contained within the kidney. In stage II, the tumor is larger than 7 centimeters and contained within the kidney.

In stage III, the tumor is any size, and (1) cancer is found only in the kidney and in one or more of the nearby lymph nodes and/or (2) the cancer is found in the main blood vessels of the kidney or in the fatty tissue around the kidney. In stage IV, the cancer has spread beyond the fatty tissue around the kidney and may be found in (1) the adrenal gland above the kidney with cancer or in nearby lymph nodes or (2) to other organs such as the lungs, liver, bones, or brain and may also be in the nearby lymph nodes.

Although RCC is treated by curative nephrectomy in early stage diseases, 20–30% of patients will ultimately develop metastatic lesions [12]. By the time patients develop locally metastatic RCC lesions, distant metastases to lungs, bone, or other sites may already be present in as many as 50% of patients. Prognosis is poor for patients who have metastatic disease, and the median overall survival (OS) is 7 to 11 months.

There are two types of clinical presentation. For patients who present with a mass confined to the kidney and no metastatic disease, laparoscopic or open partial or total nephrectomy is an option. In patients with concordant presentation (kidney mass plus metastatic disease) and who have a good or intermediate prognosis according to the Memorial Sloan Kettering Cancer Center prognostic criteria, the treatment option is nephrectomy followed by systemic therapy; for those patients with poor prognosis, the treatment option is systemic therapy without nephrectomy. Primary therapies include sunitinib, pazopanib, interferon-α, axitinib and temsirolimus, which will be outlined in this chapter.

Histology

The majority of cases are clear cell RCC (cRCC), which are characterized by the dysfunction of the von Hippel–Lindau (VHL) gene and a hypoxic response resulting from the upregulation of hypoxia inducible factor-1 (HIF-1) and -2 (HIF-2) (Figure 8.1) [13]. Von Hippel–Lindau mutation, deletion, or loss of expression leads to the

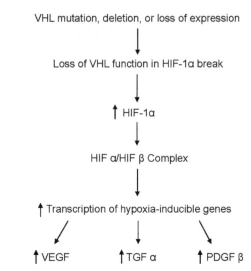

FIGURE 8.1 VHL tumor suppressor gene in clear cell renal cell cancer. VHL = Von Hippel–Lindau tumor suppressor; HIF = hypoxia-inducible factors; HIF-1α = hypoxia-inducible factor 1 alpha; HIF α = hypoxia-inducible factor alpha; HIF β = hypoxia-inducible factor beta; VEGF = vascular endothelial growth factor; TGF α = transforming growth factor alpha; PDGF β = platelet-derived growth factor beta.

upregulation of HIF-1α, which results in the transcription of hypoxia-inducible genes. This results in increased vascular endothelial growth factor (VEGF), increased platelet-derived growth factor-β (PDGF-β) and increased transforming growth factor (TGF).

The mammalian target of rapamycin (mTOR) pathway also aids in the pathogenesis of cancer. It regulates key proteins, including cell cycle regulators, pro-angiogenic factors and amino acid and glucose transports (Figure 8.2). Activation of mTOR is linked to increased protein synthesis by modulating elements that are important in a number of cellular processes, including growth, proliferation, angiogenesis, nutrient uptake and metabolism. At the translational level, mTOR stimulates and regulates the synthesis of several proteins through its phosphorylation of S6K1 and 4E-BP1. Additionally, mTOR activation stimulates cell growth through

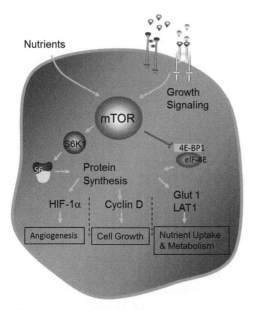

Nutrients

Growth Signaling

mTOR

S6K1

S6

4E-BP1
eIF-4E

Protein Synthesis

HIF-1α | Cyclin D | Glut 1
LAT1

Angiogenesis | Cell Growth | Nutrient Uptake & Metabolism

FIGURE 8.2 mTOR activation supports cancer cell growth. mTOR = mammalian target of rapamycin; S6K1 = ribosomal protein S6 kinase beta-1; 4E-BP1 = eukaryotic translation initiation factor 4E-binding protein 1; eIF-4E = eukaryotic initiation factor 4E; HIF-1α = hypoxia-inducible factor 1 alpha; Glut 1 = glucose transporter 1; LAT1 = large neutral amino acid transporter. This figure is reproduced in color in the color plate section.

cyclin D1, an important component of a cell cycle checkpoint for DNA replication, increases the production of the HIF-1α protein and stimulates increased expression of glucose and amino acid transporters. Increased transporter expression allows the cell to take up additional metabolic fuel and extracellular nutrients; the net result is uncontrolled cell growth.

Treatment

For initial treatment of stage I tumors, surgical resection is the accepted therapy. This may be simple or radical, and the latter may include the removal of the kidney, adrenal gland, perirenal fat and/or Gerota fascia with or without a regional lymph node dissection. For patients who are not candidates for surgery, external-beam radiation therapy (EBRT) or arterial embolization can result in palliation of symptoms. Patients who have bilateral stage I neoplasms (concurrent or subsequent) are often treated with bilateral nephrectomy with dialysis or transplantation. However, when feasible, a bilateral partial nephrectomy or unilateral partial nephrectomy with contralateral radical nephrectomy may be preferred [14].

For the treatment of localized disease or stage II tumors, radical resection is the standard of care. This includes the removal of the kidney, adrenal gland, perirenal fat and Gerota fascia with or without a regional lymph node dissection. A lymphadenectomy may also be considered, but its effectiveness has not yet been definitively proven. Although there is not conclusive evidence that an EBRT given before or after a nephrectomy will improve survival in comparison to nephrectomy alone, it may be of benefit in selected patients who have more extensive tumors for palliation of symptoms. Patients who are not candidates for surgery may receive an arterial embolization for palliation of symptoms.

For patients who have RCC with nodal spread (stage III), surgery is curable in a small minority of cases. The standard of care includes a radical nephrectomy and lymph node dissection. An arterial embolization may be employed preoperatively to reduce blood loss for patients receiving a nephrectomy or who are not candidates for surgery and are seeking palliation of symptoms.

Patients who have progressing, recurring, or relapsing disease have a poor prognosis. Patients with stage IV RCC are incurable. Limited treatment options are available for patients who develop metastatic RCC. Adjuvant therapy has not proved effective, cytotoxic chemotherapy and radiotherapy are generally ineffective, and immunotherapy with the cytokines interleukin-2 or interferon-alpha (IFN-α) produces objective responses in only 10–15% of patients (Table 8.1).

TABLE 8.1 Response Rate for Chemotherapy and Cytokine Treatment

	Drug	Response rate
Cytokines	Interleukin-2 (high dose) [68,69]	≤20% response rate
	Interleukin-2 (low dose) [68]	15% response rate
	Interferon-α [70]	15% response rate
Chemotherapy	Floxuridine [71]	10% response rate
	Gemcitabine + fluorouracil [72]	17% response rate PFS 6.6 months
	Gemcitabine + capecitabine [73]	8.4% response rate PFS 4.6 months OS 17.9 months
	Vinblastine [74]	4% response rate
	5-Fluoro 2′-deoxyuridine + interferon-α	19% response rate

When cytokines are administered alongside chemotherapy, response rates are only slightly higher, and survival does not appear to be prolonged. Additionally, the large cytokine doses often result in severe systemic toxicity. Thus, there is a need for treatments that have increased clinical benefit with minimal adverse events for patients with RCC.

Recent translational research has led to new therapies that target important signaling molecules critical in the pathogenesis of RCC (Figure 8.3). These therapies work by focusing on molecular or cellular changes that are specific to RCC and thus have the potential to be more effective than immunotherapy treatments while causing less adverse events to the patient. Currently, there are three main types of molecular-targeted therapies used to treat RCC: small molecule tyrosine kinase inhibitors (TKI), mammalian target of rapamycin (mTOR) inhibitors and monoclonal antibodies including vascular endothelial growth factor-A (VEGF-A). This review will examine these drugs that target

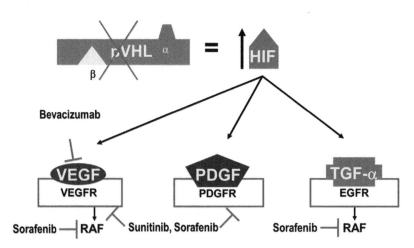

FIGURE 8.3 Targets of therapeutic agents − IFN alpha? pVHL = Von Hippel−Lindau tumor suppressor; HIF = hypoxia-inducible factors; VEGF = vascular endothelial growth factor; VEGFR = vascular endothelial growth factor receptor; PDGF = platelet-derived growth factor; PDGFR = platelet-derived growth factor receptor; TGF-α = transforming growth factor alpha; EGFR = epidermal growth factor receptor; RAF = a serine/threonine-specific protein kinase. This figure is reproduced in color in the color plate section.

TKI, mTOR and VEGF-A pathways and discuss the associated adverse events (Table 8.2).

MECHANISMS OF ACTION

Tyrosine Kinase Inhibitors

Tyrosine kinases are enzymes responsible for the activation of signal transduction cascades through a phosphate group from adenosine triphosphate to a protein in the cell. These kinases act as an "on" and "off" switch for many cellular functions. Tyrosine kinases include enzymes such as vascular endothelial growth factor receptor (VEGFR), platelet-derived growth factor receptor (PDGFR), epidermal growth factor receptor (EGFR), stem cell factor receptor and colony-stimulating factor-1 receptor.

Renal cell cancer is a highly vascularized tumor, which is associated with high expression of VEGF. VEGF is a signal protein produced by cells that stimulate angiogenesis and vascularization of tumors. It is also a key mediator of angiogenesis and is currently the only known angiogenic factor present through the entire tumor life cycle [15]. VEGF is involved in both vasculogenesis (the formation of the circulatory system) and angiogenesis (the growth of blood vessels from pre-existing vasculature), and enhances microvascular permeability. It binds to VEGFR-1, VEGFR-2 and VEGFR-3. The binding of VEGF to its main receptor, VEGFR-2, results in a number of biological effects, which include vasculogenesis, angiogenesis and apoptosis [16].

Activation of EGFR can lead to tumor growth through uncontrolled cell division as well as the inhibition of apoptosis, stimulation of angiogenesis and metastasis [17–19]. EGFR is often overexpressed in tumors [18] and it is expressed in 50–90% of RCC tumors [20]. PDGFR regulates cell proliferation, cellular differentiation, and cell growth [21]. Tyrosine kinase inhibitors work by reducing enzyme activity through the inhibition of the molecules that bind to tyrosine kinases.

Mammalian Target of Rapamycin

The mTOR molecule is a protein kinase that acts as a biological switch that senses nutrients in the microenvironment available for cell growth (Figure 8.3). mTOR responds to external signals such as cytokines, hormones and growth factors as well as to cellular stresses such as hypoxia, pH or osmotic alterations, heat shock, oxidative stress and DNA damage. mTOR is found in the growth factor-activated PI3k, protein kinase B (Akt) signaling pathway, which is downstream of Akt, and it causes abnormal activation of Akt caused by genetic alterations that increase the function of the catalytic (p110) of PI3k [22] or reduce the function of PTEN tumor suppressor protein [23]. A second pathway through which mTOR is activated involves the cAMP-dependent protein kinase (AMP kinase) and the tuberous sclerosis complex 1 and 2 proteins, which results in the suppression of mTOR kinase through nutrient and energy depletion.

Two distinct TOR complexes have been identified — TORC1 and TORC2 — which phosphorylate and activate Akt [24,25]. TORC1 controls the translation of cyclin D, c-Myc and other key proteins involved in cell proliferation as well as regulating the expression and stability of HIF-1α (Table 8.2) [26–28]. TORC2 regulates cell morphology and adhesion; it also phosphorylates and activates the Akt oncogene, which stimulates angiogenesis and tumorigenesis [21,29]. The mTOR pathway has been found to affect prognosis of patients with localized and metastatic RCC [30]. Activation of the mTOR pathway occurs most significantly in cRCC, high-grade tumors and tumors with poor prognosis features. Laboratory analysis indicates that PI3k/Akt activation may be a key predictor of sensitivity to mTOR inhibitor therapy [23].

TABLE 8.2 Targeted Therapy for Renal Cell Carcinoma

	Drug (year approved in US)	Dose	Mechanism of action effect	Approved indication in the USA	Response rate	Notable side-effects
Tyrosine kinase	Sorafenib (2005)	400 mg BID	Decreases vasculogenesis and angiogenesis	Advanced RCC	PFS, 5.5 months	Skin rash, hand–foot syndrome, diarrhea
	Sunitinib (2006)	50 mg QD	Decreases the effect of VEGF, PDGFR-beta, C-kit, FLT3	Advanced RCC	PFS, 10.9 months	GI (major), bleeding, hypertension
	Pazopanib (2009)	800 mg QD	Targets VEGFR1,2, and 3, PDGFR-alpha/beta, c-kit	Advanced RCC	OR, 30% PFS, 9.2 months	Diarrhea, hypertension, hair color changes, elevated liver enzymes
	Axitinib (2012)	5 mg BID	Targets VEGFR1,2, and 3, PDGFR, c-kit	Advanced RCC following failure of one prior systemic therapy	PFS, 6.7 months	Diarrhea, hypertension, fatigue
mTOR	Temsirolimus (2007)	25 mg QWK	Decreases proliferation, angiogenesis, survival and growth of tumor cells	Advanced RCC	OS, 10.9 months PFS, 5.5 months	Rash, asthenia, mucositis
	Everolimus (2009)	10 mg QD	Inhibits mTORC1 negative feedback loop	Advanced RCC after failure of treatment with sunitinib or sorafenib	PFS, 4.9 months OR, 2%	Stomatitis, infection, asthma, pneumonitis
VEGF	Bevacizumab (2009)	10 mg/kg QOD	Decrease vasculogenesis and angiogenesis	Metastatic RCC	PFS, 10.2 months	Bleeding, hypertension, proteinuria; arterial and venous thrombosis

Vascular Endothelial Growth Factor-A

Renal cell carcinomas have high levels of VEGF-A expression [31]. VEGF-A is a protein of the PDGF and VEGF family. It is a glycosylated mitogen that specifically targets endothelial cells to mediate increased vascular permeability; induce angiogenesis, vasculogenesis and endothelial cell growth; promote cell migration; and inhibit apoptosis [32,33]. The tyrosine kinase receptors Flt-1 (fms-like tyrosine kinase)/VEGFR-1 and KDR (kinase insert domain-containing receptor)/VEGFR-2, which are expressed on vascular endothelium, activate VEGF-A [34].

MOLECULAR-TARGETED DRUGS

Tyrosine Kinase Inhibitors

Sorafenib (Nexavar)

Sorafenib is a dual-action Raf kinase and VEGF inhibitor that arrests tumor cell proliferation and angiogenesis. Although originally developed as a Raf kinase inhibitor, subsequent studies have shown this compound to inhibit a variety of tyrosine kinases involved in tumor progression, including VEGFR, EGFR and PDGFR kinases [35,36].

Sorafenib was approved for treating RCC based on a multicenter, international, randomized double-blind, placebo-controlled phase III study of 903 patients with advanced RCC who received one prior systemic therapy [37]. Patients received sorafenib 400 mg BID or a placebo. Median PFS (progression-free survival) was 5.5 months for the sorafenib arm vs. 2.8 months for the placebo arm. Objective response consisting of a partial response was reported in 10% of patients in the sorafenib arm and 2% of patients in the placebo arm.

Common grade 1 and 2 treatment-related adverse events included reversible skin rash (40%), hand−foot skin reaction (30%), diarrhea (43%), hypertension (17%), sensory neuropathic changes (13%), asymptomatic hypophosphatemia (45%) and elevated serum lipase (41%). Grade 3 and 4 adverse events were minimal and consisted of hand−foot skin reaction (5%) and grade 4 pancreatitis (<1%).

Sunitinib (Sutent)

Sunitinib is a broad-spectrum, orally available multi-targeted receptor tyrosine kinase inhibitor that has anti-proliferative effects and anti-angiogenic properties that target VEGFR, PDGFR-β, c-KIT and FLT-3 activity [38,39]. Preclinical xenograft models demonstrated sunitinib to produce potent anti-tumor activity that caused regression, growth arrest, or reduced growth of various established xenografts derived from human or rat tumor cell lines [40−42].

Sunitinib was approved for RCC following a multicenter, international, randomized phase III study of 750 patients with metastatic clear cell RCC who had no previous treatment [43]. Patients received a repeated 6-week cycle of 50 mg sunitinib for 4 weeks followed by 2 weeks without treatment or three times weekly 9 MU IFN-α. Patients in the sunibitinb arm received a starting dose of 50 mg daily for 4 weeks followed by 2 weeks off treatment. IFN-α was given 3 nonconsecutive days a week at a dose of 3 μU for the first week, 6 μU for the second week and 9 μU thereafter. Median PFS was 47.3 weeks for the sunitinib arm and 22.0 weeks for the IFN-α arm. Objective response rate in the sunitinib arm was 27.5% vs. 5.3% in the IFN-α arm.

Treatment-related adverse events included gastrointestinal events (diarrhea, nausea, mucositis, vomiting, dyspepsia, abdominal pain, gastroesophageal reflux, oral pain, glossodynia and flatulence); bleeding; hypertension; dermatologic events (rash, skin discoloration, dry skin and hair color changes); hand−foot syndrome; limb pain; decreases in cardiac ejection fraction; hypothyroidism; and peripheral edema. Grade 3/4 adverse events included hypertension, diarrhea, hand—foot syndrome, nausea, vomiting, mucositis, bleeding, hematologic abnormalities (neutropenia, thrombocytopenia and leucopenia), increased lipase, increased amylase, hyponatremia, hyperuricemia and hyperbilirubinemia.

Pazopanib (Votrient)

Pazopanib is a multi-targeted TKI of VEGFR-1, VEGFR-2, VEGFR-3, PDGFR-a/β and cKit, which blocks tumor growth and inhibits angiogenesis [44]. Pazopanib was approved following a multicenter, international, randomized, double-blind phase III study of 435 patients with metastatic RCC who were previously untreated or had received no prior cytokine therapy [45]. Patients either received pazopanib 800 mg QD or a placebo. Median PFS for the pazopanib arm ($n = 290$) was 9.2 months vs. 4.2 months in the placebo arm ($n = 145$). The objective response rate was 30% for patients in the pazopanib arm and 3% for patients in the placebo arm, and the median duration of response was 13.5 months.

Adverse events that occurred at a greater than 20% rate included diarrhea, hypertension, hair color changes, nausea, anorexia and vomiting. Common laboratory abnormalities that occurred at a greater than 10% rate in the pazopanib arm included increased transaminases (liver enzymes), hyperglycemia, leukopenia, hyperbilirubinemia, neutropenia, hypophosphatemia, thrombocytopenia, lymphocytopenia, hyponatremia (low level of sodium in the blood), hypomagnesemia (low level of magnesium in the blood) and hypoglycemia. Grade 3 and 4 severe adverse events included abnormal hepatic function, diarrhea, hypertension and proteinuria.

Axitinib (Inlyta)

Axitinib is a small molecule TKI that inhibits VEGFR-1, VEGFR-2, VEGFR-3, PDGFR and cKIT. It has been approved for the treatment of advanced RCC after failure of one prior systemic therapy.

Axitinib received FDA approval following an international, multicenter, randomized open-label, phase III study of 723 patients with advanced RCC who failed one prior systemic therapy consisting of sunitinib, temsirolimus, bevacizumab, or cytokine(s) [46]. Patients in the axitinib treatment arm ($n = 361$) received 5 mg BID orally, and patients in the sorafenib treatment arm ($n = 362$) received 400 mg BID. Patients in the axitinib treatment arm had a median PFS of 6.7 months compared to 4.7 months for patients in the sorafenib treatment arm. Patients in the axitinib treatment arm who were previously treated with cytokines had a greater PFS in comparison to patients who were previously treated with sunitinib. Common axitinib-related adverse events included diarrhea, hypertension and fatigue.

Mammalian Target of Rapamycin

Temsirolimus (CCI-779)

Temsirolimus works by inhibiting mTOR and interfering with the synthesis of the proteins that regulate proliferation, tumor angiogenesis, growth and survival of tumor cells. Temsirolimus results in cell cycle arrest and reduces the synthesis of VEGF [47].

Temsirolimus was approved by the FDA in 2007 based on results of a multicenter, international, randomized, open-label, phase III study of 626 previously untreated patients with advanced RCC [48]. Patients were assigned to one of three arms: IFN-α ($n = 207$) 3 MIU alone three times weekly, temsirolimus ($n = 209$) 25 mg alone weekly, or the combination of 15 mg temsirolimus weekly plus 6 MIU IFN-α weekly ($n = 210$). Patients receiving temsirolimus had intravenous infusion over 30—60 minutes once a week until either disease progression or unacceptable toxicity. The temsirolimus alone arm had an OS (overall survival) of 10.9 months and a PFS of 5.5 months vs. an OS of 7.3 months and a PFS of 3.1 months in the IFN-α alone arm. The combination of temsirolimus and IFN-α did not reveal any statistically significant clinical benefit over temsirolimus alone, and it was associated with an increase in adverse events.

Adverse events that occurred at a greater than 30% rate included rash, asthenia, mucositis, nausea, edema and anorexia. Grade 3 and 4 severe adverse events included asthenia, dyspnea, rash and pain. Common laboratory abnormalities that occurred at a greater than 30% rate included anemia, hyperglycemia, hyperlipidemia, hypertriglyceridemia, elevated serum alkaline phosphatase, elevated serum creatinine, lymphopenia, hypophosphatemia, thrombocytopenia, elevated serum aspartate transaminase and leukopenia. Grade 3 and 4 severe laboratory abnormalities included hypertriglyceridemia, anemia, hypophosphatemia, hyperglycemia, lymphopenia and neutropenia. Temsirolimus has been associated with lung toxicity, particularly in patients who had abnormal pre-treatment pulmonary functions or with a history of pulmonary disease [49].

Everolimus (Afinitor)

Everolimus targets the mTORC1 protein and not the mTORC2 protein, which can lead to the hyperactivation of the kinase AKT by inhibiting the mTORC1 negative feedback loop and not the mTORC2 positive feedback loop to AKT.

Everolimus was approved following a multicenter, international, randomized, double-blind phase III study of 416 metastatic RCC patients who failed treatment with sunitinib or sorafenib [50]. Patients were treated with everolimus 10 mg daily or a placebo. Median PFS was 4.9 months for patients who received everolimus ($n = 277$) and 1.9 months for patients who received the placebo ($n = 139$). The objective response rate was 2% for the everolimus arm and 0% for the placebo arm.

Common adverse events experienced by ≥30% included stomatitis, infections, asthenia, fatigue, cough and diarrhea. Grade 3 and 4 events included infections, dyspnea, fatigue, stomatitis, dehydration, pneumonitis, abdominal pain and asthenia. Common abnormal laboratories included anemia, hypercholesterolemia, hypertriglyceridemia, hyperglycemia, lymphopenia and elevated creatinine. Grade 3 and 4 severe laboratory abnormalities included phopenia, hyperglycemia, anemia, hypophosphatemia and hypercholesterolemia. Deaths experienced only on the everolimus arm included respiratory failure (0.7%), infection (0.7%) and acute renal failure (0.4%).

Vascular Endothelial Growth Factor-A

Bevacizumab (Avastin)

Bevacizumab is a recombinant humanized monoclonal antibody that selectively binds to all isoforms of VEGF and neutralizes VEGF by blocking it from binding to its receptors on the surface of endothelial cells. This inhibits tumor angiogenesis thereby inhibiting tumor growth and metastasis.

Bevacizumab was approved following a multicenter, international, randomized, double-blind, placebo-controlled, phase III study involving 649 patients with metastatic RCC who had undergone nephrectomy [51]. Patients received IFN-α 9 MIU subcutaneously three times a week and bevacizumab 10 mg/kg every 2 weeks or IFN-α plus placebo. The median PFS was 10.2 months for patients who received bevacizumab plus IFN-α ($n = 327$) vs. 5.4 months for patients who received IFN-α plus a placebo ($n = 322$). This trial did not demonstrate a statistically significant advantage for OS for patients treated with bevacizumab plus IFN-α vs. patients who received IFN-α plus placebo. This study received additional support from a second randomized, open-label study of bevacizumab plus IFN-α compared with IFN-α alone in patients with metastatic RCC. Median PFS in this study for patients treated with the bevacizumab combination was 8.4 months vs. 4.9 months for patients who received IFN-α. No improvement in OS was observed.

Patients who received the combination bevacizumab plus IFN-α treatment arm had a higher overall incidence of toxicities as well as more severe toxicities in comparison to the IFN-α alone treatment arm. Thirty-one percent of patients treated with the combination reported serious adverse events vs. 19% in the IFN-α alone treatment arm. Grade 3 and 4 adverse events were reported in 63% of patients treated with the combination in comparison to 47% treated with IFN-α alone. The most common grade 3 and 4 bevacizumab-related adverse events included bleeding, hypertension, proteinuria and venous or arterial thrombosis. Twenty percent of patients developed proteinuria after a median onset of 5.6 months, and bevacizumab was permanently discontinued in 30% of those patients. Because bevacizumab inhibits the growth of blood vessels, there is concern that it may interfere with the production of new blood vessels needed in wound healing or inhibit the circulation around blocked or atherosclerotic blood vessels, which may worsen heart conditions such as coronary artery disease or peripheral artery disease [48,49,51,52].

SUMMARY

The maximum dosage of molecular-targeted therapies is based on the inhibition of biologic targets in the tumor and surrogate tissues as they relate to safety assessments. Dosages are developed in phase I and phase II studies to find the maximum tolerable dose. In phase III trials, survival benefit is defined in randomized trials [28]. Most adverse events of molecular-targeted therapies for RCC are reversible and may be managed through dose adjustments or interruptions to maintain optimal dosing.

Nausea and Vomiting

Nausea and vomiting can be managed as outlined by anti-emetic guidelines.

Diarrhea

Diarrhea may be initially managed with loperamide, but it may require diphenoxylate hydrochloride/atropine sulfate if the initial treatment does not yield a response.

Hypertension

Hypertension associated to VEGF/VEGFR inhibitors is dose dependent, but the mechanism is unknown [53—55]. Blood pressure increases may be seen within the first day of treatment, but it is most commonly seen within 3—4 weeks of TKI initiation [56—58]. Anti-hypertensive therapy is recommended if a patient develops stage I hypertension ($\geq$140/90 mm Hg) or have increases in blood pressure $\geq$20 mm Hg from baseline [59]. Currently, there are no recommendations for the use of anti-hypertensive medications with VEGF/VEGFR inhibitor-associated hypertension. In choosing an agent, the patient's co-morbid conditions should be considered [60]. Anti-hypertensive agents commonly utilized to manage TKI-induced hypertension include angiotensin-converting enzymes (ACE), calcium channel blockers and beta blockers. Dose optimization or the addition of a second anti-hypertensive agent may be required. If blood pressure cannot be controlled with a combination of hypertension agents, dose modification or ultimately discontinuation may be required.

Hypothyroidism

Antiangiogenic agents such as sunitinib and sorafenib are commonly reported to cause a disruption in thyroid homeostatasis [61—63]. However, the mechanism is unknown. It has been postulated that VEGFR inhibition may directly induce thyroiditis and hypothyroidism [64]. VEGFR inhibition may also result in capillary regression around the thyroid follicles. Management of TKI-induced hypothyroidism should follow standard guidelines [65].

Cutaneous Reactions

Antiangiogenic agents commonly cause rash, hand–foot syndrome and mucositis/stomatitis. Hand–foot syndrome is characterized by palmoplantar lesions that arise in areas of friction or trauma (hands and feet) and may significantly affect activities of daily living and, ultimately, quality of life [37]. The mechanism that leads to dermal toxicity is unknown. However, in a sunitinib study, direct anti-VEGFR and/or PDGF receptor effects on dermal endothelial cells may have led to skin toxicity that was characterized by dermal vascular modifications, scattered keratinocyte necrosis and intraepidermal cleavage [66]. Petroleum jelly-based products such as Vaseline and Aquaphor provide moisture, so should be applied liberally to affected areas [67]. During treatment, patients should also utilize shock-absorbing shoe inserts to relieve painful pressure points. In addition, wicking socks that absorb moisture from the plantar surface have also been found to be helpful. In severe cases, treatment may be dose reduced or discontinued.

Hyperglycemia and Hyperlipidemia

Hyperglycemia and hyperlipidemia management should follow standard guidelines.

Therapies that target molecular pathways hold promise in the treatment of RCC. Managing adverse effects while still maintaining optimal dosage level will provide the opportunity for clinical benefit. Further development may include sequential therapy and/or the combination of strategies.

References

[1] Siegel R, Naishadham D, Jemal A. Cancer statistics, 2012. CA Cancer J Clin 2012;62(1):10–29.

[2] Ferlay J, Shin HR, Bray F, Forman D, Mathers C, Parkin DM. Estimates of worldwide burden of cancer in 2008: GLOBOCAN 2008. Int J Cancer 2010;127(12): 2893–917.

[3] Chow WH, Dong LM, Devesa SS. Epidemiology and risk factors for kidney cancer. Nat Rev Urol 2010;7(5):245–57.

[4] Hunt JD, van der Hel OL, McMillan GP, Boffetta P, Brennan P. Renal cell carcinoma in relation to cigarette smoking: meta-analysis of 24 studies. Int J Cancer 2005;114(1):101–8.

[5] Oh SW, Yoon YS, Shin SA. Effects of excess weight on cancer incidences depending on cancer sites and histologic findings among men: Korea National Health Insurance Corporation Study. J Clin Oncol 2005;23(21):4742–54.

[6] Pischon T, Lahmann PH, Boeing H, et al. Body size and risk of renal cell carcinoma in the European Prospective Investigation into Cancer and Nutrition (EPIC). Int J Cancer 2006;118(3):728–38.

[7] Reeves GK, Pirie K, Beral V, et al. Cancer incidence and mortality in relation to body mass index in the Million Women Study: cohort study. BMJ 2007; 335(7630):1134.

[8] Adams KF, Leitzmann MF, Albanes D, et al. Body size and renal cell cancer incidence in a large US cohort study. Am J Epidemiol 2008;168(3):268–77.

[9] Renehan AG, Tyson M, Egger M, Heller RF, Zwahlen M. Body-mass index and incidence of cancer: a systematic review and meta-analysis of prospective observational studies. Lancet 2008;371(9612): 569–78.

[10] Chow WH, Gridley G, Fraumeni Jr JF, Jarvholm B. Obesity, hypertension, and the risk of kidney cancer in men. N Engl J Med 2000;343(18):1305–11.

[11] Choi MY, Jee SH, Sull JW, Nam CM. The effect of hypertension on the risk for kidney cancer in Korean men. Kidney Int 2005;67(2):647–52.

[12] Godley PA, Taylor M. Renal cell carcinoma. Curr Opin Oncol 2001;13(3):199–203.

[13] Kaelin Jr WG. The von Hippel–Lindau protein, HIF hydroxylation, and oxygen sensing. Biochem Biophys Res Commun 2005;338(1):627–38.

[14] Novick AC, Streem S, Montie JE, et al. Conservative surgery for renal cell carcinoma: a single-center experience with 100 patients. J Urol 1989;141(4):835–9.

[15] Folkman J. Antiangiogenesis agents. Philadelphia: Lippincott Williams and Wilkins; 2005.

[16] Carmeliet P. VEGF as a key mediator of angiogenesis in cancer. Oncology 2005;69(Suppl. 3):4–10.

[17] Langner C, Ratschek M, Rehak P, Schips L, Zigeuner R. Are heterogenous results of EGFR immunoreactivity in renal cell carcinoma related to non-standardised criteria for staining evaluation? J Clin Pathol 2004;57(7):773–5.

[18] Mendelsohn J, Baselga J. Status of epidermal growth factor receptor antagonists in the biology and treatment of cancer. J Clin Oncol 2003;21(14):2787–99.

[19] Price JT, Wilson HM, Haites NE. Epidermal growth factor (EGF) increases the in vitro invasion, motility and adhesion interactions of the primary renal carcinoma cell line, A704. Eur J Cancer 1996;32A(11): 1977–82.

[20] Harari PM. Epidermal growth factor receptor inhibitor strategies in oncology. Endocr Relat Cancer 2004;11:689–708.

[21] Williams LT. Signal transduction by the platelet-derived growth factor receptor. Science 1989; 243(4898):1564–70.

[22] Kang S, Bader AG, Vogt PK. Phosphatidylinositol 3-kinase mutations identified in human cancer are oncogenic. Proc Natl Acad Sci U S A 2005;102(3):802–7.

[23] Neshat MS, Mellinghoff IK, Tran C, et al. Enhanced sensitivity of PTEN-deficient tumors to inhibition of FRAP/mTOR. Proc Natl Acad Sci U S A 2001;98(18): 10314–9.

[24] Inoki K, Guan KL. Complexity of the TOR signaling network. Trends Cell Biol 2006;16(4):206–12.

[25] Sarbassov DD, Guertin DA, Ali SM, Sabatini DM. Phosphorylation and regulation of Akt/PKB by the rictor-mTOR complex. Science 2005;307(5712):1098–101.

[26] Fingar DC, Richardson CJ, Tee AR, Cheatham L, Tsou C, Blenis J. mTOR controls cell cycle progression through its cell growth effectors S6K1and 4EBP1/eukaryotic translation factor 4E. Mol Cell Biol 2004;24(1):200–16.

[27] Hudson CC, Liu M, Chiang GG, et al. Regulation of hypoxia-inducible factor 1a expression and function by the mammalian target of rapamycin. Mol Cell Biol 2002;22:7004–14.

[28] Thomas GV, Tran C, Mellinghoff IK, et al. Hypoxia-inducible factor determines sensitivity to inhibitors of mTOR in kidney cancer. Nat Med 2006;12(1):122–7.

[29] Corradetti MN, Guan KL. Upstream of the mammalian target of rapamycin: do all roads pass through mTOR? Oncogene 2006;25(48):6347–60.

[30] Pantuck AJ, Seligson DB, Klatte T, et al. Prognostic relevance of the mTOR pathway in renal cell carcinoma: implications for molecular patient selection for targeted therapy. Cancer 2007;109(11):2257–67.

[31] Lonser RR, Glenn GM, Walther M, et al. Von Hippel–Lindau disease. Lancet 2003;361:2059–67.

[32] Ferrara N. Role of vascular endothelial growth factor in physiologic and pathologic angiogenesis: therapeutic implications. Semin Oncol 2002;29(6 Suppl. 16): 10–4.

[33] Cao R, Eriksson A, Kubo H, Alitalo K, Cao Y, Thyberg J. Comparative evaluation of FGF-2-, VEGF-A-, and VEGF-C-induced angiogenesis, lymphangiogenesis, vascular fenestrations, and permeability. Circ Res 2004;94(5):664–70.

[34] George ML, Tutton MG, Janssen F, et al. VEGF-A, VEGF-C, and VEGF-D in colorectal cancer progression. Neoplasia 2001;3(5):420–7.

[35] Wilhelm SM, Carter C, Tang L, et al. BAY 43-9006 exhibits broad spectrum oral antitumor activity and targets the RAF/MEK/ERK pathway and receptor tyrosine kinases involved in tumor progression and angiogenesis. Cancer Res 2004;64(19):7099–109.

[36] Strumberg D, Richly H, Hilger RA, et al. Phase I clinical and pharmacokinetic study of the Novel Raf kinase and vascular endothelial growth factor receptor inhibitor BAY 43-9006 in patients with advanced refractory solid tumors. J Clin Oncol 2005;23(5):965–72.

[37] Escudier B, Eisen T, Stadler WM, et al. Sorafenib in advanced clear-cell renal-cell carcinoma. N Engl J Med 2007;356(2):125–34.

[38] Mendel DB, Laird AD, Xin X, et al. Development of a preclinical pharmacokinetic/pharmacodynamic relationship for the angiogenesis inhibitor SU11248, a selective inhibitor of VEGF and PDGF receptor tyrosine kinases in clinical development. Proc Am Soc Clin Oncol 2002;21:94.

[39] O'Farrell AM, Abrams TJ, Yuen HA, et al. SU11248 is a novel FLT3 tyrosine kinase inhibitor with potent activity in vitro and in vivo. Blood 2003;101:3597–605.

[40] Mendel DB, Laird AD, Xin X, et al. In vivo antitumor activity of SU11248, a novel tyrosine kinase inhibitor targeting vascular endothelial growth factor and platelet-derived growth factor receptors: determination of a pharmacokinetic/pharmacodynamic relationship. Clin Cancer Res 2003;9(1):327–37.

[41] Bergsland EK. Vascular endothelial growth factor as a therapeutic target in cancer. Am J Health Syst Pharm 2004;61:S4–11.

[42] Traxler P, Allegrini PR, Brandt R, et al. AEE788: a dual family epidermal growth factor receptor/ErbB2 and vascular endothelial growth factor receptor tyrosine kinase inhibitor with antitumor and antiangiogenic activity. Cancer Res 2004;64(14):4931–41.

[43] Motzer RJ, Hutson TE, Tomczak P, et al. Sunitinib versus interferon alfa in metastatic renal-cell carcinoma. N Engl J Med 2007;356(2):115–24.

[44] Sonpavde G, Hutson TE. Pazopanib: a novel multitargeted tyrosine kinase inhibitor. Curr Oncol Rep 2007;9(2):115–9.

[45] Sternberg CN, Davis ID, Mardiak J, et al. Pazopanib in locally advanced or metastatic renal cell carcinoma: results of a randomized phase III trial. J Clin Oncol 2010;28(6):1061–8.

[46] Rini BI, Escudier B, Tomczak P, et al. Comparative effectiveness of axitinib versus sorafenib in advanced renal cell carcinoma (AXIS): a randomised phase 3 trial. Lancet 2011;378(9807):1931–9.

[47] Wan X, Shen N, Mendoza A, Khanna C, Helman LJ. CCI-779 inhibits rhabdomyosarcoma xenograft growth by an antiangiogenic mechanism linked to the targeting of mTOR/Hif-1alpha/VEGF signaling. Neoplasia 2006;8(5):394—401.

[48] Hudes G, Carducci M, Tomczak P, et al. Temsirolimus, interferon alfa, or both for advanced renal-cell carcinoma. N Engl J Med 2007;356(22):2271—81.

[49] Duran I, Siu LL, Oza AM, et al. Characterisation of the lung toxicity of the cell cycle inhibitor temsirolimus. Eur J Cancer 2006;42(12):1875—80.

[50] Motzer RJ, Escudier B, Oudard S, et al. Phase 3 trial of everolimus for metastatic renal cell carcinoma: final results and analysis of prognostic factors. Cancer 2010;116(18):4256—65.

[51] Escudier B, Pluzanska A, Koralewski P, et al. Bevacizumab plus interferon alfa-2a for treatment of metastatic renal cell carcinoma: a randomised, double-blind phase III trial. Lancet 2007;370(9605):2103—11.

[52] Semenza GL. A new weapon for attacking tumor blood vessels. N Engl J Med 2008;358(19):2066—7.

[53] Ravaud A, Sire M. Arterial hypertension and clinical benefit of sunitinib, sorafenib and bevacizumab in first and second-line treatment of metastatic renal cell cancer. Ann Oncol 2009;20(5):966—7; author reply 7.

[54] Rini BI, Cohen DP, Lu DR, et al. Hypertension as a biomarker of efficacy in patients with metastatic renal cell carcinoma treated with sunitinib. J Natl Cancer Inst 2011;103(9):763—73.

[55] Rini BI, Schiller JH, Fruehauf JP, et al. Diastolic blood pressure as a biomarker of axitinib efficacy in solid tumors. Clin Cancer Res 2011;17(11):3841—9.

[56] Maitland ML, Kasza KE, Karrison T, et al. Ambulatory monitoring detects sorafenib-induced blood pressure elevations on the first day of treatment. Clin Cancer Res 2009;15(19):6250—7.

[57] Veronese ML, Mosenkis A, Flaherty KT, et al. Mechanisms of hypertension associated with BAY 43-9006. J Clin Oncol 2006;24(9):1363—9.

[58] Chu TF, Rupnick MA, Kerkela R, et al. Cardiotoxicity associated with tyrosine kinase inhibitor sunitinib. Lancet 2007;370(9604):2011—9.

[59] Maitland ML, Bakris GL, Black HR, et al. Initial assessment, surveillance, and management of blood pressure in patients receiving vascular endothelial growth factor signaling pathway inhibitors. J Natl Cancer Inst 2010;102(9):596—604.

[60] Izzedine H, Ederhy S, Goldwasser F, et al. Management of hypertension in angiogenesis inhibitor-treated patients. Ann Oncol 2009;20(5):807—15.

[61] Rini BI, Tamaskar I, Shaheen P, et al. Hypothyroidism in patients with metastatic renal cell carcinoma treated with sunitinib. J Natl Cancer Inst 2007;99(1):81—3.

[62] Tamaskar I, Bukowski R, Elson P, et al. Thyroid function test abnormalities in patients with metastatic renal cell carcinoma treated with sorafenib. Ann Oncol 2008;19(2):265—8.

[63] Miyake H, Kurahashi T, Yamanaka K, et al. Abnormalities of thyroid function in Japanese patients with metastatic renal cell carcinoma treated with sorafenib: a prospective evaluation. Urol Oncol 2010;28(5):515—9.

[64] Faris JE, Moore AF, Daniels GH. Sunitinib (sutent)-induced thyrotoxicosis due to destructive thyroiditis: a case report. Thyroid 2007;17:1147—9.

[65] Hennessey JV, Scherger JE. Evaluating and treating the patient with hypothyroid disease. J Fam Pract 2007;56(8 Suppl Hot Topics):S31—9.

[66] Faivre S, Delbaldo C, Vera K, et al. Safety, pharmacokinetic, and antitumor activity of SU11248, a novel oral multitarget tyrosine kinase inhibitor, in patients with cancer. J Clin Oncol 2006;24(1):25—35.

[67] Robert C, Soria JC, Spatz A, et al. Cutaneous side-effects of kinase inhibitors and blocking antibodies. Lancet Oncol 2005;6(7):491—500.

[68] Yang JC, Topalian SL, Parkinson D, et al. Randomized comparison of high-dose and low-dose intravenous interleukin-2 for the therapy of metastatic renal cell carcinoma: an interim report. J Clin Oncol 1994;12(8):1572—6.

[69] Fyfe G, Fisher RI, Rosenberg SA, Sznol M, Parkinson DR, Louie AC. Results of treatment of 255 patients with metastatic renal cell carcinoma who received high-dose recombinant interleukin-2 therapy. J Clin Oncol 1995;13(3):688—96.

[70] Coppin C, Porzsolt F, Awa A, Kumpf J, Coldman A, Wilt T. Immunotherapy for advanced renal cell cancer. Cochrane Database Syst Rev 2005;1(1): CD001425.

[71] Bjarnason GA, Hrushesky WJ, Diasio R. Flat versus circadian modified 14 day infusion of FUDR for advanced renal cell cancer (RCC): a phase-III study. Proc Am Soc Clin Oncol 1994;1994:233.

[72] Rini BI, Vogelzang NJ, Dumas MC, Wade 3rd JL, Taber DA, Stadler WM. Phase II trial of weekly intravenous gemcitabine with continuous infusion fluorouracil in patients with metastatic renal cell cancer. J Clin Oncol 2000;18(12):2419—26.

[73] Tannir NM, Thall PF, Ng CS, et al. A phase II trial of gemcitabine plus capecitabine for metastatic renal cell cancer previously treated with immunotherapy and targeted agents. J Urol 2008;180(3):867—72; discussion 72.

[74] Fossa SD, Droz JP, Pavone-Macaluso MM, Debruyne FJ, Vermeylen K, Sylvester R. Vinblastine in metastatic renal cell carcinoma: EORTC phase II trial 30882. The EORTC Genitourinary Group. Eur J Cancer 1992;28A(4—5):878—80.

9

Renal Tumors in Children

Kelly L. Vallance[1], Jeffrey S. Dome[2]

[1]Cook Children's Medical Center, Fort Worth, TX, USA [2]Children's National Medical Center, Washington, DC, USA

RENAL TUMORS IN CHILDREN/ ADOLESCENTS

Renal malignancies account for 6% of pediatric cancer diagnoses with 7.7 per million under age 15 and 6.1 per million under age 20. In the USA approximately 500–550 children and adolescents are diagnosed with renal tumors yearly. The majority of these are nephroblastoma (Wilms tumor). Non-Wilms tumors, which account for less than 10% of primary renal neoplasms and less than 1% of all childhood cancers, include renal cell carcinoma (RCC), clear cell sarcoma of the kidney (CCSK), malignant rhabdoid tumor of the kidney (MRTK), cystic nephroma, mesoblastic nephroma and renal medullary carcinoma. Figure 9.1 depicts the latest SEER Incidence rates per million and Figure 9.2 shows the distribution of renal tumors in children aged 0 to 19 years [1].

WILMS TUMOR

Wilms tumor accounts for the majority of renal tumors in children and has an overall durable survival rate exceeding 85%. A multimodal treatment approach is necessary including surgery, chemotherapy and radiation therapy. Wilms tumor has contributed greatly to our biological understanding of cancer and its treatment has evolved through consecutive studies conducted by two collaborative groups: the National Wilms Tumor Study group (NWTSG), now the Children's Oncology Group (COG), in North America and the International Society of Pediatric Oncology (SIOP) in Europe. Although the survival rate has exceeded 80% since the mid-1980s, recent trials have focused on reducing the duration of therapy and exposure to agents associated with late effects, mainly doxorubicin and radiation therapy. Despite a reduction in therapy, the excellent survival rate has been preserved. However, there remain subsets of patients who have a less favorable prognosis, including those with bilateral Wilms tumor and anaplastic Wilms tumor.

Epidemiology

The incidence of Wilms tumor is highest in the first several years of life, peaking at 3–4 years and steadily decreasing with age; it is

Renal Disease in Cancer Patients
http://dx.doi.org/10.1016/B978-0-12-415948-8.00009-X

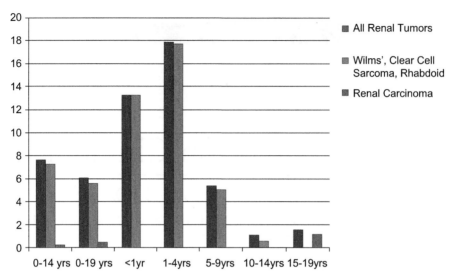

FIGURE 9.1   **SEER cancer incidence rates by international classification of childhood cancer per 1,000,000 from 2004 to 2008.**

rare in adults. The median age at presentation is 44 months in unilateral disease and 31 months in bilateral disease. Wilms tumor presents as bilateral disease in 5–10% of cases and 12% of unilateral cases have evidence of multifocal disease within the kidney [2]. The male to female ratio is 0.92:1.00 in unilateral disease and 0.6:1.00 in bilateral disease. There is a slightly higher incidence in African-Americans compared to Caucasians, with lower incidence in Asians [2]. Most cases are sporadic, but 1–2% of cases are familial [3].

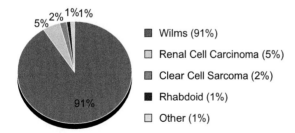

FIGURE 9.2   **Types of renal tumors in children and adolescents.** SEER data 1975–1995.

History

The first description of a childhood renal tumor is attributed to T. Rance in 1814, who described a 17-month-old female with a metastatic kidney tumor. However, John Hunter had collected and prepared specimens of bilateral Wilms tumor associated with cryptorchidism prior to 1793. The first histological description well documented was by Eberth in 1872. In 1894 German pathologist Birch-Hirschfeld published an overview of 47 nephrectomies describing pathological variants of renal cancers in children [4]. Surgeon Carl Max Wihelm Wilms reviewed the literature, presented new cases and concluded that all these tumors arose from the same germ cell. Wilms published a monograph in 1899 on "mixed tumors of the kidney" and became the namesake of this disease [5].

Clinical Presentation

The classic presentation is a painless mass noticed by parents in their toddler. Additional symptoms are listed in Table 9.1 [6,7].

TABLE 9.1 Clinical Presentation of Wilms Tumor

Distention/Palpable mass	80%
Abdominal pain	40%
Hematuria	<25%
Fever	10–30%
Hypertension	25%
Congenital anomaly/syndrome	7–10%

Diagnostic Evaluation/Initial Workup

For a new patient with a suspected abdominal tumor, the history should include a detailed family history of renal masses and genetic syndromes or developmental delay (Table 9.2). Physical exam should note evidence of hemihypertrophy or limb length discrepancy, genitourinary anomalies, aniridia, or other features of Wilms tumor-associated syndromes. There may also be an increased prevalence of congenital heart defects in Wilms patients up to 1.8% [8,9].

Special attention should also be given to blood pressure and possible hypertensive sequelae. Twenty-five percent of children have hypertension at diagnosis due to increased renin production or less commonly due to compression of renal vasculature. If antihypertensive agents are indicated, angiotensin converting enzyme (ACE) inhibitors are usually effective [10]. Occasionally, children may have hypertensive encephalopathy or other complications and need to be stabilized prior to surgery. Hypertension usually resolves after nephrectomy.

Gross hematuria is noted in less than 20% and microscopic hematuria in less than 25% of patients [11]. Clotting abnormalities have been demonstrated in Wilms patients at presentation, including an acquired von Willebrand disease in 1–2%; so, prothrombin time and partial thromboplastin time should be measured if bleeding

TABLE 9.2 Initial Evaluation Specific to Renal Tumors in Children

History	Any trauma or possibility of rupture Family history of congenital anomalies, tumors, syndromes
Physical	Vitals: Close attention to blood pressure Mass characteristics Congenital anomalies especially GU anomalies and aniridia Hemihypertrophy/Limb discrepancies Developmental delay Hepatomegaly
Laboratory evaluations	CBC, chemistry panel, LFTs Urinalysis for gross/microscopic hematuria Coagulation studies/von Willebrand if clinically indicated
Imaging	CT or MRI abdomen and pelvis – evaluate contralateral kidney Chest CT for pulmonary metastasis Ultrasound abdomen + Doppler of IVC/renal veins (assess for thrombus if not definitive on CT/MRI scan) MRI brain in CCSK and rhabdoid tumor Bone scan/Skeletal survey in CCSK and rhabdoid tumor PET-CT no clear role in renal tumors yet
Genetic testing	Chromosome analysis (karyotype) or FISH for WT1 if concern for syndrome, or presence of aniridia, hemihypertrophy, GU malformation

GU, genitourinary; CBC, complete blood count; LFTs, liver function tests; IVC, inferior vena cava; CT, computed tomography; MRI, magnetic resonance imaging; CCSK, clear cell sarcoma of kidney; RCC, renal cell carcinoma; PET, positron emission tomography; FISH, fluorescence in-situ hybridization; WT1, Wilms tumor 1 gene.

occurs or prior to invasive procedures with clinical suspicion [12,13].

Either computed tomography (CT) or magnetic resonance imaging (MRI) of the abdomen establishes the organ of origin for any abdominal mass. CT scans are more rapidly obtained, usually without sedation, and post-contrast imaging may help delineate vascular involvement of the tumor [14]. If the renal veins and inferior vena cava (IVC) are not adequately visualized on CT/MRI imaging, most clinicians recommend abdominal ultrasound with Doppler of IVC/renal veins to assess for tumor thrombus and extension. CT scans may also help to provide information about preoperative tumor rupture [15].

It is critical to fully rule out synchronous tumor or nephrogenic rests (Wilms tumor precursor lesions) in the contralateral kidney. This can be done by CT or MRI. MRI of kidneys may help to provide more information and distinguish between nephrogenic rests or tumor [16,17].

Whether to perform chest CT or chest X-ray (CXR) to assess for pulmonary metastases has long been the subject of debate. Chest CT scans are more sensitive than CXR, but there is considerable variability among radiologists in reading CT scans [18,19]. A recent study suggested that 82% of isolated nodules and 69% of multiple nodules seen on CT scan but not CXR that were biopsied contained tumor tissue [20]. Moreover, patients with CT-only nodules who were treated without doxorubicin had a higher risk of relapse compared to patients treated with doxorubicin, suggesting that CT scans indeed provide prognostic information in the workup of Wilms tumor. Based on this finding, CT chest has become part of the workup of Wilms tumor on COG studies. Smets et al. recently reported on the outcomes of patients with CT-only nodules on the SIOP-2001 study [21]. Patients with CT-only nodules had inferior relapse-free and overall survival compared to patients without nodules, further indicating that CT scanning adds value to the initial workup of Wilms tumor [18–20,22].

MRI of the brain, bone scan and bone marrow biopsy are not part of the initial workup of Wilms tumor because Wilms tumor seldom spreads to these sites. Brain MRI and bone scan should be performed as part of the initial staging for clear cell sarcoma of the kidney and malignant rhabdoid tumor of the kidney [23,24]. Brain MRI and bone scan should be considered for patients with renal cell carcinoma who have neurologic symptoms or bone pain.

There is no standard role of positron emission tomography (FDG-PET) CT in Wilms tumor. One limiting factor is the normal excretion of FDG through the kidney which makes interpretation at initial diagnosis difficult. PET also has limited sensitivity in identifying lung nodules less than 1 cm in diameter [25]. There may be a potential role for PET in the restaging of relapsed Wilms by detecting areas of occult disease and in assessing response to therapy [26]. In a small cohort, Misch et al. reported a possible difference in activity between favorable and anaplastic pathology; however, this has not been shown in additional reports [26,27]. False positives are seen with PET and some children may have additional imaging studies or surgery to further delineate questionable areas on PET. Further investigation for the role of PET is needed.

Differential Diagnoses

In addition to the main pediatric renal cancers such as Wilms tumor, RCC, CCSK, MRTK, congenital mesoblastic nephroma and renal medullary carcinoma, several benign tumors should be considered in the differential diagnosis of a renal mass in a child. Benign lesions include cystic nephroma, metanephric lesions (adenoma and stromal tumor) and angiolipomas. Nephrogenic rests and nephroblastomatosis may be difficult to distinguish from tumor on imaging. One should also consider other malignancies including leukemic infiltration of kidney, lymphoma, sarcoma, rhabdomyosarcoma and neuroblastoma. Non-malignant etiologies of a renal mass include infection, hydronephrosis and polycystic kidney disease [6].

Pathology

Classic nephroblastoma has three subtypes of cells which arise from embryonic nephroblastic cells: blastemal, epithelial and stromal

(Figure 9.3). Sheets or nests of small undifferentiated blue cells are the blastemal component [28]. The epithelial component may appear as tubules and glomeruli and, occasionally, as mucinous or squamous epithelium. The stromal component may appear as supportive mesenchyme with occasional immature spindle cells, skeletal muscle, cartilage, adipose, or osteoid [29]. Tumors can present with primarily one or two subtypes and may be difficult to differentiate from other malignancies.

Anaplastic Wilms Tumor

Anaplasia is found in 5–8% of Wilms tumors. Criteria for anaplasia include nuclei with a diameter three times that of adjacent cells, hyperchromasia due to increased chromatin and multipolar/mitotic figures (Figure 9.4) [30]. Focal anaplasia requires anaplastic foci to be only within primary renal tumor and to be completely surrounded by non-anaplastic cells. Patients with focal anaplasia have a better prognosis than those with diffuse anaplasia [31].

Diagnostic criteria for diffuse anaplasia involves having any of the following [31]:

- Anaplasia in any extra-renal site
- Presence of anaplasia on random biopsy
- Anaplasia and extreme nuclear unrest in additional areas
- Anaplasia on more than one tumor slide, unless known to be from the same immediate section from sample

Diffuse anaplasia confers a significantly worse prognosis than favorable histology. Wilms tumors with diffuse anaplasia appear to resist chemotherapy intrinsically and tend to present at advanced stages compared to those with favorable histology [30,32].

Nephrogenic Rests

Another important pathological feature is the presence and location of nephrogenic rests. Nephrogenic rests are comprised of persistent embryonal nephroblastic tissue in the kidney and are precursors to Wilms tumor. They are noted incidentally in 1% of perinatal autopsies, in 35% of children with unilateral Wilms tumor

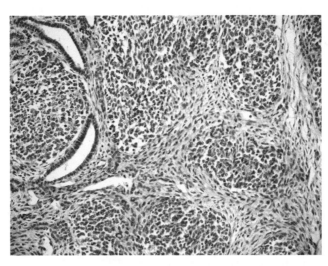

FIGURE 9.3 Triphasic favorable histology Wilms tumor consisting of blastemal, epithelial and stromal components. This figure is reproduced in color in the color plate section.

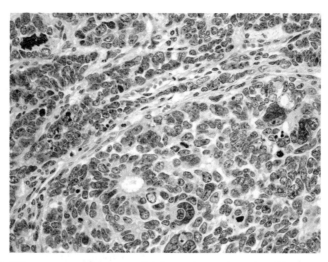

FIGURE 9.4 Anaplastic Wilms tumor with large nuclei, hyperchromasia and multipolar mitotic figures. This figure is reproduced in color in the color plate section.

and in almost all children with bilateral Wilms tumor. Nephroblastomatosis refers to the presence of multiple or diffuse nephrogenic rests [33].

Most nephrogenic rests will stay dormant or spontaneously regress, while few become hyperplastic and grow without evidence of malignancy. Very few undergo malignant transformation into Wilms tumor. Nephrogenic rests can be considered intralobar (ILNR) or perilobar (PLNR) with different typical characteristics (Table 9.3, Figures 9.5 and 9.6). It is difficult to distinguish hyperplastic rests from Wilms tumor on imaging and even biopsy. A fibrous pseudocapsule develops in Wilms and not around nephrogenic rests, and MRI imaging may help to distinguish Wilms from rests [6,16,34]. The development of metachronous tumors occurred in 10% of infants treated on NWTS protocols who had nephrogenic rests compared to 1.2% of all patients combined [35]. Close follow-up is needed in patients with nephrogenic rests, especially infants who have already developed Wilms tumor [36].

Diffuse hyperplastic perilobar nephroblastomatosis (DHPLN) is defined by hyperplastic nephroblastic tissue along the cortical surface of one or both kidneys. Perlman et al. reviewed

51 cases and found that 32% developed Wilms tumor with a higher rate of anaplasia, compared to 5% in patients with sporadic Wilms tumors. Close surveillance is recommended for early

TABLE 9.3 Characteristics of Nephrogenic Rests

	Intralobar (ILNR)	Perilobar (PLNR)
Location	Central/Random	Peripheral
Interface with kidney	Non-discrete	Well circumscribed
Histological component	Stroma	Blastemal or epithelial
Number of rests	Solitary	Multiple
Syndromes associated*	WAGR, Denys–Drash	BWS, hemihypertrophy
Development of Wilms	Younger age, median 16 mo	Older age, median 36 mo
Bilateral development	Metachronous	Synchronous

* Although ILNR are classically associated with WT1 mutations and PLNR are associated with genetic and epigenetic changes at the BWS locus, there is some overlap and patients that may have both types of rests are not mutually exclusive.

WAGR, Wilms tumor, aniridia, genitourinary anomalies, and mental retardation; BWS, Beckwith–Wiedemann syndrome.

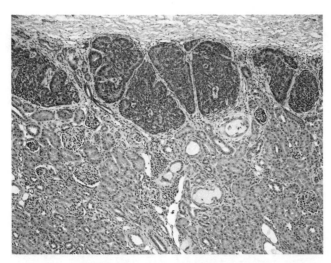

FIGURE 9.5 **Perilobar nephrogenic rests in patient with Beckwidth–Weideman syndrome.** Undifferentiated cells make up the small multiple nephrogenic rests just beneath renal capsule with sharp demarcation from cortex. This figure is reproduced in color in the color plate section.

detection of tumor development in DHPLN and nephron-sparing strategies should play a role in treatment and surgery [37].

Biology and Genetics

The study of Wilms tumor genetics has contributed much to the overall understanding of cancer biology, including the roles of tumor suppressor genes and genomic imprinting [38]. We know that Wilms genetics are more complex than the initial Knudson two-hit hypothesis proposed in 1972 [39]. An overview of the genes important in Wilms' tumor is presented below and a model of Wilms tumor development is depicted in Figure 9.8 [40].

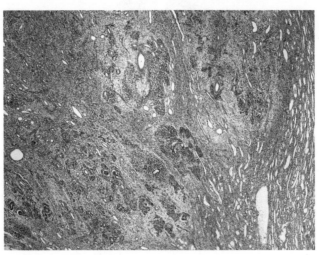

FIGURE 9.6 **Intralobar nephrogenic rests with irregular margins with nephrons intermingled within the rest with prominent stroma.** This figure is reproduced in color in the color plate section.

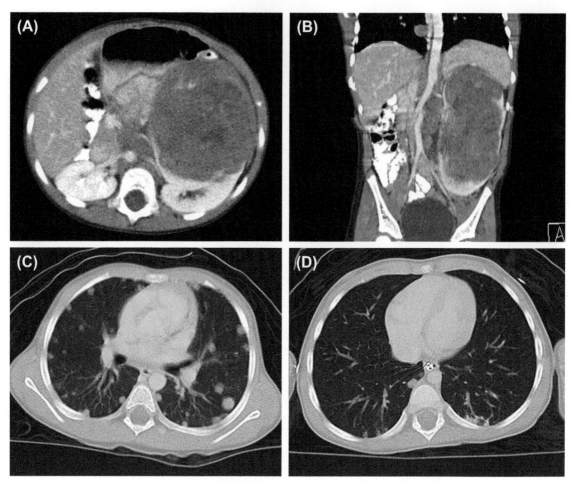

FIGURE 9.7 (A) Axial computed tomography scan of abdomen with large right Wilms tumor in 3-year-old female demonstrating classic radiologic "claw sign" in which the rind of tissue suggests the kidney as site of origin. (B) Coronal view of same patient at presentation. (C) Multiple pulmonary metastases in the same patient at diagnosis. (D) Lung metastasis improved but still present after 6 weeks of chemotherapy.

WT1

The initial and most widely studied gene identified in association with Wilms tumor is *WT1*, located at chromosome 11p13. This locus was first identified based on its deletion in individuals with WAGR syndrome (Wilms tumor, aniridia, genitourinary anomalies and mental retardation) [41,42]. *WT1* encodes a transcription factor that regulates genes critical in renal and gonadal development. Individuals with WAGR syndrome have an estimated 30% risk of developing Wilms tumor. Whereas WAGR syndrome is associated with deletions of *WT1*, the Denys—Drash and Frasier syndromes are associated with intra-genic mutations. These syndromes are summarized in Table 9.4. Although *WT1* clearly predisposes to Wilms tumor, only about 15—20% of sporadic/non-syndromic Wilms tumors have *WT* mutations, suggesting that Wilms tumor has multiple genetic etiologies [43,44].

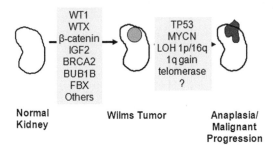

Model of Wilms Tumor Development

FIGURE 9.8 **Model of Wilms tumor development.** This figure is reproduced in color in the color plate section.

IGF2

The *IGF2* gene at chromosome 11p15 is one of the genes at the chromosomal locus implicated in Beckwith—Wiedemann syndrome (BWS), which has long been associated with Wilms tumor and other malignancies including hepatoblastoma, rhabdomyosarcoma and adrenocortical carcinoma [45,46] (Table 9.4). Patients with BWS and isolated hemi-hypertrophy, part of the BWS spectrum, have a 5—10% lifetime risk of developing Wilms tumor. The BWS locus has several genes that have genomic imprinting, preferential expression from one allele, which is regulated by epigenetic changes such as DNA methylation. Although several genes at 11p15 have been implicated in BWS, the one that is most frequently altered in individuals who develop Wilms tumor is *IGF2*, which is normally expressed exclusively from the paternal allele [47].

Studies of somatic Wilms tumor have shown that approximately 70% of Wilms tumors have IGF2 overexpression, either through loss of imprinting (LOI) or loss of heterozygosity (LOH) with duplication of the paternal allele, leading to a double dose of IGF2 [47—50].

CTNNB1 (β-catenin) and WTX

Activating mutations of *CTNNB1* (*β-catenin*) have been detected in about 15% of Wilms tumors, usually in association with *WT1* mutations [51,52]. β-catenin is a central effector in the Wnt signaling pathway, which regulates cell growth and also has been implicated in kidney development. A new Wilms tumor gene on the X-chromosome (*WTX*) was recently found to be mutated in 20—30% of sporadic Wilms tumors [53,54]. Interestingly, in girls the mutations are found exclusively on the active X-chromosome, providing a twist on the two-hit hypothesis, since only one hit is needed. *WTX* also participates in the Wnt pathway [55]. Although *CTNNB1* and *WTX* mutations were initially thought to be mutually exclusive, further study has shown that some Wilms tumors contain mutations of both genes, suggesting that their functions are not completely redundant [47,52].

TP53

TP53, the most commonly mutated gene in human cancer, is a tumor suppressor gene that plays a central role in the cellular response to DNA damage. *TP53* mutations are common in anaplastic Wilms tumors (up to 75%) and are rare in favorable histology [56,57]. The *TP53* mutation is usually restricted to the areas of anaplasia within a tumor suggesting that it is likely a clonal growth among favorable histology cells [58].

Surveillance of Wilms Tumor-associated Conditions

Experts in the field generally recommend surveillance of patients at risk for development of Wilms tumor to detect tumors at a lower stage, thereby decreasing therapy and potentially enabling nephron-sparing surgery. Scott et al. published pragmatic screening guidelines based on their research and a thorough review of literature and expert opinions. Recommendations include routine surveillance in children with associated conditions with a >5% increased risk in addition to genetic counseling/testing. Recommended screening includes renal ultrasound

TABLE 9.4   High Risk Conditions for Wilms Tumors

Estimated risk	Condition/Syndrome	Locus/Gene mutation	Clinical phenotype	Risk
HIGH >20%				
	WAGR (Wilms–aniridiia–GU anomalies–mental retardation)	11p13/*WT1*deletion	Aniridia: (partial/complete). Mental retardation GU defects: ambiguous genitalia, cryptorchidism Renal: 40% of renal failure by age 20	30%
	Denys–Drash	11p13/*WT1* truncating or missense mutation	Widely variable GU defects: hypospadias to pseudohermaphroditism Renal: diffuse mesangial sclerosis presents w/HTN and proteinurea. Often requires dialysis/transplant by age 10	>90%
	Familial Wilms tumor 1 Familial Wilms tumor 2	17q12-21 19q13.4	Autosomal dominant penetration only 30% Little known	20% 70%
	Perlman syndrome	Unknown/Autosomal recessive	Overgrowth syndrome: dysmorphic facies, developmental delay, cryptorchidism Renal: dysplasia, nephroblastomatosis, renal hamartomas	30%
	Mosaic variegated aneuploidy	15q15/Biallelic *BUB1B*	Cancer predisposition syndrome: microcephaly, growth retardation, developmental delay, heart defects, cataracts Other risk: rhabdomyosarcoma and leukemias	25%
	Fanconi anemia D1	13q12/Biallelic *BCRA2*	Cancer predisposition syndrome: short stature, radial bone defects, marrow failure, skin pigmentation Other risk: brain tumors, MDS, AML, solid tumors in adults	20%
MODERATE 5–20%				
	Frasier syndrome	11p13/*WT1* point mutations	Nephropathy with gonadal dysgenesis and gonadoblastoma. Ambiguous genitalia, streak gonads Renal: focal segmental glomerulosclerosis develops to renal failure in age 20–30s	8%
	Beckwith–Wiedemann	11p15 uniparental disomy Isolated *H19* hypermethylation *IGF2, p57, LIT1*	Overgrowth syndrome: organomegaly, macroglossia, omphalocele, hemihypertrophy, exophthalmos, GU anomalies Other risk: hepatoblastoma and adrenal carcinoma	5%
	Simpson–Golabi–Behmel	Xq26/*GPC3* mutations	Overgrowth syndrome: X-linked, coarse facial features, skeletal and cardiac anomalies Renal: dysplasia or nephromegaly reported in 30%	7.5%

LOW <5%

Syndrome	Gene/locus	Features	Risk
Bloom	15q26/ *BLM*	Chromosomal instability disorder: autosomal recessive, short stature, photosensitivity, cancer development in 50%	3%
Isolated hemihypertrophy (IHH)	Without 11p15	True risk difficult to assess	2%
2q37 deletions	2q37/terminal deletion	Developmental delay, heart defects, dysmorphic facies, skeletal abnormalities	3%
Mulibrey nanism (muscle–liver–brain–eye)	TRIM37/ various mutations	Short stature, typical facies, retinal yellow dots, pericardial constriction, hepatic hamartomas	<3%
Li–Fraumeni syndrome	17p13/ *p53*	Familial cancer predisposition: autosomal dominant, high risk for breast cancer, sarcomas, adrenocortical and brain tumors	Low
Sotos syndrome	5q35/*NSD1* point mutations or deletions	Overgrowth syndrome. Dysmorphic facies, mental retardation, cerebral gigantism. Other risk: neuroblastoma and acute lymphocytic leukemia	Low
Hereditary hyperparathyroidism–jaw tumor syndrome	1q21-q31/*HRPT2*	Autosomal dominant, fibro-osseous jaw lesion, parathyroid tumor. Renal: renal cysts, epithelial–stromal tumors, cortical adenomas, papillary renal cell carcinoma	Low
Trisomy 18 (Edwards syndrome)	18	Multiple congenital abnormalities. Renal: horseshoe kidneys, perilobar nephrogenic rests, nephroblastomatosis	Low
Trisomy 13 (Patau syndrome)	13	Multiple congenital anomalies. Median survival one week. Renal: renal tract abnormalities	Low

every 3—4 months until 5 years of age with extension of ultrasounds to 7 years of age in BWS, SGBS and some familial Wilms tumors [59]. Alpha fetoprotein should also be screened in children with BWS due to increased risk of hepatoblastoma [60]. Children with complete or partial aniridia should have a baseline karyotype and FISH analysis for *WT1* and *PAX6* gene with surveillance offered if *WT1* deletion is present [59]. Based on review of patients with DHPLN, experts recommend imaging surveillance of patients with high-risk nephroblastomatosis alternating MRI with ultrasound every 3 months until nephrogenic rests resolve, then ultrasound every 3 months until 7 years of age [37].

Staging

Routes and frequency of distant and local metastasis are listed in Table 9.5. Figure 9.7 shows CT evaluations of a patient with Stage IV disease. The COG staging system for Wilms tumor is based on initial nephrectomy at diagnosis with surgical, pathological and radiographic metastatic evaluation (Table 9.6). The SIOP staging is based on a combination of pre-chemotherapy imaging for metastases and post-chemotherapy surgical and pathological evaluation (Table 9.7).

Prognostic Factors

Histology remains the most important indicator of prognosis. Patients with diffuse anaplasia fare worse than focal anaplasia, and those with focal anaplasia fare worse than those with favorable histology [31]. In SIOP trials, tumors at resection post-initial chemotherapy that are blastemal predominant have increased recurrence risk [61,62].

Stage, which is based on anatomic extent of the tumor and the completeness of surgical resection, remains extremely important in prognosis and recommended therapy.

Weight of the tumor had prognostic significance in the early NWTS trials, but is not used

TABLE 9.5 Routes of Spread in Wilms Tumors

Routes of spread (% Presenting)		Stage
Local spread	Renal capsule penetration	II
	Renal sinus or ureter invasion	II*
		II*
	Blood vessels	III#
	— Renal vein into IVC (4—10%)	III
	— Thoracic IVC or atrium (rare)	
	Regional lymph nodes (15—20%)	
Hematogenous metastases (12%)	Lung (80%)	IV
	Liver (15%)	
	Brain/bone/bone marrow (rare)	
Bilateral disease	Synchronous disease	V
	— 5—7% at diagnosis	
	Metachronous disease	
	— 1.2% by 4 years post diagnosis	
	— 10% infants with perilobar rests at diagnosis	

*Regional extension or thrombus in blood vessels within the nephrectomy site is Stage II unless tumor removed in greater than one piece then Stage III.
#Extension within inferior vena cava (IVC) into thorax or heart is Stage III.

in current treatment stratification except for patients less than 24 months of age with a Stage I favorable histology Wilms tumor weighing less than 550 grams (so-called "very low risk" Wilms tumor) [63].

Age is inversely related to prognosis, likely due to increased rates of favorable histology and lower stage in infants and children younger than 2 years and the higher rates of anaplasia and advanced stage in older children [30,32,64]. Wilms tumor in adults accounts for less than 1% of all renal tumors. Adults historically have had significantly worse prognosis than children, possibly due to delay in therapy after diagnosis and lower tolerance for vincristine [65—67]. Recent studies indicate that the outcomes for adults approach those of children

TABLE 9.6 Children's Oncology Group Staging for Wilms Tumor, Rhabdoid Tumor of Kidney and Clear Cell Sarcoma of the Kidney

Staging	Description
Stage I	Tumor limited to kidney and completely resected with renal capsule intact. The tumor was not ruptured or biopsied prior to removal. No involvement of vessels of renal sinus. No evidence of tumor at or beyond the margins. To enroll on therapeutic protocols as Stage I, regional lymph nodes must be sampled.
Stage II	Tumor is completely resected with no evidence of tumor beyond margins. The tumor extends beyond kidney, evidenced by one of the following criteria: — Regional extension of tumor (penetration of renal capsule or extensive invasion of soft tissues of renal sinus) — Blood vessels within nephrectomy outside of renal parenchyma, including renal sinus, contain tumor
Stage III	Any of the following conditions: — Residual nonhematogenous tumor present following surgery confined to abdomen — Lymph nodes within abdomen or pelvis are involved — Tumor penetration through peritoneal surface — Tumor implants on peritoneal surface — Gross or microscopic disease postoperatively — Tumor not resectable due to local infiltration of vital structures — Tumor spillage before or during surgery. (Note: Spillage confined to flank is no longer considered Stage II) — Tumor treated with preoperative chemotherapy (with or without biopsy) before resection — Tumor is removed in greater than one piece — E.g. tumor thrombus within renal vein removed separately or tumor cells found in adrenal gland separately excised — Extension of tumor within vena cava and into thoracic vena cava and heart are considered Stage III
Stage IV	Hematogenous metastasis (lung, liver, bone, etc.) or lymph nodes outside of abdomen and pelvis.
Stage V	Bilateral renal involvement by tumor at diagnosis. Each side should be staged individually on basis of extent of disease.

when they are treated according to pediatric protocols. SIOP and COG have recently published treatment recommendations for the management of adults with Wilms tumor [68].

Molecular markers with prognostic implications include loss of heterozygosity (LOH) 1p and 16q, gain at 1q, telomerase expression and certain gene expression profiles. LOH at chromosomes 1p and 16q were prospectively analyzed as part of the NWTS-5 trial. LOH at both 1p and 16q was associated with decreased event-free and overall survival. Based on this observation, current COG studies are assessing whether augmenting therapy for patients with LOH at both 1p and 16q (which occurs in

approximately 5% of tumors) will improve outcomes [69,70]. Of note, the genes implicated at 1p and 16q remain to be determined. Because 1p and 16q are associated with 1q gain, it is possible that 1q gain is the key determinant of biological behavior [71,72].

High telomerase RNA expression is related to risk of recurrence in favorable histology after adjustment for age and stage [73]. Perlman et al. demonstrated that in patients who received surgery alone, gene expression profiles reveal different subgroups with different risks of recurrence [74]. A subgroup with WT1 mutation and 11p15 LOH had a higher rate of relapse [75]. New research in gene expression profiling

TABLE 9.7   International Society of Pediatric Oncology Working Classification of Renal Tumors

Staging	Description
Stage I	Tumor limited to kidney or surrounded with fibrous pseudocapsule. Completely resected with clear margins. Tumor may: — Invade the capsule or pseudocapsule but does not reach outer surface — Protrude into pelvic system and invade ureter but not infiltrate walls — Involve intrarenal vessels but may not have renal sinus vessel involvement — Have necrotic tumor or chemotherapy-induced changes in renal sinus or hilar fat at resection
Stage II	Tumor is completely excised with clear margins but has any of the following: — Extension beyond kidney or penetrates through the capsule into perirenal fat — Infiltration of the renal sinus or invades blood/lymphatic vessels outside renal parenchyma — Invasion of adjacent organs or vena cava
Stage III	Any of the following conditions: — Incomplete excision; gross or microscopic disease remains — Any abdominal lymph node involvement — Tumor rupture before or intraoperatively — Tumor thrombi at resection margins in ureter or vessel which are transected — Open biopsy prior to chemotherapy or surgery* — Presence of necrotic tissue of chemotherapy-induced changes in lymph node or at resection margins
Stage IV	Hematogenous spread to lung, liver, bone, brain, or lymph nodes outside abdomen and pelvis.
Stage V	Bilateral tumors at diagnosis.

* Fine needle or percutaneous core needle biopsy do not upstage tumor.

is identifying genetic signatures that may help define risk categories for relapse in favorable histology Wilms [76–78].

Treatment

Historical Perspective

Surgical resection was the mainstay of therapy and nephrectomies were described in the literature in 1894 [4]. Of the 47 patients with nephrectomy in this manuscript, 19 died from surgical complications and 21 relapsed following their surgeries. In Paris, in 1915, Anna Heimann described treatment of Wilms tumor with radiotherapy and, due to its extreme radiosensitivity, pre- and postoperative radiation was used for several decades [4]. Surgical resection offered the best chance for cure; however, some cures were described by radiotherapy alone [79]. In the 1950s and 1960s chemotherapy treatment

with vincristine and dactinomycin were found to be effective. In the 1970s, doxorubicin was added to the treatment of patients with higher-risk features [4].

A multimodality approach evolved through the efforts of the NWTS/COG and SIOP cooperative groups over the next 40 years have resulted in today's recommended therapy and excellent cure rates. The NWTS/COG recommends upfront nephrectomy with treatment based on clinical, radiological, surgical and pathological elements at diagnosis. In contrast, the SIOP trials use 4–6 weeks of preoperative chemotherapy with staging and postoperative therapy based on initial presentation and response to initial chemotherapy.

The main conclusions from the NWTS trials are described in Table 9.8 and outline the evolution of multimodality treatment for Wilms tumor. The NWTS trials have led to our current

TABLE 9.8 National Wilms Tumor Study (NWTS) 1–5 Main Conclusions

Study	Stage	Main conclusions
NWTS-1 (1969–1973)	I	Postoperative XRT unnecessary
	II–III	Combination VCR and AMD better than single drug
NWTS-2 (1974–1978)	I	6 months VCR and AMD comparable to 15 months. XRT not needed
	II–IV	Adding DOX increased 2 year RFS
NWTS-3 (1979–1986)	I	11 weeks VCR and AMD comparable 6 months
	II	DOX and XRT unnecessary
	III	Can decrease XRT from 20 Gy to 10 Gy with DOX use
	IV	No benefit to adding cyclophosphamide for favorable histology disease; benefit seen for anaplastic histology
NWTS-4 (1986–1994)	I–IV	"Pulse-intensive" dactinomycin and doxorubicin lowered hematologic toxicity; matched efficacy
	II–IV	6 months chemotherapy adequate
NWTS-5 (1995–2001)	I–V	Loss of heterozygosity at 1p and 16q predicted recurrence
	I	<24 months and <550g RFS 84% and OS 98%; nephrectomy only arm closed

XRT, radiation; DOX, doxorubicin; VCR, vincristine; AMD, dactinomycin; Gy, gray; RFS, relapse-free survival; OS, overall survival.
Modified from Metzger and Dome. The Oncologist 2005;10:815–26.

standard of care and set the foundation for the current COG trials. The main accomplishments of NWTS trials 1 through 5 included reduction of radiation therapy, decreased use of anthracyclines, decreased duration of therapy and identification of crucial biological markers and risk factors to allow a risk-based stratification and treatment model [80–84].

Current Surgical Guidelines

The recommended surgical approach to Wilms tumor is unilateral radical ureteronephrectomy with lymph node sampling. Transperitoneal, transabdominal, or thoracoabdominal incision is preferred for adequate visualization and removal of the tumor intact. If there is any question on preoperative imaging of contralateral tumor involvement, inspection of the contralateral kidney and biopsy should be considered. Otherwise, due to the high quality of modern imaging studies,

evaluation of the contralateral kidney is no longer required. Every attempt should be made at removing tumor, kidney, hilar structures and ureter en bloc to avoid spillage. If the tumor is removed in more than one piece, the stage is considered Stage III. It is important to biopsy suspicious regional lymph nodes. Otherwise, it is important to sample nodes randomly from hilar/para-aortic/para-caval nodes. Studies have shown that lack of lymph node sampling is an adverse prognostic factor, probably due to understaging of tumors [85]. For bilateral tumors, preoperative chemotherapy followed by partial nephrectomy is favored. In North America, resection of renal tumors is usually delayed in the following circumstances:

- Extension of tumor thrombus above the hepatic veins
- Contiguous structure involvement that would require removal of organs (spleen, pancreas, or colon)

TABLE 9.9 Event-free Survival (EFS) and Overall Survival (OS) for Renal Tumors

Stage	Favorable histology		Diffuse anaplastic Wilms		Clear cell sarcoma	Rhabdoid	Renal cell
	EFS (%)	OS (%)	EFS (%)	OS (%)	OS (%)	OS (%)	OS (%)
I	94.2	98.4	68.4	78.9	100	33.3	92.4
II	84.4	97.2	82.6	81.5	97.3	46.9	84.6
III	86.5	94.4	64.7	66.7	86.9	21.8	72.7
IV	75.1	85.2	33.3	33.3	45	8.4	13.9
V	61	80.8	25.1	41.6			

Favorable histology, diffuse anaplastic and bilateral Wilms results of NWTS-5 [32,70,86].
Clear cell sarcoma results of NWTS-4 [87].
Renal cell carcinoma results were from a systematic review of the literature [88].

- Increased risk for unnecessary perioperative morbidity, diffuse tumor spill, or residual tumor
- Pulmonary compromise due to pulmonary metastases
- Bilateral disease

Current Chemotherapy Guidelines

Event-free survival (EFS) and overall survival (OS) from the most recently reported NWTS trials are shown in Table 9.9. The survival for patients with favorable histology was excellent using Regimen EE4A (Stage I/II) and Regimen DD4A (Stage III/IV), so these regimens provide a reasonable standard of care (Figure 9.9). The regimens used in SIOP protocols also have produced excellent outcomes (Figure 9.10).

Outcomes for Stage I anaplastic Wilms tumor were inferior to Stage I favorable histology when treated with Regimen EE4A, suggesting that additional therapy may be warranted for that group. Outcomes for Stage II–IV anaplastic Wilms tumor were better than historical controls when treated with Regimen I, so this regimen provides a reasonable standard of care for patients not on study (Figure 9.9).

Current Radiation Therapy Guidelines

Flank/abdominal radiation is utilized in Stage III and IV disease and typically is administered soon after nephrectomy during week 1 of treatment. If resection is delayed, radiation should be given after surgery, usually at week 7 or week 13. Radiation is also given to metastatic sites. Whole lung radiation is given for patients with lung metastases on the NWTS/COG studies. Radiation doses from NWTS-5 are indicated in Table 9.10. The SIOP radiation guidelines differ from NWTS guidelines in that the flank/abdominal radiation dose is higher and a boost is provided for patients with positive lymph nodes (Table 9.11). Additionally, patients who achieve a complete response of their lung nodules after either surgical resection or chemotherapy do not receive radiation therapy. It should be noted that the SIOP approach of not giving lung radiation to any patient cannot be directly translated to patients treated on NWTS/COG protocols without further study because the anthracycline dose used on SIOP studies is considerably higher. Withholding lung XRT for patients whose lung nodules disappear after 6 weeks of chemotherapy is a current study question in the COG.

Week		1	2	3	4	5	6	7	8	9	10	11	12	13	14	15	16	17	18	19	20	21	22	23	24	25
EE-4A	S	A			A			A			A			A			A			A						
	U	V	V	V	V	V	V	V	V	V	V	V		V²			V²			V²						
DD-4A	R	A						A						A						A						A
	G				D						D						D²						D²			
	E	V	V	V	V	V	V	V	V	V	V			V²			V²			V²			V²			V²
	R	XRT																								
I	Y	D						D						D						D						D
		V	V	V		V	V	V	V	V		V	V	V²	V²					V²						V²
		Cy			Cy⁵			Cy			Cy⁵			Cy			Cy⁵			Cy			Cy⁵			Cy
					E						E						E						E			
		XRT																								

V-Vincristine — <30kg 0.05 mg/kg/day x1; ≥30kg 1.5 mg/m²/day x1
V²-Vincristine — <30kg 0.067mg/kg/day x1; ≥30kg 2 mg/m²/day x1; Max dose 2mg
Infants <1 year all doses are 50% of mg/kg dose

A-Dactinomycin — <30kg 0.045 mg/kg/day x1; ≥30kg 1.35 mg/m²/day x1; Max dose 2.3mg
D-Doxorubicin — <30kg 1.5 mg/kg/day x1; ≥30kg 45 mg/m²/day x1
D²-Doxorubicin — <30kg 1 mg/kg/day x1; ≥30kg 30 mg/m²/day x1

Cy-Cyclophosphamide — <30kg 14.7 mg/kg/day x3; ≥30kg 440 mg/m²/day x3
Cy⁵- Cyclophosphamide — <30kg 14.7 mg/kg/day x5; ≥30kg 440 mg/m²/day x5
E-Etoposide — <30kg 3.3 mg/kg/day x5; ≥30kg 100 mg/m²/day x5
XRT- Radiation Therapy

FIGURE 9.9 National Wilms Study Group chemotherapy regimens.

Bilateral Disease

Bilateral Wilms tumor (BWT) is present in 4 to 13% of Wilms patients and can be synchronous (5–7%) or metachronous (1–2%) [2,36,88]. Synchronous tumors present simultaneously and metachronous disease refers to the sequential development of an additional contralateral primary tumor, usually within 4 years of initial diagnosis. Patients with a Wilms tumor predisposition syndrome or a family history of Wilms tumor have a higher risk of BWT than non-syndromic patients, though most patients with syndromes do not have BWT. Likewise, most patients with BWT do not have known Wilms predisposition syndromes [6,36].

The outcomes in children with bilateral Wilms tumor are significantly lower than in

Pre-operative Chemotherapy			Regimen	Post-Operative Chemotherapy																			
Week	1 2 3 4 5 6			Week: 1	2	3	4	5 6 7 8 9 10	12	14	16	18	20	22	24	26	28	30	32	34		
Localized	A A / V V V V	S U R G E R Y	VA	A⁵ / V	V	V	V															
			AVA	A⁵ V V V V	A⁵ V V V	A⁵ V V	A⁵ V V	A⁵ V V	V V													
				D	D	D	D	D														
Metastatic	A A A / V V V V V V / D D	S U R G E R Y	EICA	E C I D	E C	E C I	E C	I D	E C	I		E C		I		E C	I		I D		

Post-operative Therapy:
Stage 1	Low Risk	None
Stage 1	Intermediate and Anaplastic	VA x4 or 18 weeks*
Stage II-III	Intermediate	AVA x 27 weeks
Stage IV	Complete response 9 weeks	AVA x27 weeks
Stage IV	Residual disease at 9 weeks	EICA x34 weeks
Stage I-IV	High Risk/Anaplastic	EICA x34 weeks

VA Vincristine, Dactinomycin
AVA Dactinomycin, Vincristine, Doxorubicin
EICA Etoposide, Ifosfamide, Carboplatin, Doxorubicin
Doses reduced 2/3 for weight <12kg

V-Vincrisine — 1.5 mg/m²/day x1 — Max dose 2mg
A-Dactinomycin — 0.015mg/kg/day x3 — Max dose 0.5mg
A⁵-Dacinomycin — 0.015mg/kg/day x5
D-Adriamycin — 50 mg/m²/day x1
E-Etoposide — 100 mg/m²/day x5
C-Carboplatin — 600mg/ m²/day x1
I- Ifosfamide — 3,000mg/m²/day x2

FIGURE 9.10 International Society of Pediatric Oncology Study 93-01 chemotherapy regimens.

TABLE 9.10 National Wilms Tumor Group Study 5 Radiation Guidelines

Stage	XRT site	Dose (Gy)
I	N/A	N/A
II	N/A	N/A
III	Flank*	10.8
	Whole abdomen**	10.8
	Whole abdomen***	21
IV	Lung (<12 months)	12 (10.5)
	Brain	21.6 + 10.8 boost
	Liver	19.8
	Bone	25.2
	Lymph node	19.8

* Stage III due to positive lymph nodes, local spillage or biopsy.
** Stage III due to preop rupture, diffuse intraoperative rupture, or cytology positive ascities.
*** Stage III with diffuse unresectable peritoneal implants.

children with unilateral tumors. SIOP has reported a 10-year OS of 69% in synchronous BWT, while the most recent NWTS-5 study treated 158 patients with BWT with 4-year EFS of 61% and an OS of 80% [88]. The cumulative incidence of end stage renal disease (ESRD) in NWTS patients from 1969 to 2002 was 0.7%,

TABLE 9.11 International Society of Pediatric Oncology Study 93-01 Radiation Guidelines

Stage	XRT site	Intermediate risk (Gy)	High risk* (Gy)
I	None	None	None
II LN⁻	Tumor bed	None	30 + 5 boost**
LN⁺	Tumor bed	15 + 15 boost**	30 + 5 boost**
III	Tumor bed	15 + 15 boost**	30 + 5 boost**
IV	Lung	12	12
	Lung CR***	None	

* High risk patients have diffuse anaplasia or blastemal type.
** XRT boost to sites of residual disease and/or positive lymphatic chain.
*** If no residual lung disease at week 9 due to surgery or chemotherapy, Stage IV patients do not receive lung XRT.
XRT, radiation therapy; LN⁻, lymph node negative; LN⁺, lymph node positive; Gy, gray.

but was 4% in patients with synchronous bilateral Wilms tumor and 19.3% in patients with metachronous Wilms tumor. The risk factors for ESRD included stromal predominant lesions, presence of intralobar rests and age less than 2 years at presentation [89]. Bilateral partial nephrectomies have been shown to result in improved long-term renal function without significant increase in recurrence rate [90]. Most cases of ESRD result from tumor progression or metachronous tumor formation, necessitating surgical resection, rather than treatment-related complications such as radiation nephritis.

Relapsed Disease

Fewer than 15% of patients with favorable histology relapse with current treatment regimens, but 50% of those with anaplastic Wilms tumor recur [38]. Most recurrences present within 2 years from completing therapy and are in the lungs, initial tumor bed, or liver [91]. Favorable outcome after a first relapse is expected for those patients with Stage I/II at diagnosis, prior treatment with only two drug chemotherapy, no initial radiation, favorable histology, lung-only site of relapse and time from nephrectomy to relapse longer than 12 months [92].

Data from NWTS and SIOP identify the most important prognostic indicators to be anaplasia or SIOP high-risk histology and initial treatment including doxorubicin [93]. Three risk categories for recurrent Wilms tumor with relevant treatment strategies are seen in Table 9.12.

In the USA, fewer than 75 children with Wilms tumor relapse each year, so large prospective studies have been difficult to perform. Most data on relapsed treatment are derived from small retrospective series. Surgical removal, if feasible, may help to reduce tumor burden but its benefit has not been proven in prospective studies. The resection of all pulmonary metastases is thought to be unlikely to improve post-relapse outcomes compared to treatment of whole-lung radiation and chemotherapy based on NWTS data [94]. Complete surgical resection of recurrent disease was found to increase survival in a retrospective analysis by Dome et al., although it is possible that the ability to perform surgical resection was an indicator of lower disease burden, which may account for the improved outcomes in patients who underwent surgery. This review also found a higher probability of survival with radiation used in locations of relapse which had not been included in prior radiation therapy fields [91]. Bilateral whole-lung irradiation is commonly used with any relapse to the lung.

Published chemotherapy regimens used in standard-risk relapse include the NWTS-5 relapse protocol Stratum B/Regimen I with nine alternating courses of vincristine, doxorubicin, plus cyclophosphamide and cyclophosphamide plus etoposide [95] (Table 9.12). The United Kingdom Children's Study Group (UKCCSG) has used vincristine, dactinomycin and doxorubicin in patients who had received therapy with vincristine alone and doxorubicin plus cyclophosphamide alternating with cyclophosphamide plus etoposide for patients who had received prior two-drug therapy [96]. High-risk relapse patients have received dose-intensive chemotherapy on NWTS-5 with alternating cyclophosphamide plus etoposide and carboplatin plus etoposide with an OS of 48% [92]. Other series have published an OS of 60% with ifosfamide, carboplatin and etoposide (ICE) although there are reports of persistent nephrotoxicity [97,98]. A Phase 2 trial of topotecan had a 48% response rate in heavily pretreated children [99]. High-dose chemotherapy with autologous stem cell rescue has been used, but currently there is no consensus on its benefit over conventional chemotherapy [96,100,101]. UKCCSG performed a nonrandomized risk stratified trial for relapsed renal tumors which recently completed accrual and results are pending [96]. Very high-risk patients have a very poor prognosis with current salvage therapy [32,91]. These patients should be offered novel

TABLE 9.12   Risk Stratification in Relapse Patients and Treatment Strategies

Risk group (% of relapses)	Patient characteristics	Expected EFS	Salvage regimens
Standard risk (30%)	Favorable histology only treated with VCR and/or AMD	70–80%	Doxorubicin, etoposide and alkylating agent (ifosfamide or cyclophosphamide) in combination with radiation Example: NWTS Regimen I
High risk (45–40%)	Favorable histology treated with three or more agents	40–50%	Conventional chemotherapy: — Cyclophosphamide, etoposide, carboplatin (CCE) or ifosfamide/carboplatin/etoposide (ICE) — Topotecan added to CCE or ICE may be considered
Very-high risk (10–15%)	Recurrent anaplastic or SIOP blastemal-predominant histology	10–15%	Overall very poor response to chemotherapy Refer to institution with research trials on novel agents High dose chemotherapy with autologous stem cell rescue

VCR, vincristine; AMD, dactinomycin; EFS, event free survival; NWTSG, National Wilms Tumor Study Group; SIOP, International Society of Pediatric Oncology.

agents on Phase 1 or 2 trials if families are interested.

NON-WILMS RENAL TUMORS

Renal Cell Carcinoma

Renal cell carcinoma (RCC) represents 2−5% of pediatric renal tumors and less than 2% of all RCC occur under the age of 21 [102]. Pediatric RCC is a distinct entity from adult RCC. Whereas most adult RCC are the clear cell subtype and associated with mutations of the von Hippel−Lindau (VHL) gene, this subtype is seen in only a minority of children and adolescents. Approximately 50% of pediatric RCC are associated with various translocations involving the TFE3 or TFEB genes. These translocations result in overexpression of TFE3 and TFEB proteins and can be detected by immunohistochemistry. Other histologic types of RCC seen in the pediatric population are papillary and sarcomatoid [103,104]. A specific subtype of RCC occurs in patients as a secondary malignancy after neuroblastoma [102].

Prognosis is closely related to stage at diagnosis. About 20% of RCC are metastatic at diagnosis, most often to lungs, bone, liver, or brain. Of note, lymph node involvement in children does not appear to portend the poor prognosis that it does in adults [105]. The treatment for pediatric RCC remains to be determined. For localized disease (Stages I and II), the outcomes are excellent (OS of 92.4% for Stage I and 84.6% for Stage II) without adjuvant therapy. For Stage III disease with lymph node involvement and Stage IV disease, outcomes are less favorable (OS of 72.7% and 13.9%, respectively); however, there is no established role for adjuvant therapy. For metastatic disease, various regimens have been used, but it is important to realize that effective therapies for adult clear cell RCC have not been well studied in pediatric RCC. There are reports that tyrosine kinase inhibitors have some efficacy for translocation RCC [106,107].

Clear Cell Sarcoma of the Kidney

Clear cell sarcoma of the kidney (CCSK) is the second most common renal malignancy in children under 15 years old, with peak incidence between 1 and 4 years of age and twice the frequency in boys [108]. It has a different metastatic pattern than Wilms tumor and may spread to bone and brain, in addition to lymph nodes and lung [108]. The initial workup, therefore, should include a bone scan and imaging of brain. No cases of bilateral CCSK tumor have been reported.

Histology of classic CCSK consists of nests of pale-stained ovoid to spindle tumor cells separated by vascular septa. There are many variants of CCSK (myxoid, sclerosing, cellular, epithelioid, pallisading, spindle-cell, storiform and anaplastin) and it remains frequently misdiagnosed [6,108]. Vimentin stains positive but there is no identified characteristic immunohistochemical pattern [109].

The NWTS-5 Regimen I produced excellent results with an EFS of 77.6% at 4 years [87] (Table 9.9). In addition to chemotherapy, patients received radiation therapy to the flank and to metastatic sites. Relapsed disease frequently involved brain metastasis and 20% of the relapses occurred after 3 years. A series of eight patients with brain metastases who received ICE chemotherapy in combination with surgery and radiation had a 75% RFS at 30 months [110].

Malignant Rhabdoid Tumor

Malignant rhabdoid tumor (MRT) was originally thought to be an unfavorable histological variant of Wilms tumor until it was presented as a separate entity named for its resemblance to rhabdomyoblasts [111]. MRT accounts for 2% of pediatric renal tumors, with 60%

presenting before 12 months. Metastases occur in 80% of patients, primarily to lung, liver and brain. Hypercalcemia may be present due to elevated parathormone levels [112].

Histologically, MRT is described as monomorphic cells with vesicular nuclei with characteristic eosinophillic paranuclear cytoplasm inclusions [103,113]. Molecular studies in renal and extra-renal rhabdoid tumor show inactivation of *HSNF5/INI-1* tumor suppressor gene on chromosome 22q11-12 [114]. Germline mutations in *HSNF5/INI-1* have been identified, confirming familial associations with MRT and brain atypical teratoid/rhabdoid tumors [115,116].

The NWTS trials have not been successful with finding an effective regimen for MRT. Overall prognosis is historically dismal due to advanced stage at diagnosis, aggressive clinical behavior and poor response to chemotherapy. NWTS-5 attempted a Regimen RTK with carboplatin/etoposide alternating with cyclophosphamide which had an OS of only 25.8% [117]. Several case reports document successful treatment with ifosfamide and etoposide alternating with vincristine, doxorubicin and cyclophosphamide [118–120].

Mesoblastic Nephroma

Congenital mesoblastic nephroma (CMN) accounts for 3–10% of pediatric renal tumors and is most common in infants less than 2 months of age [24,121]. It often presents with a large abdominal mass and sometimes hematuria. Cases can be diagnosed by prenatal ultrasound and occasionally polyhydramnios and premature delivery occur [122]. A parathyroid hormone-like substance or a prostaglandin has been reported to cause hypercalcemia and hypertension may be present due to increased renin [123,124].

CMN histology can be classic, cellular or a combination of the two (mixed). Initially thought to be a congenital form of Wilms tumor, CMN originates from proliferating nephrogenic mesenchyme with immunohistochemical features of myofibroblastic differentiation [125]. A translocation t(12;15)(p13;25) fusing *ETV6* and *NTRK3* is present in the cellular variant which is the same gene-fusion transcript found in infantile fibrosarcoma [126].

Nephrectomy alone cures 95% of patients. Rarely CMN may have an extensive local recurrence or distant metastases to lungs, liver, heart, or brain [127]. Risk factors for recurrence include age greater than 3 months, cellular variant, local spillage, or positive surgical margins. Patients with these risk factors may benefit from adjuvant chemotherapy [127–130]. In several small series, vincristine, dactinomycin, cyclophosphamide, or ICE combinations were shown to be effective [131,132].

Renal Medullary Carcinoma

Renal medullary carcinoma (RMC) is a very rare entity primarily affecting young adults with sickle cell trait. Clinical presentation includes gross hematuria, abdominal pain and occasionally weight loss or fever [133]. It originates in the medulla of the kidney and grows rapidly with invasion of the lymphatics. Eighty-one percent of patients are Stage IV and 18% are Stage III at diagnosis [134].

Tumor cells have eosinophilic cytoplasm with prominent nucleoli with intracytoplasmic inclusions. It appears as a very infiltrative tumor with nests, tubules and strands in a desmoplastic stroma [135]. Chronic hypoxia has been suggested to contribute to development of cell proliferation in the renal medulla to explain the occurrence in sickle cell trait [103,136].

Overall RMC patients have a poor prognosis with advanced disease at diagnosis. Recent reports, however, show improved survival with radical nephrectomy in localized disease and promising results from chemotherapy regimens including cisplatin, gemcitabine and paclitaxel [134,137,138].

SURVEILLANCE AFTER COMPLETION OF THERAPY

There is no standard recommendation for surveillance imaging after completion of therapy. Chest radiograph and abdominal ultrasound have been used for many years, but recent protocols include CT or MRI scans in the follow-up imaging. Whether these higher resolution imaging techniques improve outcome after recurrence remains questionable. The imaging surveillance schedule used by the authors for patients not on clinical trials is shown in Table 9.13.

TABLE 9.13   Recommended Imaging Surveillance

Condition	Schedule of imaging
Favorable histology Wilms tumor	CXR and abdominal u/s every 3 months for 2 years; then every 6 months for 2 years; then every 12 months for 1 year. In Stage III and IV CT chest/abdomen may be alternated with CXR/abdominal u/s for the first two years after completion of therapy
Anaplastic Wilms tumor and renal cell carcinoma (RCC)	CT chest/abdomen (or CT chest/MRI abdomen) every 3 months for 2 years; then CXR/abd u/s every 6 months for 2 years and every 12 months for 1 year. For RCC, add MRI brain and bone scans if patient is symptomatic
Rhabdoid tumor	Image as for anaplastic Wilms tumor and add MRI of the brain every 3 months for 1 year; then every 6 months for 1 year
Clear cell kidney sarcoma	Image as for anaplastic Wilms tumor and add MRI of the brain and bone scan every 3 months for 1 year; then every 6 months for 2 years
Bilateral Wilms tumor	After completion of imaging for 2 years continue imaging at least abdominal u/s every 3 months until 7 years of age

CXR, chest X-ray; abd u/s, abdominal ultrasound; CT, computed tomography; MRI, magnetic resonance imaging.

Late Effects/Toxicities

With excellent cure rates, survivors of pediatric renal tumors are increasing in number. In an assessment of patients enrolled on NWTS from 1969 to 1995, there was a 24-fold higher risk of death in the first 5 years following treatment than in the general population. After 5 years there was an almost 13-fold increase for years 5–10 and beyond 10 years a 3–4-fold increase in risk of death [139]. The Childhood Cancer Survivor Study (CCSS) recently published health outcomes of 1256 survivors of Wilms tumor at 25 years or longer from diagnosis. The cumulative incidence of chronic health conditions in these survivors was 65.4% while 24.2% had severe health conditions [140]. Most late effects seen in Wilms tumor survivors are toxicities and complications related to the treatment, though some effects are related to underlying genetic predisposition syndromes.

Cardiac

CONGESTIVE HEART FAILURE

A study from the NWTSG found a cumulative frequency of congestive heart failure of 4.4% of patients at 20 years. The frequency increased to 17% in patients treated for relapse. Relative risk for girls developing CHF was higher than boys at 4.5. For each additional $100 \, mg/m^2$ of doxorubicin, the estimated risk of CHF increased 3.2-fold. Treatment on current COG protocols uses a cumulative anthracycline dose of $150 \, mg/m^2$ compared to the historical $300 \, mg/m^2$ in prior NWTS trials. We expect the frequency of CHF to decrease as future survivors will have been treated with lower cumulative doses. An additional risk factor for the development of CHF was radiation: 10 Gy of whole lung irradiation and left abdominal radiation increased the relative risk of CHF by 1.6 and 1.8, respectively [141,142].

CARDIAC DYSFUNCTION

The lifetime risk of cardiac dysfunction or major ventricular overload has been reported as 39% in childhood survivors over 15 years who had doxorubicin. Concerning to these authors was that there was no evidence of a plateau in the cumulative incidence of heart disease in these patients [143]. Asymptomatic increased afterload and decreased contractility were found in 25% of Wilms tumor survivors with doxorubicin exposure, and the risk was higher in those who had been treated with radiation to the chest/heart [144]. The COG guidelines for frequency of evaluation of cardiac function are depicted in Table 9.14.

Renal

END STAGE RENAL DISEASE (ESRD)

The cumulative incidence for ESRD was 0.6% in unilateral Wilms patients without predisposing conditions and 12% in bilateral disease [145]. In contrast ESRD developed in 62% of patients with Denys–Drash, 38% of patients with WAGR and 11% of those with genitourinary anomalies including cryptorchidism and hypospadias [146]. Hypertension was not found to be significantly more common in renal cancer survivors [147,148]. Some studies suggest that survivors have subclinical renal damage and some have reported chronic renal insufficiency in 19–73% [98,149]. No evidence of long-term renal impairment was found in 40 survivors at a median of 8.8 years [148]. Mild or moderate renal dysfunction is likely more common in survivors of relapsed, very high-risk disease who had more intensive chemotherapy, especially with ifosfamide and platinum agents [98]. The COG guidelines for long-term follow-up of patients with a single kidney are shown in Table 9.15.

TABLE 9.14 Recommended Frequency of ECHO or MUGA Scan

Age at treatment	Radiation with cardiac potential	Anthracycline dose (mg/m^2) doxorubicin equivalent dose	Recommended frequency
<1 year old	Yes	Any	Every year
	No	<200 mg/m^2	Every 2 years
		≥200 mg/m^2	Every year
1–4 years old	Yes	Any	Every year
	No	<100 mg/m^2	Every 5 years
		≥100 mg/m^2 to <300 mg/m^2	Every 2 years
		≥300 mg/m^2	Every year
≥5 years old	Yes	<300 mg/m^2	Every 2 years
		≥300 mg/m^2	Every year
	No	<200 mg/m^2	Every 5 years
		≥200 to <300 mg/m^2	Every 2 years
		≥300 mg/m^2	Every year
Any age with decrease in serial function			Every year

Recommendations from Children's Oncology Group Long Term Follow-up Guidelines.

TABLE 9.15 Long-term Follow-up Recommendations for Survivors with Single Kidney

Annual*	Medical exam with blood pressure and urinalysis
Baseline at 2 years off therapy	Electrolytes, BUN, creatinine
Nephrology referral	Hypertension, proteinurea, or signs of kidney dysfunction
General education	Maintain good hydration
	Close monitoring for urinary tract infections
	Use non-steroidal anti-inflammatory drugs with caution
	Prevent injury to single kidney whenever possible
	Avoid contact sports or consider kidney guard (provider recommendations vary)

For additional individual recommendations based on specific chemotherapy and radiation toxicity risks refer to COG Guidelines (www.survivorshipguidelines.org). See Table 9.14 for cardiac monitoring recommendations.

Fertility/Pregnancy

MALE FERTILITY

Gonadal dysfunction and infertility may result from alkylator exposure. Alkylating agents are used primarily in high-risk favorable histology Wilms tumor, anaplastic Wilms tumor and recurrent Wilms tumor. There are no effects of radiation on male survivors on the outcome of pregnancies that they father [150].

FEMALE FERTILITY

The gonadal toxicity of alkylators is exacerbated by radiation to the abdomen or pelvis if the ovaries are exposed. Absent or hypoplastic ovaries, abnormal ovarian function and premature menopause have been reported as late effects of treatment [151,152].

OBSTETRICAL COMPLICATIONS

Females with radiation for renal tumors have a higher risk for fetal malposition, premature labor, low birth weight infants and spontaneous abortions [153,154]. A recent review of 1021 pregnancies in female survivors of Wilms tumor or partners of male survivors found that females with flank radiation had an increased risk of hypertension complicating pregnancy and were more likely to have malposition, premature births and low birth weight infants [155]. All pregnancies in women with a history of abdominal or pelvic radiation should be considered high risk.

Pulmonary

Mild to moderate restrictive lung function tests have been found in survivors. They are thought to be related to thoracic hypoplasia and are worse the younger the age at treatment [156]. Diffuse interstitial fibrosis has not been reported. Only three of 819 deaths in survivors of Wilms tumor treated on NWTS trials were attributed to pulmonary causes [139].

Second Malignancies

In the NWTS studies the rate of second malignant neoplasm (SMN) was 1.6% at 15 years. This is eight times higher than expected in the general population. Patients who received doxorubicin and radiation had a 36-fold increase in SMN compared to the general population. In a comparable SIOP study, the cumulative incidence of SMNs was reported at 0.65% [157]. The recent CCSS study of Wilms tumor survivors at 25 years found the SMN rate to be 3% [140]. Secondary tumors diagnosed in the NWTS cohort included acute leukemia, lymphomas, gastrointestinal and peritoneal tumors, central nervous system tumors, sarcomas, melanoma and breast cancer [139]. The majority of solid tumor SMNs occurred within radiation fields. Treatment for relapse increased the risk more than four-fold in the NWTS cohort [158].

Other

Other late effects have been associated with radiation therapy, including hypoplastic breast tissue and spinal/thoracic wall abnormalities such as scoliosis and small chest [159]. Loss of height is dependent on the dose of radiation to the spine, but is not likely to be factor with modern dosing.

References

[1] Howlader N, Noone A, Krapcho M, Neyman N, Aminou R, Waldron W, et al. SEER Cancer Statistics Review. 1975–2008. Bethesda, MD: National Cancer Institute, http://seer.cancer.gov/csr/1975_2008/; 2011, based on November 2010 SEER data submission, posted to the SEER website.

[2] Breslow N, Olshan A, Beckwith JB, Green DM. Epidemiology of Wilms tumor. Med Pediatr Oncol 1993;21(3):172–81.

[3] Breslow NE, Olson J, Moksness J, Beckwith JB, Grundy P. Familial Wilms' tumor: a descriptive study. Med Pediatr Oncol 1996;27(5):398–403.

[4] Oak S, Parelkar S, editors. Wilms' Tumor: Saga of a Century. 2nd ed. New Delhi, India: Jaypee Brothers Medical Publishers Ltd; 2002.

[5] Beckwith JB. The John Lattimer lecture. Wilms tumor and other renal tumors of childhood: an update. J Urol 1986;136(1 Pt 2):320–4.

[6] Pizzo P, Poplack D, editors. Principles and Practice of Pediatric Oncology. 6th ed. Philadelphia: Lippincott Williams & Wilkins; 2011.

[7] Lanzkowsky P, editor. Manual of Pediatric Hematology and Oncology. 4th ed. USA: Elsevier Academic Press; 2005.

[8] Stiller CA, Lennox EL, Wilson LM. Incidence of cardiac septal defects in children with Wilms' tumour and other malignant diseases. Carcinogenesis 1987;8(1):129–32.

[9] Bonaiti-Pellie C, Chompret A, Tournade MF, Hochez J, Moutou C, Zucker JM, et al. Genetics and epidemiology of Wilms' tumor: the French Wilms' tumor study. Med Pediatr Oncol 1992;20(4):284–91.

[10] Maas MH, Cransberg K, van Grotel M, Pieters R, van den Heuvel-Eibrink MM. Renin-induced hypertension in Wilms tumor patients. Pediatr Blood Cancer 2007;48(5):500–3.

[11] Amar AM, Tomlinson G, Green DM, Breslow NE, de Alarcon PA. Clinical presentation of rhabdoid tumors of the kidney. J Pediatr Hematol Oncol 2001;23(2):105–8.

[12] Leung RS, Liesner R, Brock P. Coagulopathy as a presenting feature of Wilms tumour. Eur J Pediatr 2004;163(7):369–73.

[13] Blanchette V, Coppes MJ. Routine bleeding history and laboratory tests in children presenting with a renal mass. Pediatr Blood Cancer 2009;52(3):314–5.

[14] Khanna G, Rosen N, Anderson JR, Ehrlich PF, Dome JS, Gow KW, et al. Evaluation of diagnostic performance of CT for detection of tumor thrombus in children with Wilms tumor: a report from the Children's Oncology Group. Pediatr Blood Cancer 2012;58(4):551–5.

[15] Brisse HJ, Schleiermacher G, Sarnacki S, Helfre S, Philippe-Chomette P, Boccon-Gibod L, et al. Preoperative Wilms tumor rupture: a retrospective study of 57 patients. Cancer 2008;113(1):202–13.

[16] Gylys-Morin V, Hoffer FA, Kozakewich H, Shamberger RC. Wilms tumor and nephroblastomatosis: imaging characteristics at gadolinium-enhanced MR imaging. Radiology 1993;188(2):517–21.

[17] Owens CM, Brisse HJ, Olsen OE, Begent J, Smets AM. Bilateral disease and new trends in Wilms tumour. Pediatr Radiol 2008;38(1):30–9.

[18] Owens CM, Veys PA, Pritchard J, Levitt G, Imeson J, Dicks-Mireaux C. Role of chest computed tomography at diagnosis in the management of Wilms' tumor: a study by the United Kingdom Children's Cancer Study Group. J Clin Oncol 2002; 20(12):2768–73.

[19] Wilimas JA, Kaste SC, Kauffman WM, Winer-Muram H, Morris R, Luo X, et al. Use of chest computed tomography in the staging of pediatric Wilms' tumor: interobserver variability and prognostic significance. J Clin Oncol 1997;15(7):2631–5.

[20] Ehrlich PF, Hamilton TE, Grundy P, Ritchey M, Haase G, Shamberger RC, et al. The value of surgery in directing therapy for patients with Wilms' tumor with pulmonary disease; A report from the National Wilms' Tumor Study Group (National Wilms' Tumor Study 5). J Pediatr Surg 2006;41(1):162–7; discussion 162–7.

[21] Smets AM, Tinteren HV, Bergeron C, Camargo BD, Graf N, Pritchard-Jones K, et al. The contribution of chest CT-scan at diagnosis in children with unilateral Wilms' tumour. Results of the SIOP 2001 study. Eur J Cancer 2012;48(7):1060–5.

[22] Vujanic GM, Sandstedt B, Harms D, Boccon-Gibod L, Delemarre JF. Rhabdoid tumour of the kidney: a clinicopathological study of 22 patients from the International Society of Paediatric Oncology (SIOP) nephroblastoma file. Histopathology 1996;28(4):333–40.

[23] van den Heuvel-Eibrink MM, Grundy P, Graf N, Pritchard-Jones K, Bergeron C, Patte C, et al. Characteristics and survival of 750 children diagnosed with a renal tumor in the first seven months of life: A collaborative study by the SIOP/GPOH/SFOP,

NWTSG, and UKCCSG Wilms tumor study groups. Pediatr Blood Cancer 2008;50(6):1130−4.

[24] Jadvar H, Connolly LP, Fahey FH, Shulkin BL. PET and PET/CT in pediatric oncology. Semin Nucl Med 2007;37(5):316−31.

[25] Moinul Hossain AK, Shulkin BL, Gelfand MJ, Bashir H, Daw NC, Sharp SE, et al. FDG positron emission tomography/computed tomography studies of Wilms' tumor. Eur J Nucl Med Mol Imaging 2010;37(7):1300−8.

[26] Misch D, Steffen IG, Schonberger S, Voelker T, Furth C, Stover B, et al. Use of positron emission tomography for staging, preoperative response assessment and posttherapeutic evaluation in children with Wilms tumour. Eur J Nucl Med Mol Imaging 2008;35(9):1642−50.

[27] Beckwith JB. Wilms' tumor and other renal tumors of childhood: a selective review from the National Wilms' Tumor Study Pathology Center. Hum Pathol 1983;14(6):481−92.

[28] Beckwith JB, Palmer NF. Histopathology and prognosis of Wilms tumors: results from the First National Wilms' Tumor Study. Cancer 1978;41(5):1937−48.

[29] Beckwith JB, Zuppan CE, Browning NG, Moksness J, Breslow NE. Histological analysis of aggressiveness and responsiveness in Wilms' tumor. Med Pediatr Oncol 1996;27(5):422−8.

[30] Faria P, Beckwith JB, Mishra K, Zuppan C, Weeks DA, Breslow N, et al. Focal versus diffuse anaplasia in Wilms tumor − new definitions with prognostic significance: a report from the National Wilms Tumor Study Group. Am J Surg Pathol 1996;20(8):909−20.

[31] Dome JS, Cotton CA, Perlman EJ, Breslow NE, Kalapurakal JA, Ritchey ML, et al. Treatment of anaplastic histology Wilms' tumor: results from the fifth National Wilms' Tumor Study. J Clin Oncol 2006;24(15):2352−8.

[32] Beckwith JB. Precursor lesions of Wilms tumor: clinical and biological implications. Med Pediatr Oncol 1993;21(3):158−68.

[33] Smets AM, de Kraker J. Malignant tumours of the kidney: imaging strategy. Pediatr Radiol 2010; 40(6):1010−8.

[34] Hennigar RA, O'Shea PA, Grattan-Smith JD. Clinicopathologic features of nephrogenic rests and nephroblastomatosis. Adv Anat Pathol 2001;8(5): 276−89.

[35] Coppes MJ, Arnold M, Beckwith JB, Ritchey ML, D'Angio GJ, Green DM, et al. Factors affecting the risk of contralateral Wilms tumor development: a report from the National Wilms Tumor Study Group. Cancer 1999;85(7):1616−25.

[36] Perlman EJ, Faria P, Soares A, Hoffer F, Sredni S, Ritchey M, et al. Hyperplastic perilobar nephroblastomatosis: long-term survival of 52 patients. Pediatr Blood Cancer 2006;46(2):203−21.

[37] Kalapurakal JA, Dome JS, Perlman EJ, Malogolowkin M, Haase GM, Grundy P, et al. Management of Wilms' tumour: current practice and future goals. Lancet Oncol 2004;5(1):37−46.

[38] Knudson Jr AG, Strong LC. Mutation and cancer: a model for Wilms' tumor of the kidney. J Natl Cancer Inst 1972;48(2):313−24.

[39] Dome JS, Coppes MJ. Recent advances in Wilms tumor genetics. Curr Opin Pediatr 2002;14(1):5−11.

[40] Miller RW, Fraumeni Jr JF, Manning MD. Association of Wilms' tumor with aniridia, hemihypertrophy and other congenital malformations. N Engl J Med 1964;270:922−7.

[41] Riccardi VM, Sujansky E, Smith AC, Francke U. Chromosomal imbalance in the Aniridia-Wilms' tumor association: 11p interstitial deletion. Pediatrics 1978;61(4):604−10.

[42] Rivera MN, Haber DA. Wilms' tumour: connecting tumorigenesis and organ development in the kidney. Nat Rev Cancer 2005;5(9):699−712.

[43] Scott RH, Stiller CA, Walker L, Rahman N. Syndromes and constitutional chromosomal abnormalities associated with Wilms tumour. J Med Genet 2006;43(9):705−15.

[44] DeBaun MR, Tucker MA. Risk of cancer during the first four years of life in children from The Beckwith−Wiedemann Syndrome Registry. J Pediatr 1998;132(3 Pt 1):398−400.

[45] Lapunzina P. Risk of tumorigenesis in overgrowth syndromes: a comprehensive review. Am J Med Genet C Semin Med Genet 2005;137C(1):53−71.

[46] Dome JS, Coppes MJ. Recent advances in Wilms tumor genetics. Curr Opin Pediatr 2002;14(1):5−11.

[47] Steenman MJ, Rainier S, Dobry CJ, Grundy P, Horon IL, Feinberg AP. Loss of imprinting of IGF2 is linked to reduced expression and abnormal methylation of H19 in Wilms' tumour. Nat Genet 1994;7(3):433−9.

[48] Rainier S, Johnson LA, Dobry CJ, Ping AJ, Grundy PE, Feinberg AP. Relaxation of imprinted genes in human cancer. Nature 1993;362(6422):747−9.

[49] Reeve AE. Role of genomic imprinting in Wilms' tumour and overgrowth disorders. Med Pediatr Oncol 1996;27(5):470−5.

[50] Koesters R, Ridder R, Kopp-Schneider A, Betts D, Adams V, Niggli F, et al. Mutational activation of the beta-catenin proto-oncogene is a common event in the development of Wilms' tumors. Cancer Res 1999;59(16):3880−2.

[51] Maiti S, Alam R, Amos CI, Huff V. Frequent association of beta-catenin and WT1 mutations in Wilms tumors. Cancer Res 2000;60(22):6288–92.

[52] Rivera MN, Kim WJ, Wells J, Driscoll DR, Brannigan BW, Han M, et al. An X chromosome gene, WTX, is commonly inactivated in Wilms tumor. Science 2007;315(5812):642–5.

[53] Ruteshouser EC, Robinson SM, Huff V. Wilms tumor genetics: mutations in WT1, WTX, and CTNNB1 account for only about one-third of tumors. Genes Chromosomes Cancer 2008;47(6):461–70.

[54] Major MB, Camp ND, Berndt JD, Yi X, Goldenberg SJ, Hubbert C, et al. Wilms tumor suppressor WTX negatively regulates WNT/beta-catenin signaling. Science 2007;316(5827):1043–6.

[55] Malkin D, Sexsmith E, Yeger H, Williams BR, Coppes MJ. Mutations of the p53 tumor suppressor gene occur infrequently in Wilms' tumor. Cancer Res 1994;54(8):2077–9.

[56] Beniers AJ, Efferth T, Fuzesi L, Granzen B, Mertens R, Jakse G. p53 expression in Wilms' tumor: a possible role as prognostic factor. Int J Oncol 2001;18(1):133–9.

[57] Bardeesy N, Beckwith JB, Pelletier J. Clonal expansion and attenuated apoptosis in Wilms' tumors are associated with p53 gene mutations. Cancer Res 1995;55(2):215–9.

[58] Scott RH, Walker L, Olsen OE, Levitt G, Kenney I, Maher E, et al. Surveillance for Wilms tumour in at-risk children: pragmatic recommendations for best practice. Arch Dis Child 2006;91(12): 995–9.

[59] Everman DB, Shuman C, Dzolganovski B, O'Riordan MA, Weksberg R, Robin NH. Serum alpha-fetoprotein levels in Beckwith–Wiedemann syndrome. J Pediatr 2000;137(1):123–7.

[60] Vujanic GM, Sandstedt B. The pathology of Wilms' tumour (nephroblastoma): the International Society of Paediatric Oncology approach. J Clin Pathol 2010;63(2):102–9.

[61] Weirich A, Ludwig R, Graf N, Abel U, Leuschner I, Vujanic GM, et al. Survival in nephroblastoma treated according to the trial and study SIOP-9/GPOH with respect to relapse and morbidity. Ann Oncol 2004;15(5):808–20.

[62] Gratias EJ, Dome JS. Current and emerging chemotherapy treatment strategies for Wilms tumor in North America. Paediatr Drugs 2008;10(2):115–24.

[63] Green DM, Beckwith JB, Weeks DA, Moksness J, Breslow NE, D'Angio GJ. The relationship between microsubstaging variables, age at diagnosis, and tumor weight of children with stage I/favorable histology Wilms' tumor. A report from the National Wilms' Tumor study. Cancer 1994;74(6):1817–20.

[64] Izawa JI, Al-Omar M, Winquist E, Stitt L, Rodrigues G, Steele S, et al. Prognostic variables in adult Wilms tumour. Can J Surg 2008;51(4):252–6.

[65] Mitry E, Ciccolallo L, Coleman MP, Gatta G, Pritchard-Jones K. EUROCARE Working Group. Incidence of and survival from Wilms' tumour in adults in Europe: data from the EUROCARE study. Eur J Cancer 2006;42(14):2363–8.

[66] Reinhard H, Semler O, Burger D, Bode U, Flentje M, Gobel U, et al. Results of the SIOP 93-01/GPOH trial and study for the treatment of patients with unilateral nonmetastatic Wilms tumor. Klin Padiatr 2004;216(3):132–40.

[67] Segers H, van den Heuvel-Eibrink MM, Pritchard-Jones K, Coppes MJ, Aitchison M, Bergeron C, et al. Management of adults with Wilms' tumor: recommendations based on international consensus. Expert Rev Anticancer Ther 2011;11(7):1105–13.

[68] Grundy PE, Telzerow PE, Breslow N, Moksness J, Huff V, Paterson MC. Loss of heterozygosity for chromosomes 16q and 1p in Wilms' tumors predicts an adverse outcome. Cancer Res 1994;54(9):2331–3.

[69] Grundy PE, Breslow NE, Li S, Perlman E, Beckwith JB, Ritchey ML, et al. Loss of heterozygosity for chromosomes 1p and 16q is an adverse prognostic factor in favorable-histology Wilms tumor: a report from the National Wilms Tumor Study Group. J Clin Oncol 2005;23(29):7312–21.

[70] Hing S, Lu YJ, Summersgill B, King-Underwood L, Nicholson J, Grundy P, et al. Gain of 1q is associated with adverse outcome in favorable histology Wilms' tumors. Am J Pathol 2001;158(2):393–8.

[71] Lu YJ, Hing S, Williams R, Pinkerton R, Shipley J, Pritchard-Jones K, et al. Chromosome 1q expression profiling and relapse in Wilms' tumour. Lancet 2002;360(9330):385–6.

[72] Dome JS, Bockhold CA, Li SM, Baker SD, Green DM, Perlman EJ, et al. High telomerase RNA expression level is an adverse prognostic factor for favorable-histology Wilms' tumor. J Clin Oncol 2005; 23(36):9138–45.

[73] Sredni ST, Gadd S, Huang CC, Breslow N, Grundy P, Green DM, et al. Subsets of very low risk Wilms tumor show distinctive gene expression, histologic, and clinical features. Clin Cancer Res 2009;15(22): 6800–9.

[74] Perlman EJ, Grundy PE, Anderson JR, Jennings LJ, Green DM, Dome JS, et al. WT1 mutation and 11P15 loss of heterozygosity predict relapse in very low-risk Wilms tumors treated with surgery alone: a

children's oncology group study. J Clin Oncol 2011;29(6):698–703.

[75] Williams RD, Hing SN, Greer BT, Whiteford CC, Wei JS, Natrajan R, et al. Prognostic classification of relapsing favorable histology Wilms tumor using cDNA microarray expression profiling and support vector machines. Genes Chromosomes Cancer 2004;41(1):65–79.

[76] Takahashi M, Yang XJ, Lavery TT, Furge KA, Williams BO, Tretiakova M, et al. Gene expression profiling of favorable histology Wilms tumors and its correlation with clinical features. Cancer Res 2002;62(22):6598–605.

[77] Huang CC, Gadd S, Breslow N, Cutcliffe C, Sredni ST, Helenowski IB, et al. Predicting relapse in favorable histology Wilms tumor using gene expression analysis: a report from the Renal Tumor Committee of the Children's Oncology Group. Clin Cancer Res 2009;15(5):1770–8.

[78] Gross RE, Neuhauser EB. Treatment of mixed tumors of the kidney in childhood. Pediatrics 1950;6(6):843–52.

[79] Sutow WW, Breslow NE, Palmer NF, D'Angio GJ, Takashima J. Prognosis in children with Wilms' tumor metastases prior to or following primary treatment: results from the first National Wilms' Tumor Study (NWTS-1). Am J Clin Oncol 1982;5(4):339–47.

[80] Green DM, Breslow NE, Evans I, Moksness J, Finklestein JZ, Evans AE, et al. The effect of chemotherapy dose intensity on the hematological toxicity of the treatment for Wilms' tumor. A report from the National Wilms' Tumor Study. Am J Pediatr Hematol Oncol 1994;16(3):207–12.

[81] Green DM, Breslow NE, Beckwith JB, Finklestein JZ, Grundy PE, Thomas PR, et al. Comparison between single-dose and divided-dose administration of dactinomycin and doxorubicin for patients with Wilms' tumor: a report from the National Wilms' Tumor Study Group. J Clin Oncol 1998;16(1):237–45.

[82] Breslow NE, Ou SS, Beckwith JB, Haase GM, Kalapurakal JA, Ritchey ML, et al. Doxorubicin for favorable histology, Stage II–III Wilms tumor: results from the National Wilms Tumor Studies. Cancer 2004;101(5):1072–80.

[83] Green DM. The treatment of stages I–IV favorable histology Wilms' tumor. J Clin Oncol 2004;22(8):1366–72.

[84] Shamberger RC, Guthrie KA, Ritchey ML, Haase GM, Takashima J, Beckwith JB, et al. Surgery-related factors and local recurrence of Wilms tumor in National Wilms Tumor Study 4. Ann Surg 1999;229(2):292–7.

[85] Green DM, Breslow NE, Beckwith JB, Ritchey ML, Shamberger RC, Haase GM, et al. Treatment with

nephrectomy only for small, stage I/favorable histology Wilms' tumor: a report from the National Wilms' Tumor Study Group. J Clin Oncol 2001;19(17):3719–24.

[86] Seibel NL, Li S, Breslow NE, Beckwith JB, Green DM, Haase GM, et al. Effect of duration of treatment on treatment outcome for patients with clear-cell sarcoma of the kidney: a report from the National Wilms' Tumor Study Group. J Clin Oncol 2004;22(3):468–73.

[87] Ehrlich PF. Bilateral Wilms' tumor: the need to improve outcomes. Expert Rev Anticancer Ther 2009;9(7):963–73.

[88] Lange J, Peterson SM, Takashima JR, Grigoriev Y, Ritchey ML, Shamberger RC, et al. Risk factors for end stage renal disease in non-WT1-syndromic Wilms tumor. J Urol 2011;186(2):378–86.

[89] Davidoff AM, Giel DW, Jones DP, Jenkins JJ, Krasin MJ, Hoffer FA, et al. The feasibility and outcome of nephron-sparing surgery for children with bilateral Wilms tumor. The St Jude Children's Research Hospital experience: 1999–2006. Cancer 2008;112(9):2060–70.

[90] Dome JS, Liu T, Krasin M, Lott L, Shearer P, Daw NC, et al. Improved survival for patients with recurrent Wilms tumor: the experience at St. Jude Children's Research Hospital. J Pediatr Hematol Oncol 2002;24(3):192–8.

[91] Malogolowkin M, Cotton CA, Green DM, Breslow NE, Perlman E, Miser J, et al. Treatment of Wilms tumor relapsing after initial treatment with vincristine, actinomycin D, and doxorubicin. A report from the National Wilms Tumor Study Group. Pediatr Blood Cancer 2008;50(2):236–41.

[92] Spreafico F, Pritchard Jones K, Malogolowkin MH, Bergeron C, Hale J, de Kraker J, et al. Treatment of relapsed Wilms tumors: lessons learned. Expert Rev Anticancer Ther 2009;9(12):1807–15.

[93] Green DM, Breslow NE, Ii Y, Grundy PE, Shochat SJ, Takashima J, et al. The role of surgical excision in the management of relapsed Wilms' tumor patients with pulmonary metastases: a report from the National Wilms' Tumor Study. J Pediatr Surg 1991;26(6):728–33.

[94] Green DM, Cotton CA, Malogolowkin M, Breslow NE, Perlman E, Miser J, et al. Treatment of Wilms tumor relapsing after initial treatment with vincristine and actinomycin D: a report from the National Wilms Tumor Study Group. Pediatr Blood Cancer 2007;48(5):493–9.

[95] Hale J, Hobson R, Moroz V, Sartori P. Results of UK Children's Cancer and Leukemia Group (CCLG) protocol for relapsed Wilms tumor (UKWR): unified relapse strategy improves outcome. Proceeding of

the 40th Meeting of International Society of Paediatric Oncology 2008;62:O154.

[96] Abu-Ghosh AM, Krailo MD, Goldman SC, Slack RS, Davenport V, Morris E, et al. Ifosfamide, carboplatin and etoposide in children with poor-risk relapsed Wilms' tumor: a Children's Cancer Group report. Ann Oncol 2002;13(3):460−9.

[97] Daw NC, Gregornik D, Rodman J, Marina N, Wu J, Kun LE, et al. Renal function after ifosfamide, carboplatin and etoposide (ICE) chemotherapy, nephrectomy and radiotherapy in children with Wilms tumour. Eur J Cancer 2009;45(1):99−106.

[98] Metzger ML, Stewart CF, Freeman 3rd BB, Billups CA, Hoffer FA, Wu J, et al. Topotecan is active against Wilms' tumor: results of a multi-institutional phase II study. J Clin Oncol 2007; 25(21):3130−6.

[99] Kremens B, Gruhn B, Klingebiel T, Hasan C, Laws HJ, Koscielniak E, et al. High-dose chemotherapy with autologous stem cell rescue in children with nephroblastoma. Bone Marrow Transplant 2002;30(12):893−8.

[100] Spreafico F, Bisogno G, Collini P, Jenkner A, Gandola L, D'Angelo P, et al. Treatment of high-risk relapsed Wilms tumor with dose-intensive chemotherapy, marrow-ablative chemotherapy, and autologous hematopoietic stem cell support: experience by the Italian Association of Pediatric Hematology and Oncology. Pediatr Blood Cancer 2008;51(1):23−8.

[101] Bruder E, Passera O, Harms D, Leuschner I, Ladanyi M, Argani P, et al. Morphologic and molecular characterization of renal cell carcinoma in children and young adults. Am J Surg Pathol 2004;28(9):1117−32.

[102] Ahmed HU, Arya M, Levitt G, Duffy PG, Mushtaq I, Sebire NJ. Part I: Primary malignant non-Wilms' renal tumours in children. Lancet Oncol 2007;8(8):730−7.

[103] Popov SD, Sebire NJ, Pritchard-Jones K, Vujanic GM. Renal tumors in children aged 10−16 years: a report from the United Kingdom Children's Cancer and Leukaemia Group. Pediatr Dev Pathol 2011; 14(3):189−93.

[104] Geller JI, Dome JS. Retroperitoneal lymph node dissection for pediatric renal cell carcinoma. Pediatr Blood Cancer 2009;52(3):430.

[105] Escudier B. Advanced renal cell carcinoma: current and emerging management strategies. Drugs 2007; 67(9):1257−64.

[106] Escudier B. Sunitinib for the management of advanced renal cell carcinoma. Expert Rev Anticancer Ther 2010;10(3):305−17.

[107] Argani P, Perlman EJ, Breslow NE, Browning NG, Green DM, D'Angio GJ, et al. Clear cell sarcoma of the kidney: a review of 351 cases from the National Wilms Tumor Study Group Pathology Center. Am J Surg Pathol 2000;24(1):4−18.

[108] Looi LM, Cheah PL. An immunohistochemical study comparing clear cell sarcoma of the kidney and Wilms' tumor. Pathology 1993;25(2):106−9.

[109] Radulescu VC, Gerrard M, Moertel C, Grundy PE, Mathias L, Feusner J, et al. Treatment of recurrent clear cell sarcoma of the kidney with brain metastasis. Pediatr Blood Cancer 2008;50(2):246−9.

[110] Haas JE, Palmer NF, Weinberg AG, Beckwith JB. Ultrastructure of malignant rhabdoid tumor of the kidney. A distinctive renal tumor of children. Hum Pathol 1981;12(7):646−57.

[111] Agrons GA, Kingsman KD, Wagner BJ, Sotelo-Avila C. Rhabdoid tumor of the kidney in children: a comparative study of 21 cases. AJR Am J Roentgenol 1997;168(2):447−51.

[112] Weeks DA, Beckwith JB, Mierau GW, Luckey DW. Rhabdoid tumor of kidney. A report of 111 cases from the National Wilms' Tumor Study Pathology Center. Am J Surg Pathol 1989;13(6):439−58.

[113] Versteege I, Sevenet N, Lange J, Rousseau-Merck MF, Ambros P, Handgretinger R, et al. Truncating mutations of hSNF5/INI1 in aggressive paediatric cancer. Nature 1998;394(6689):203−6.

[114] Biegel JA, Tan L, Zhang F, Wainwright L, Russo P, Rorke LB. Alterations of the hSNF5/INI1 gene in central nervous system atypical teratoid/rhabdoid tumors and renal and extrarenal rhabdoid tumors. Clin Cancer Res 2002;8(11):3461−7.

[115] Savla J, Chen TT, Schneider NR, Timmons CF, Delattre O, Tomlinson GE. Mutations of the hSNF5/INI1 gene in renal rhabdoid tumors with second primary brain tumors. J Natl Cancer Inst 2000;92(8):648−50.

[116] Tomlinson GE, Breslow NE, Dome J, Guthrie KA, Norkool P, Li S, et al. Rhabdoid tumor of the kidney in the National Wilms' Tumor Study: age at diagnosis as a prognostic factor. J Clin Oncol 2005;23(30):7641−5.

[117] Gururangan S, Bowman LC, Parham DM, Wilimas JA, Rao B, Pratt CB, et al. Primary extracranial rhabdoid tumors. Clinicopathologic features and response to ifosfamide. Cancer 1993;71(8): 2653−9.

[118] Waldron PE, Rodgers BM, Kelly MD, Womer RB. Successful treatment of a patient with stage IV rhabdoid tumor of the kidney: case report and review. J Pediatr Hematol Oncol 1999;21(1):53−7.

[119] Wagner L, Hill DA, Fuller C, Pedrosa M, Bhakta M, Perry A, et al. Treatment of metastatic rhabdoid tumor of the kidney. J Pediatr Hematol Oncol 2002;24(5):385−8.

[120] Glick RD, Hicks MJ, Nuchtern JG, Wesson DE, Olutoye OO, Cass DL. Renal tumors in infants less than 6 months of age. J Pediatr Surg 2004;39(4):522−5.

[121] Chen WY, Lin CN, Chao CS, Yan-Sheng Lin M, Mak CW, Chuang SS, et al. Prenatal diagnosis of congenital mesoblastic nephroma in mid-second trimester by sonography and magnetic resonance imaging. Prenat Diagn 2003;23(11):927−31.

[122] Rousseau-Merck MF, de Keyzer Y, Bourdeau A, Cournot G, Mercier F, Nezelof C. PTH mRNA transcription analysis in infantile tumors associated with hypercalcemia. Cancer 1988;62(2):303−8.

[123] Vido L, Carli M, Rizzoni G, Calo L, Dalla Palma P, Parenti A, et al. Congenital mesoblastic nephroma with hypercalcemia. Pathogenetic role of prostaglandins. Am J Pediatr Hematol Oncol 1986; 8(2):149−52.

[124] O'Malley DP, Mierau GW, Beckwith JB, Weeks DA. Ultrastructure of cellular congenital mesoblastic nephroma. Ultrastruct Pathol 1996;20(5):417−27.

[125] Knezevich SR, Garnett MJ, Pysher TJ, Beckwith JB, Grundy PE, Sorensen PH. ETV6-NTRK3 gene fusions and trisomy 11 establish a histogenetic link between mesoblastic nephroma and congenital fibrosarcoma. Cancer Res 1998;58(22):5046−8.

[126] Ahmed HU, Arya M, Levitt G, Duffy PG, Sebire NJ, Mushtaq I. Part II: Treatment of primary malignant non-Wilms' renal tumours in children. Lancet Oncol 2007;8(9):842−8.

[127] Gormley TS, Skoog SJ, Jones RV, Maybee D. Cellular congenital mesoblastic nephroma: what are the options. J Urol 1989;142(2 Pt 2):479−83. discussion 489.

[128] Beckwith JB, Weeks DA. Congenital mesoblastic nephroma; When should we worry? Arch Pathol Lab Med 1986;110(2):98−9

[129] Steinfeld AD, Crowley CA, O'Shea PA, Tefft M. Recurrent and metastatic mesoblastic nephroma in infancy. J Clin Oncol 1984;2(8):956−60.

[130] Furtwaengler R, Reinhard H, Leuschner I, Schenk JP, Goebel U, Claviez A, et al. Mesoblastic nephroma — a report from the Gesellschaft fur Padiatrische Onkologie und Hamatologie (GPOH). Cancer 2006;106(10):2275−83.

[131] McCahon E, Sorensen PH, Davis JH, Rogers PC, Schultz KR. Non-resectable congenital tumors with the ETV6-NTRK3 gene fusion are highly responsive to chemotherapy. Med Pediatr Oncol 2003;40(5):288−92.

[132] Wesche WA, Wilimas J, Khare V, Parham DM. Renal medullary carcinoma: a potential sickle cell nephropathy of children and adolescents. Pediatr Pathol Lab Med 1998;18(1):97−113.

[133] Strouse JJ, Spevak M, Mack AK, Arceci RJ, Small D, Loeb DM. Significant responses to platinum-based chemotherapy in renal medullary carcinoma. Pediatr Blood Cancer 2005;44(4):407−11.

[134] Avery RA, Harris JE, Davis Jr CJ, Borgaonkar DS, Byrd JC, Weiss RB. Renal medullary carcinoma: clinical and therapeutic aspects of a newly described tumor. Cancer 1996;78(1):128−32.

[135] Davis Jr CJ, Mostofi FK, Sesterhenn IA. Renal medullary carcinoma. The seventh sickle cell nephropathy. Am J Surg Pathol 1995;19(1):1−11.

[136] Bell MD. Response to paclitaxel, gemcitabine, and cisplatin in renal medullary carcinoma. Pediatr Blood Cancer 2006;47(2):228.

[137] Selby DM, Simon C, Foley JP, Thompson IM, Baddour RT. Renal medullary carcinoma: can early diagnosis lead to long-term survival? J Urol 2000; 163(4):1238.

[138] Cotton CA, Peterson S, Norkool PA, Takashima J, Grigoriev Y, Green DM, et al. Early and late mortality after diagnosis of Wilms tumor. J Clin Oncol 2009;27(8):1304−9.

[139] Termuhlen AM, Tersak JM, Liu Q, Yasui Y, Stovall M, Weathers R, et al. Twenty-five year follow-up of childhood Wilms tumor: a report from the Childhood Cancer Survivor Study. Pediatr Blood Cancer 2011;57(7):1210−6.

[140] Green DM, Grigoriev YA, Nan B, Takashima JR, Norkool PA, D'Angio GJ, et al. Congestive heart failure after treatment for Wilms' tumor: a report from the National Wilms' Tumor Study group. J Clin Oncol 2001;19(7):1926−34.

[141] Green DM, Grigoriev YA, Nan B, Takashima JR, Norkool PA, D'Angio GJ, et al. Correction to "Congestive heart failure after treatment for Wilms' tumor". J Clin Oncol 2003;21(12):2447−8.

[142] Pein F, Sakiroglu O, Dahan M, Lebidois J, Merlet P, Shamsaldin A, et al. Cardiac abnormalities 15 years and more after adriamycin therapy in 229 childhood survivors of a solid tumour at the Institut Gustave Roussy. Br J Cancer 2004;91(1): 37−44.

[143] Sorensen K, Levitt GA, Bull C, Dorup I, Sullivan ID. Late anthracycline cardiotoxicity after childhood cancer: a prospective longitudinal study. Cancer 2003;97(8):1991−8.

[144] Breslow NE, Collins AJ, Ritchey ML, Grigoriev YA, Peterson SM, Green DM. End stage renal disease in patients with Wilms tumor: results from the National Wilms Tumor Study Group and the United States Renal Data System. J Urol 2005;174(5):1972−5.

[145] Breslow NE, Takashima JR, Ritchey ML, Strong LC, Green DM. Renal failure in the Denys−Drash and Wilms' tumor−aniridia syndromes. Cancer Res 2000; 60(15):4030−2.

[146] Kantor AF, Li FP, Janov AJ, Tarbell NJ, Sallan SE. Hypertension in long-term survivors of childhood renal cancers. J Clin Oncol 1989;7(7):912–5.

[147] Bailey S, Roberts A, Brock C, Price L, Craft AW, Kilkarni R, et al. Nephrotoxicity in survivors of Wilms' tumours in the North of England. Br J Cancer 2002;87(10):1092–8.

[148] Bardi E, Olah AV, Bartyik K, Endreffy E, Jenei C, Kappelmayer J, et al. Late effects on renal glomerular and tubular function in childhood cancer survivors. Pediatr Blood Cancer 2004;43(6):668–73.

[149] Green DM, Peabody EM, Nan B, Peterson S, Kalapurakal JA, Breslow NE. Pregnancy outcome after treatment for Wilms tumor: a report from the National Wilms Tumor Study Group. J Clin Oncol 2002;20(10):2506–13.

[150] Wallace WH, Shalet SM, Hendry JH, Morris-Jones PH, Gattamaneni HR. Ovarian failure following abdominal irradiation in childhood: the radiosensitivity of the human oocyte. Br J Radiol 1989;62(743):995–8.

[151] Chiarelli AM, Marrett LD, Darlington G. Early menopause and infertility in females after treatment for childhood cancer diagnosed in 1964–1988 in Ontario, Canada. Am J Epidemiol 1999;150(3):245–54.

[152] Li FP, Gimbrere K, Gelber RD, Sallan SE, Flamant F, Green DM, et al. Outcome of pregnancy in survivors of Wilms' tumor. JAMA 1987;257(2):216–9.

[153] Kalapurakal JA, Peterson S, Peabody EM, Thomas PR, Green DM, D'Angio GJ, et al. Pregnancy outcomes after abdominal irradiation that included or excluded the pelvis in childhood Wilms tumor survivors: a report from the National Wilms Tumor Study. Int J Radiat Oncol Biol Phys 2004;58(5):1364–8.

[154] Green DM, Lange JM, Peabody EM, Grigorieva NN, Peterson SM, Kalapurakal JA, et al. Pregnancy outcome after treatment for Wilms tumor: a report from the national Wilms tumor long-term follow-up study. J Clin Oncol 2010;28(17):2824–30.

[155] Attard-Montalto SP, Kingston JE, Eden OB, Plowman PN. Late follow-up of lung function after whole lung irradiation for Wilms' tumour. Br J Radiol 1992;65(780):1114–8.

[156] Carli M, Frascella E, Tournade MF, de Kraker J, Rey A, Guzzinati S, et al. Second malignant neoplasms in patients treated on SIOP Wilms tumour studies and trials 1,2,5, and 6. Med Pediatr Oncol 1997;29(4):239–44.

[157] Breslow NE, Takashima JR, Whitton JA, Moksness J, D'Angio GJ, Green DM. Second malignant neoplasms following treatment for Wilm's tumor: a report from the National Wilms' Tumor Study Group. J Clin Oncol 1995;13(8):1851–9.

[158] Wright KD, Green DM, Daw NC. Late effects of treatment for Wilms tumor. Pediatr Hematol Oncol 2009;26(6):407–13.

[159] Hogeboom CJ, Grosser SC, Guthrie KA, Thomas PR, D'Angio GJ, Breslow NE. Stature loss following treatment for Wilms tumor. Med Pediatr Oncol 2001;36(2):295–304.

10

Renal Effects of Leukemia and Lymphoma

Kevin W. Finkel

UTHealth Science Center at Houston — Medical School, Houston, TX, USA
and University of Texas MD Anderson Cancer Center, Houston, TX, USA

INTRODUCTION

The development of renal disease is common in patients with lymphoma and leukemia. As with all hospitalized patients, those with lymphoma and leukemia are at risk for developing acute kidney injury (AKI) from hypotension, sepsis, or administration of radiocontrast, antifungal and antibacterial agents. With the presence of cancer, renal injury can also result from chemotherapy, immunosuppressive drugs, hematopoietic stem cell transplantation, or tumor lysis syndrome. Furthermore, patients are at risk for renal syndromes specific to the presence of lymphoma or leukemia. Various types of paraneoplastic glomerulonephritides are associated with lymphoma and leukemia and are described elsewhere in this book. This chapter will focus on infiltrative diseases of the kidney.

LYMPHOMA

Background

Although a variety of cancers can metastasize to the kidneys and invade the parenchyma, the most common malignancies to do so are lymphomas and leukemia. The true incidence of renal involvement is unknown since it is usually a silent disease and only occasionally causes renal impairment. Autopsy studies suggest renal involvement occurs in 90% of patients with lymphoma while radiographic evidence is significantly lower [1].

Clinical Features

Renal involvement in lymphoma is often clinically silent so patients can present with slowly progressive renal failure attributed to other etiologies. Therefore a high index of suspicion is needed to make a diagnosis. Patients do present with AKI but this is rare and is most commonly seen in highly malignant and disseminated disease [2–5]. Other presentations include proteinuria in both the nephrotic and non-nephrotic range, as well as a variety of glomerular lesions including pauci-immune crescentric glomerulonephritis [6]. Patients may present with flank pain and hematuria.

The cause of impaired renal function from lymphomatous infiltration is poorly understood.

Based on biopsy series, patients who present with AKI have predominantly bilateral interstitial infiltration of the kidneys with lymphoma cells and uniformly have increased renal size on radiographic imaging [7]. These findings suggest that increased interstitial pressure results in reduced intrarenal blood flow with subsequent renal tubular injury. Patients who present with proteinuria, on the other hand, often have intraglomerular infiltration with lymphoma [7]. It is not known how proteinuria develops in these cases but the local release of permeability factors and cytokines has been suggested [8,9].

Diagnosis

The diagnosis of renal failure resulting from lymphomatous infiltration is necessarily one of exclusion because more common explanations are often present. The diagnosis may be suspected from clinical features and imaging studies. Renal ultrasonography may reveal diffusely enlarged kidneys sometimes with multiple focal lesions. However, most times radiology will be unrevealing. In a study of 668 consecutive patients with lymphoproliferative disease who underwent diagnostic imaging with CT scan, only 3% with non-Hodgkin lymphoma were found to have kidney abnormalities [10]. Both diffuse enlargement and solitary lesions were detected. This discrepancy between radiological and autopsy/histopathological results may be due to the fact that renal involvement is often indolent and only detectable in histopathological examination. Due to increased metabolic activity within lymphomatous deposits, positron emission tomography may be a more sensitive imaging technique [11,12]. Although definitive diagnosis depends on renal biopsy, this procedure often is impossible because of the presence of contraindications. In such cases the following criteria support the diagnosis of renal failure as a result of lymphomatous infiltration: (1) renal enlargement without obstruction; (2) absence of other causes of renal failure; and (3) rapid improvement of renal failure after radiotherapy or systemic chemotherapy.

Treatment

The treatment of lymphomatous involvement of the kidney is directed at the underlying malignancy. There are numerous case reports of improvement in renal function after initiation of anti-tumor therapy. In indolent malignant disease that is usually treated by observation alone, kidney involvement is an indication for starting systemic therapy.

CYTOTOXIC NEPHROPATHY/ HEMOPHAGOCYTIC SYNDROME

Background

Hemophagocytic syndrome (HPS) is a reactive disorder that results from intense macrophage activation and cytokine release [13]. It is characterized by histiocytic proliferation, hemophagocytosis, fever, hypotension, hepatosplenomegaly, generalized lymphadenopathy and hypofibrinogenemia. It is the result of an intense cytokine storm similar to the systemic inflammatory response syndrome seen in patients with severe sepsis. Hemophagocytic syndrome was first described as a familial disorder of immune dysfunction in children. It is inherited in an autosomal recessive pattern with an estimated incidence of 1 per 50,000 live births [14,15]. Familial HPS is a fatal disease if untreated with a mean survival rate of 2 months [15]. It typically presents in infancy or early adolescence and can be triggered by infection.

It is now recognized that there are numerous forms of secondary HPS that can develop in a variety of diseases including malignant lymphoma, juvenile rheumatoid arthritis, severe bacterial and viral infections, and in patients receiving prolonged parenteral nutrition with soluble lipids [16].

Clinical Features

The clinical presentation of HPS is non-specific and can be confused with sepsis given their overlapping features. The most common symptoms are fever, hepatosplenomegaly and cytopenias [17]. Other findings may include liver dysfunction, coagulopathy with hypofibrinogenemia and neurological dysfunction. Less frequently patients can develop diffuse lymphadenopathy, jaundice, skin rash, respiratory failure and AKI. Histopathological examination of tissue reveals diffuse accumulation of lymphocytes and macrophages with occasional hemophagocytosis. There have been recent reports of HPS in association with occult peripheral T-cell lymphomas causing severe AKI [18]. Renal biopsy specimens are characterized by an unusually severe degree of interstitial edema with limited interstitial cellular infiltrate. Natural-killer (NK) cells tend to be low while a number of cytokines, including interferon-α, soluble interleukin-2 receptor, tumor necrosis factor-α, interleukin-6 and macrophage colony-stimulating factor are upregulated [18].

Diagnosis

Diagnosis should be suspected in any patient with malignant lymphoma who develops unexplained multiple organ dysfunction including AKI. Diagnostic criteria for diagnosing familial HPS were first developed in 1991 and later modified in 2004 (Table 10.1) [17]. However, many of the criteria have poor specificity for differentiating HPS from malignant lymphoma. Fever, splenomegaly, anemia, thrombocytopenia and hypofibrinogenemia are common to both. Therefore, bone marrow aspiration may be required for definitive diagnosis.

TABLE 10.1   Diagnostic Criteria for Familial Hemophagocytic Syndrome

1. Fever

2. Splenomegaly

3. Cytopenia ≥2 cell lines

4. Hypertriglyceridemia or hypofibrinogenemia

5. Hemophagocytosis (bone marrow, spleen, or lymph node)

6. Low or absent NK cell activity

7. Elevated serum ferritin

8. Elevated soluble interleukin-2 receptor

Modified from [17].

Treatment

Treatment of familial HPS includes cytotoxic agents, intravenous immunoglobulin (IVIG), therapeutic plasma exchange and hematopoietic stem cell transplantation [17]. It is not clear whether such regimens are effective in secondary cases of HPS due to lymphoma. Early initiation of chemotherapy is likely to be the best option. Case reports have described the use of high dose steroid and IVIG but most patients expired with multiple organ failure [19].

LEUKEMIA

Background

Leukemia cells can infiltrate any organ and the kidneys are the most frequent extramedullary site of infiltration. Autopsy studies reveal that 60–90% of patients have renal involvement [20]. On biopsy cells are usually located in the renal interstitium although occasional glomerular lesions are noted [7,21]. Increased interstitial pressure leads to vascular and tubular compression and subsequent tubular injury. Occasional nodular lesions are found but this is more common with lymphoma.

Clinical Features

Leukemic infiltration of the kidneys is often an indolent and clinically silent disease. Most often it is incidentally noted after autopsy or by detection of renal enlargement on ultrasound or CT scan. Although uncommon, many cases of AKI attributable to leukemic infiltration have been described [22–24]. Patients may also experience hematuria or proteinuria. Occasionally renal enlargement is accompanied by flank pain or fullness. Patients with significantly elevated white cell counts can develop AKI from leukostasis. Leukemic cells occlude the peritubular and glomerular capillaries thereby decreasing glomerular filtration rate. Patients may be oliguric but their renal function often improves with therapeutic leukopheresis or chemotherapy. Leukostasis has been described in both acute and chronic leukemia. There are also reports of patients with chronic lymphocytic leukemia who develop AKI from leukemic infiltration and are infected with polyomavirus (BK) [25]. Urine from patients demonstrates viral inclusions in tubular cells ("decoy" cells) and blood is positive for BK virus DNA. Therefore, in leukemia patients with AKI considered due to leukemic infiltration, evidence for coexisting BK virus infection should be sought.

Diagnosis

The diagnosis of leukemia infiltration as a cause of AKI requires a high level of vigilance since it is often clinically silent and leukemic patients usually have multiple alternative explanations for renal injury. A presumptive diagnosis can be made if there is no other obvious cause of AKI, bilateral renal enlargement is demonstrated radiographically and there is prompt improvement in renal function after chemotherapy. Screening for leukemic infiltration with radiographic imaging is not appropriate. In a study of 668 consecutive patients with lymphoproliferative disease who underwent diagnostic imaging with CT scan, only 5% with leukemia were found to have kidney abnormalities [10]. As with lymphoma, this discrepancy between radiological and autopsy/histopathological results may due to the fact that renal involvement is often indolent and only detectable in histopathological examination.

Treatment

Treatment is directed by the type of leukemia. Although some patients do not recover, in the majority of cases renal function does improve as the leukemia responds to systemic treatment.

References

[1] Schwartz JB, Shamsuddin AM. The effects of leukemic infiltrates in various organs in chronic lymphocytic leukemia. Hum Pathol 1981;12(5):432–40.

[2] Kanfer A, Vandewalle A, Morel-Maroger L, Feintuch MJ, Sraer JD, Roland J. Acute renal insufficiency due to lymphomatous infiltration of the kidneys: report of six cases. Cancer 1976;38(6):2588–92.

[3] Koolen MI, Schipper P, v Liebergen FJ, Kurstjens RM, v Unnik AJ, Bogman MJ. Non-Hodgkin lymphoma with unique localization in the kidneys presenting with acute renal failure. Clin Nephrol 1988;29(1):41–6.

[4] Malbrain ML, Lambrecht GL, Daelemans R, Lins RL, Hermans P, Zachee P. Acute renal failure due to bilateral lymphomatous infiltrates. Primary extranodal non-Hodgkin's lymphoma (p-EN-NHL) of the kidneys: does it really exist? Clin Nephrol 1994;42(3):163–9.

[5] Miyake JS, Fitterer S, Houghton DC. Diagnosis and characterization of non-Hodgkin's lymphoma in a patient with acute renal failure. Am J Kidney Dis 1990;16(3):262–3.

[6] Henriksen KJ, Hong RB, Sobrero MI, Chang A. Rare association of chronic lymphocytic leukemia/small lymphocytic lymphoma, ANCAs, and pauci-immune crescentic glomerulonephritis. Am J Kidney Dis 2011;57(1):170–4.

[7] Tornroth T, Heiro M, Marcussen N, Franssila K. Lymphomas diagnosed by percutaneous kidney biopsy. Am J Kidney Dis 2003;42(5):960–71.

[8] D'Agati V, Sablay LB, Knowles DM, Walter L. Angiotropic large cell lymphoma (intravascular malignant lymphomatosis) of the kidney: presentation as

minimal change disease. Hum Pathol Mar 1989;20(3):263—8.

[9] Agar JW, Gates PC, Vaughan SL, Machet D. Renal biopsy in angiotropic large cell lymphoma. Am J Kidney Dis 1994;24(1):92—6.

[10] Bach AG, Behrmann C, Holzhausen HJ, et al. Prevalence and patterns of renal involvement in imaging of malignant lymphoproliferative diseases. Acta Radiol 2012;53(3):343—8.

[11] Sheth S, Ali S, Fishman E. Imaging of renal lymphoma: patterns of disease with pathologic correlation. Radiographics 2006;26(4):1151—68.

[12] Metser U, Goor O, Lerman H, Naparstek E, Even-Sapir E. PET-CT of extranodal lymphoma. AJR Am J Roentgenol 2004;182(6):1579—86.

[13] Gauvin F, Toledano B, Champagne J, Lacroix J. Reactive hemophagocytic syndrome presenting as a component of multiple organ dysfunction syndrome. Crit Care Med 2000;28(9):3341—5.

[14] Henter JI, Elinder G, Ost A. Diagnostic guidelines for hemophagocytic lymphohistiocytosis. The FHL Study Group of the Histiocyte Society. Semin Oncol 1991;18(1): 29—33.

[15] Janka GE. Familial hemophagocytic lymphohistiocytosis. Eur J Pediatr 1983;140(3):221—30.

[16] Janka G, Imashuku S, Elinder G, Schneider M, Henter JI. Infection- and malignancy-associated hemophagocytic syndromes. Secondary hemophagocytic lymphohistiocytosis. Hematol Oncol Clin North Am 1998;12(2):435—44.

[17] Henter JI, Horne A, Arico M, et al. HLH-2004: Diagnostic and therapeutic guidelines for hemophagocytic lymphohistiocytosis. Pediatr Blood Cancer 2007;48(2): 124—31.

[18] Holt S, Varghese Z, Jarmulowicz M, et al. Cytokine nephropathy and multi-organ dysfunction in lymphoma. Nephrol Dial Transplant 1998;13(7): 1853—7.

[19] Hagihara M, Inoue M, Hua J, Iwaki Y. Lymphocyte-depleted Hodgkin lymphoma complicating hemophagocytic lymphohistiocytosis as an initial manifestation: a case report and review of the literature. Intern Med 2012;51(21):3067—72.

[20] Suh WM, Wainberg ZA, de Vos S, Cohen AH, Kurtz I, Nguyen MK. Acute lymphoblastic leukemia presenting as acute renal failure. Nat Clin Pract Nephrol 2007;3(2):106—10.

[21] Kowalewska J, Nicosia RF, Smith KD, Kats A, Alpers CE. Patterns of glomerular injury in kidneys infiltrated by lymphoplasmacytic neoplasms. Hum Pathol 2011;42(6):896—903.

[22] Comerma-Coma MI, Sans-Boix A, Tuset-Andujar E, Andreu-Navarro J, Perez-Ruiz A, Naval-Marcos I. Reversible renal failure due to specific infiltration of the kidney in chronic lymphocytic leukaemia. Nephrol Dial Transplant 1998;13(6):1550—2.

[23] Pagniez DC, Fenaux P, Delvallez L, Dequiedt P, Gosselin B, Tacquet A. Reversible renal failure due to specific infiltration in chronic lymphocytic leukemia. Am J Med 1988;85(4):579—80.

[24] Phillips JK, Bass PS, Majumdar G, Davies DR, Jones NF, Pearson TC. Renal failure caused by leukaemic infiltration in chronic lymphocytic leukaemia. J Clin Pathol 1993;46(12):1131—3.

[25] Boudville N, Latham B, Cordingly F, Warr K. Renal failure in a patient with leukaemic infiltration of the kidney and polyomavirus infection. Nephrol Dial Transplant 2001;16(5):1059—61.

11

Fluid and Electrolyte Abnormalities in Patients with Cancer

Ala Abudayyeh[1], Maen Abdelrahim[2], Abdulla Salahudeen[1]

[1]University of Texas MD Anderson Cancer Center, Houston, TX, USA
[2]Baylor College of Medicine and Institute of Biosciences and Technology,
Texas A&M Health Science Centre, Houston, TX, USA

INTRODUCTION

There has been increased survival of cancer patients due to advancement in chemotherapy and conditioning regimes, hematopoietic stem cell transplantation (HSCT) and general ICU care. However, challenges in cancer are still present such as increasing incidence rates and continued low survival for some cancers. Moreover, increased cancer survivorship and the use of new and stronger anti-cancer agents have left more patients with abnormalities of fluid and electrolyte balance. In this chapter we will discuss the delicate balance of electrolyte and water that the kidney maintains and the disturbances that can occur in the setting of cancer and cancer therapy. Acid–base and fluid electrolyte abnormalities are present in a sizeable proportion of patients, for example light chain loading of proximal tubules occasionally leading to severe tubular acidosis, hypokalemia and hypomagnesemia known as Fanconi's syndrome. Occasionally, ectopic secretion of hormones or hormone-like substances can lead to fluid and electrolyte disturbances; Syndrome of inappropriate antidiuretic hormone (SIADH) is the prototype that was first described in cancer patients [1,2]. A recent survey in hospitalized cancer patients reports that hyponatremia is as common as one in two patients and that it is strongly related to poor clinical outcomes [3]. Tumor lysis syndromes exclusive to cancer can be associated with severe acid–base and electrolyte abnormalities [4]. Furthermore, derangement in calcium, phosphorous and magnesium is common in cancer patients, often through unique mechanisms [5,6].

SODIUM AND WATER

The concentration of serum sodium, the primary extracellular cation, is tightly regulated, and a level lower than the lower limit of the laboratory range, usually 135 mEq/L, constitutes hyponatremia [7]. Often, the presence of hyponatremia indicates excess of total body water relative to sodium. The converse is also true in that water depletion leads to hypernatremia [7,8]. The pituitary-secreted antidiuretic hormone (ADH) (vasopressin) plays a key role in maintaining water balance primarily by regulating water excretion through the kidneys. When water content is low, the concentration of serum sodium increases vis-à-vis serum osmolality triggering the secretion of ADH. ADH in turn binds to the V2-receptors on the basolateral side of the medullary collecting tubules causing water reabsorption from the tubular lumen (Figure 11.1).

Higher serum sodium also leads to thirst stimulation resulting in increased water intake. Thus both reduced water loss and increased water intake restore water balance and thus sodium concentration. The converse is also true in that excess water intake, e.g. compulsive water drinking, can reduce serum sodium concentration that in turn shuts off the ADH secretion. This allows water loss through the kidney restoring water balance and sodium concentration. In cancer patients with dysnatremia, disruption in these efficient feedback mechanisms occurs at multiple levels leading to hyponatremia or hypernatremia.

Hyponatremia

Several drugs and conditions that are unique to cancer patients can cause hyponatremia (Table 11.1). Vincristine, vinblastine, cisplatin and cyclophosphamide are the chemotherapeutic agents most frequently associated with hyponatremia [10]. Hyponatremia has also been reported with carboplatin and ifosfamide administration, and recently with the administration

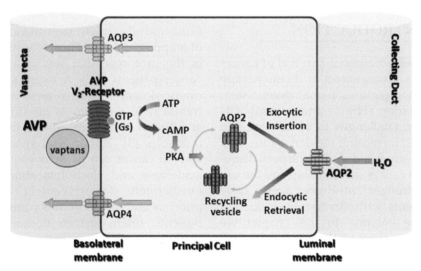

FIGURE 11.1 The principal cell of the kidney collecting duct. The V2 vasopressin receptor (V2-receptor) located in the basolateral cell surface binds to AVP present in the interstitial fluid, and activates the heterotrimeric protein G. Activated protein G increases the activity of the membrane-bound enzyme adenylyl cyclase (AC) causing an increase in the intracellular levels of cAMP. This in turn stimulates the activity of the cAMP-dependent protein kinase A (PKA), triggering a phosphorylation cascade that promotes the insertion of aquaporin 2 (AQP2) into the apical membrane of the cell. AVP-regulated AQP2 increases the water permeability of the apical membrane and allows the reabsorption of water from the hypotonic processed filtrate into the surrounding hypertonic interstitium. The water can exit the cell through the aquaporin 3 and aquaporin 4 water channels, constitutively present in the basolateral surface of the cells. Vaptans are synthetic vasopressin receptor antagonists. By interfering with AVP–V2R interaction they prevent aquaporin-mediated water reabsorption. This figure is reproduced in color in the color plate section. *Modified from Mayinger and Hensen [9].*

TABLE 11.1 Causes of Hyperkalemia and Hypokalemia in Cancer Patients

Hypokalemia	Hyperkalemia
Decreased potassium intake	Tumor lysis syndrome
Elevation in extracellular PH	Type I RTA
Increase in hematopoietic cell production	Acidosis
Hypothermia	Drugs: Bactrim, pentamidine, amiloride triameterene, cyclosporine, ACE inhibitors and ARB
Diarrhea	
Increased mineralocorticoid activity	

of immunomodulators such as interferon and interleukin-2 [10–13]. The precise mechanism by which all these drugs derange the salt and water homeostasis is generally not known. For vinca alkaloids and cisplatin and possibly with other alkylating agents, SIADH is described as a potential mechanism [14]. In one study administration of cyclophosphamide was not associated with increase in ADH levels, but study findings were consistent with potentiation by cyclophosphamide or its metabolites of ADH effects at tubular level [15]. Renal salt wasting has been described with platinum compounds, a likely mechanism for hyponatremia. While ectopic ADH secretion by small cell lung tumor is the prototype of SIADH [16], relative excess of ADH levels in the systemic circulation often occurs due to ineffective plasma volume as a result of volume depletion (vomiting and diarrhea, for example, from chemotherapy). Relative excess of ADH coupled with excessive fluid intake, often hypotonic, that often accompanies chemotherapy is probably the most common clinical scenario that leads to mild to moderate hyponatremia in hospitalized cancer patients [17]. Furthermore, cancer patients receiving chemotherapy are encouraged to drink plenty of fluid which often leads to excessive water intake. In a prospective study limited to 106 cancer patients with hyponatremia, volume depletion and SIADH accounted for nearly two-thirds of all causes of hyponatremia, although such clear separation of causes in clinical practice can be difficult as multiple factors for hyponatremia can coexist in cancer patients [17]. The cause of hyponatremia in cancer patients can often be multifactorial as illustrated in this example: A patient is on thiazide diuretic for hypertension, who is now hypovolemic due to vomiting and diarrhea from chemotherapy for diffuse B-cell lymphoma that includes cyclophosphamide. The patient is now only able to keep clear water down. In this clinical scenario, volume depletion is a strong stimulus for ADH secretion thus increasing this patient's ADH levels. Further, cyclophosphamide is known to potentiate ADH water reabsorption at the tubular level, whereas thiazide and excess water intake are well known to aggravate hyponatremia.

Pain and pain medications commonly used in cancer patients are associated with potentiation of ADH and so contribute to hyponatremia in cancer patients [18]. Antidepressants are widely used in cancer patients and they — especially the SSRIs — are well known to be associated with hyponatremia [19]. Ectopic hormones, notably ectopic ADH secretion, can cause hyponatremia and nearly one-third of hyponatremia in small cell lung cancer (SCLC) is due to SIADH [1,2]. Some patients with SCLC may have ectopic production of ANP as the cause of their hyponatremia, although in one study AVP appears to be elevated in nearly all patients with SCLC and hyponatremia [20,21]. In clinical practice the classical features of SIADH may not always be present in cancer patients, but the cardinal features such as inappropriately elevated urine osmolality >100 mOsm/kg in the setting of decreased serum osmolality (<275 mOsm/kg) and urine sodium concentration adequate to exclude hypovolemia (>20 mmol/L) often point towards absolute or relative excess of ADH [22].

HYPOALBUMINEMIA, INTRAVASCULAR VOLUME CONTRACTION AND HYPONATREMIA

Hypoalbuminemia is quite common in cancer patients especially during the treatment phase or in the terminal stage. In both occasions malnutrition is an important cause for chronic hypoalbuminemia, although acute hypoalbuminemia as a reflection of possible acute hepatic chemotoxicity can occur in patients receiving chemotherapy as noted in this case report (Figure 11.2). The patient was a 53-year-old man with myeloma-related end stage renal disease who had been on dialysis for 2 years. His myeloma had relapsed after recent chemotherapy and SCT and he was readmitted to receive additional chemotherapy consisting of cyclophosphamide, doxorubicin, bortezomib and dexamethasone. The graph shows the acute depressive effect of chemotherapy on serum albumin levels. Hypoalbuminemia can reduce the effective plasma volume triggering ADH secretion and this combined with customary high fluid intake during chemotherapy can be a potential mechanism that contributes to hyponatremia in chemo-treated cancer patients.

CLINICAL OUTCOMES IN CANCER PATIENTS WITH HYPONATREMIA

Although a large body of literature is available on the epidemiology of hyponatremia in patients with non-cancer conditions, such information in patients with cancer, especially its frequency or impact on clinical outcomes, is limited [23–27]. In a recent analysis of prospectively collected data on 3357 patients admitted to the University of Texas MD Anderson Cancer Center (MDACC) over a 3-month period in 2006, we reported a hyponatremia (sodium <135 mEq/L) rate of 48% in hospitalized cancer patients, which is almost one in two patients hospitalized [3]. This frequency is higher than

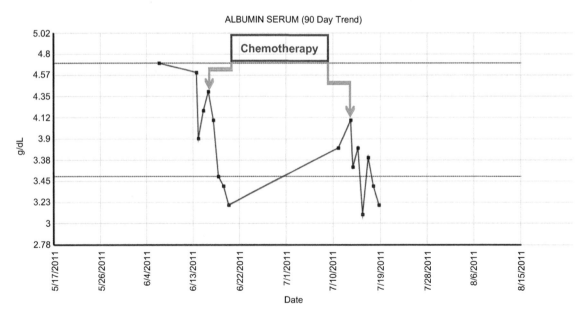

FIGURE 11.2 **Acute depressive effect of chemotherapy on serum albumin levels.** This figure is reproduced in color in the color plate section.

some of the highest frequencies reported in hospitalized non-cancer patients [27]. In our survey, eunatremia and hypernatremia were categorized as: eunatremia = 135–147 mEq/L, mild hyponatremia = 134–130 mEq/L, moderate hyponatremia = 129–120 mEq/L and severe hyponatremia = <120 mEq/L. Severe hyponatremia was noted in 1%, moderate in 10% and the majority was mild in 36%. Hyponatremia was acquired during a hospital stay in 24%. As in non-cancer patients, a strong and independent association was demonstrable between hyponatremia and clinical outcomes in hospitalized cancer patients [27–29]. The mean length of stay was found to be prolonged in hyponatremic patients: 5.6 ± 5.0 (mean $\pm$ SD) days for eunatremics, and 9.9 ± 9.2, 13.0 ± 14.1 and 11.5 ± 12.6 days for mild, moderate and severe hyponatremics, respectively. Similarly the hazard ratio for 90-day mortality (HR, 95% CI) in the multivariate model was also higher for patients with hyponatremia compared to eunatremic patients: mild vs. eunatremia 2.04 (1.42–2.91), moderate vs. eunatremia 4.74 (3.21–7.01) and severe vs. eunatremia 3.46 (1.05–11.44). In general, hyponatremia patients in our survey were sicker and often terminally ill. While there is little doubt that hyponatremia in hospitalized patients is associated with very poor clinical outcomes, what is less certain at this time is whether correction of hyponatremia especially with the availability of orally active V2-receptor antagonist will improve outcomes of these patients.

POTASSIUM

The concentration of serum potassium, the main intracellular cation, is primarily regulated by the handling of its excretion by the kidneys. Of the estimated 3500 meq of potassium (50 meq/kg) present in the intracellular space, there is 3.5–5.0 meq/L in the extracellular space because of the presence of Na^+/K^+ ATPase in

every cell membrane. Different stimuli such as insulin, ephinephrine, alkalosis and acidosis induce changes in potassium. To maintain potassium balance and serum potassium within the range, the body must excrete the daily intake of potassium (50–150 meq/day) through the kidneys. Almost all of the filtered K^+ is reabsorbed in the proximal tubule and the loop of Henle, so that less than 10% of the filtered load is delivered to the early distal tubule passively following that of Na^+ and water from the proximal tubule. The reabsorption in the thick ascending limb of the loop of Henle is mediated by the $Na^+/K^+/2Cl^-$ carrier in the luminal membrane. K^+ is secreted mainly by the principal cells in the cortical and outer medullary collecting tubule. This distal secretion can be partially counteracted by K^+ reabsorption by the intercalated cells Type A in the cortical and outer medullary collecting tubules. In Type A intercalated cells the process of potassium reabsorption may be mediated by an active H^+-K^+-ATPase pump in the luminal membrane, which results in both H^+ secretion and K^+ reabsorption. The activity of this pump is increased with K^+ depletion and is reduced with K^+ loading. Potassium secretion mainly occurs in the sodium reabsorbing principal cells in the collecting tubules. The selective sodium channels or ENaC creates an electronegative gradient in the lumen by which potassium is secreted into the lumen via K channels (ROMK) in the apical membrane. The two most important determinants are mineralocorticoid activity and distal delivery of salt and water, both have relevance in the derangement of K^+ balance in cancer patients such as aldosterone secreting tumors or reduced urine flow rate in postchemotherapy hypovolemic patients. Aldosterone causes ENaC channels to be more open and increases Na^+ reabsorption. This leads to increased electro-negativity of the lumen and further secretion of potassium. Also aldosterone increases intracellular potassium by increasing Na^+/K^+ ATPase and increases luminal membrane permeability to potassium. Distal delivery of sodium will increase sodium reabsorption and therefore create increased luminal electro-negativity and increase potassium secretion. With increased flow rate this will continue to maintain low potassium concentration in the luminal membrane and be the driving force for potassium continued secretion [30]. The converse is true in that in the prerenal state distal sodium delivery is reduced decreasing the luminal potassium secretion. Two important potassium channels have been noted in the cortical collecting duct. The renal outer medullary K^+ (ROMK) channel has a low conductance and high probability of being open under physiological conditions. The other channel is the maxi-K^+ channel which is a large conductance channel activated under increased flow. In the principal cells increased flow leads to increased intracellular calcium and therefore activates the maxi-K^+ channels. The cilium on the principal cells is believed to detect the increased flow rate and therefore lead to increased intracellular calcium. Increased potassium intake has been shown to increase ROMK and maxi-K potassium channel expression [31]. Long WNK1 antagonizes kidney-specific kinases named kidney specific with-no-lysine (KS-WNK1) effects. Long WNK1 inhibits effects of ROMK by stimulating endocytosis of the channel which is appropriate in the setting of hypokalemia. Long-WNK1 also stimulates activity of EnaC. The ratio of long WNK1 to KS-WNK1 is important in maintaining potassium balance [32]. Hypokalemia can lead to an increase in BP by decreased potassium; there is an increased ratio of WNK-1 to KS-WNK1 and therefore there is decreased ROMK channels but also increased NA/Cl channels and EnaC activity.

Plasma concentration of potassium is a determinant of potassium excretion and vice versa. A faster tubular flow rate allows tubular potassium loss leading to lower serum potassium. Alkalosis increases potassium secretion because a decrease in intracellular hydrogen results in an intracellular potassium increase and hence secretion. Aldosterone effects in the principal cells combine with the cytosolic mineralocorticoid receptor (Aldo-R) and lead to enhanced Na reabsorption and potassium secretion by increasing both the number of open Na channels and the number of Na,K-ATPase pumps. Increased aldosterone secretion is directly stimulated by increased plasma potassium concentration. Atrial natriuretic peptide, on the other hand, acts primarily in the inner medullary collecting duct by combining with its basolateral membrane receptor (ANP-R) and activating guanylate cyclase. ANP inhibits sodium reabsorption by closing the Na channels [33]. The potassium-sparing diuretics act by closing Na channels, amiloride and triamterene directly and spironolactone by competing with aldosterone.

Serum potassium is tightly regulated and as we discussed kidney plays a central role. Disturbance in serum potassium is common in cancer patients through a variety of mechanisms (Table 11.1). One of the most common clinical settings is tumor lysis syndrome (TLS), which is caused by the disintegration of malignant cells, usually following the initiation of chemotherapy or rapidly growing tumor, especially hematologic malignancies such as acute leukemia with high white cell counts at presentation or diffuse Burkitt-type non-Hodgkin lymphoma.

When these cells start to break down intracellular ions, proteins, nucleic acids and their metabolites are released into the plasma causing the characteristic metabolic abnormalities of hyperuricemia, hyperkalemia, hyperphosphatemia and hypocalcemia. Hyperkalemia is often the earliest and potentially the most serious clinical consequence. In order for patient stability there has to be increased potassium and phosphate ions and uric acid excretion. By increasing fluid intake and the use of uricosuric drugs, this may be achieved. However, crystallization of uric acid and calcium phosphate in the renal tubules leads to reduced renal excretion of potassium with consequent worsening of plasma hyperkalemia, which can contribute to hypocalcemia and as a result lead to cardiac death [34]. Potassium load will be extremely high in urate crystals and calcium phosphate precipitation leading to acute tubular necrosis (ATN). The thick ascending loop of Henle and principal cells of the collecting duct will no longer adequately secrete excess potassium. Therefore in order to increase kaliuresis, urinary flow rate should be increased using intravenous infusion of saline with sodium bicarbonate solutions. This increase will lead to activation of maxi-K channels and potassium secretion into the tubules.

Cancer patients following chemotherapy will be immunocompromised and at high risk of developing infections possibly leading to sepsis/hypotension, increased lactic acidosis and hyperkalemia. During episodes of sepsis and neutropenic fevers antifungal use is the mainstay in the critically ill which can result in Fanconi's-like syndrome and cause multiple electrolyte loss, especially potassium.

Development of both proximal and distal renal tubular acidosis associated with multiple myeloma, monoclonal gammopathies and use of ifosfamide can cause potassium disturbances. Proximal RTA in adults includes light chain-induced proximal tubular toxicity and hypokalemia/acidosis. Long-term effects can also lead to distal RTA with impaired tubular acidification and hyperkalemia (Type 1 RTA) [35]. Steroids are also used as part of the chemotherapeutic regimen or in acute sepsis can have mineralocorticoid effects leading to hypokalemia. Other causes of hyperkalemia are the following: potassium-sparing diuretics such as amiloride and triameterene; antibiotics such as bactrim, pentamidine block ENaC leading to hyperkalemia; immunosuppressive agents such as cyclosporin blocks Na^+/K^+ ATPase in the distal nephron, leading to hyperkalemia; and the use of ACEi and ARB, which can lead to hyperkalemia due to their aldosterone inhibitory effects and therefore decreased potassium secretion in the collecting tubule principal cells.

MAGNESIUM

Derangement in magnesium metabolism or body content is rare in the general patient population but fairly common in patients with cancer, often related to renal toxicity of drugs used for chemotherapy, HCT or both. We will review the renal handling of magnesium followed by its derangements in cancer patients. The average daily magnesium intake is 360 mg (15 mmol). Forty to fifty percent of dietary magnesium is reabsorbed in the gastrointestinal tract mediated by a channel encoded by the TRPM6 gene. Total body magnesium in the body is 25 g with 60−65% in the bone and the rest in the intracellular muscle and soft tissue. One percent of total body magnesium is present in the extracellular fluid compartment. Serum magnesium in a healthy individual is closely maintained at 1.50−2.30 meq/L. Only 20% is protein bound, therefore variations in serum albumin have less of an effect, unlike calcium. One to two percent of the 28 g of magnesium in an adult body is present in the extracellular fluid compartment − 350 meq is in muscle complexed to intracellular organic phosphates and proteins. Bone has 1200 meq of the magnesium content.

Regarding the renal handling of magnesium, about 95−97% of filtered magnesium is reabsorbed by the kidney with only 15−25% in the proximal tubule. The thick ascending loop of Henle absorbs 60−70% of the filtered load via a paracellular process. The lumen (+) in this segment drives this process via tight junction proteins, Claudin-16 and -19, which control paracellular permeability to magnesium. The extracellular Ca^{2+}/Mg^{2+} sensing receptor (caSR) if activated then reduces calcium and magnesium reabsorption in the thick ascending loop of Henle. Inhibition of ROMK apical potassium channels in the thick ascending loop of Henle would decrease the gradient that fuels the $Na^+/K^+/2Cl^-$ (NKCC2) cotransporter and therefore causes reduction in transepithelial voltage and paracellular permeability of magnesium and calcium. Final urinary magnesium is regulated by the distal convoluted tubule. Cellular uptake is mediated in the cortical collecting tubule by a channel in the luminal membrane called TRPM6 (transient receptor potential cation channel, subfamily M, member 6). It is believed to be a sodium/magnesium exchanger and in the presence of low intracellular sodium (10 to 15 meq/L) compared to that in the extracellular fluid, there is an increased magnesium reabsorption. Therefore the use of thiazide diuretics and amiloride which inhibit sodium chloride reabsorption in the distal tubule will lead to low intracellular sodium and increased activity of TRMP6, and therefore reabsorb magnesium as explained above. Enhanced magnesium reabsorption via TRMP6 channels is increased due to increased sex hormones, parathyroid hormone (PTH), calcitonin, glucagon, arginine, vasopressin and acid−base status [36]. Epidermal growth factor has also been implicated in increased TRMP6 activity and therefore increased magnesium reabsorption. Therefore in colorectal cancer patients treated with cetuximab and EGF receptor targeted monoclonal antibody, hypomagnesemia is common. Also, tacrolimus and cyclosporine A decrease TRMP6 expression and therefore contribute to hypomagnesemia.

Magnesium excretion is determined by the plasma magnesium concentration. Also, hypocalcemia leads to a decrease in magnesium reabsorption in the thick ascending limb and distal convoluted tubule. This is all mediated by the calcium sensing receptor in the basolateral membrane. Volume contraction increases reabsorption in the proximal tubule while volume expansion decreases. Aldosterone can increase reabsorption in the thick ascending loop and the distal convoluted tubule. Loop diuretics reduce reabsorption of magnesium because of the reduction of the lumen-positive transepithelial membrane.

Although several causes such as GI losses, malabsorption, or rare gene mutation in TRPM6 can lead to hypomagnesemia, drugs that impair magnesium reabsorption in the distal convoluted tubule and thick ascending loop of Henle are the commonest cause in cancer patients. They include cisplatin, ifosfamide, cetuximab, amphotericin B, carboplatin, aminoglycosides, foscarnet, pemtamidine and calceneurin inhibitors to mention the most clinically encountered drugs [37]. These drugs can cause severe tubular injury and take months to resolve even after cessation of the drug for hypomagnesemia. Cetuximab, a human/mouse chimeric monoclonal antibody, causes reversible urinary magnesium wasting by binding to the EGF and EGFR which are expressed in the kidney DCT and contribute to magnesium balance [37]. Long-term parenteral nutrition is required especially in GI cancers and can lead to magnesium deficiency. Other rare causes of hypomagnesemia that occur in non-cancer patients are Gitelman's syndrome where there is a mutation of the DCT Na^+/Cl^- cotransporter, pancreatitis from precipitation of calcium and magnesium in the pancreas and low PTH after thyroid−parathyroid surgery [38]. Also, increased magnesium wasting is noted in hyperthyroidisim, hyperaldosteronism and SIADH contributing to hypomagnesemia.

Hypermagnesemia is rare and usually occurs if there is excessive supplementation with laxatives, antacids, Epsom salts and magnesium-containing enemas especially in patients with impaired magnesium excretion as in AKI or CKD. In order to treat such patients effectively and prevent respiratory depression or cardiac arrhythmias, serum calcium can be increased which would act as a direct antagonist. Also, use of saline and diuretics as explained earlier can lead to increased magnesium excretion. If renal function is poor in patients with severe hypomagnesemia use of hemodialysis can help to lower magnesium to safer levels as in severe hypercalcemia.

URIC ACID

Uric acid is the end product of purine metabolism. Purine degradation involves the breakdown of the purine mononucleotides, guanylic acid (GMP), inosinic acid (IMP) and adenylic acid (AMP) into guanine and hypoxanthine. The latter two compounds are then metabolized to xanthine. Xanthine oxidase irreversibly oxidizes xanthine to produce uric acid. Humans do not have the ability to metabolize urate, therefore it needs to be eliminated via the GI tract or the kidney. In the intestines there are bacteria that would be able to degrade uric acid (uricolysis) which is a third of total urate excretion. Urinary uric acid excretion accounts for the remaining two-thirds of the daily uric acid disposal. Uric acid dissociates in to hydrogen ion and urate and it is handled exclusively by the proximal tubule in three different stages. Uric acid excretion involves glomerular filtration. In the proximal tubule the following occurs: presecretory reabsorption; secretion; and postsecretory reabsorption. Less than 5% of urate is bound to serum proteins and there is a net 90% absorption of the filtered urate in the early proximal tubule. Tubular secretion, which is the source of most of the uric acid excreted, occurs in the S2 segment of the proximal tubule, which returns 50% of the filtered urate to the tubular lumen. Finally, in the S3 segment of the proximal tubule there is reabsorption of the urate.

Two transporters belonging to the organic acid transporter (OAT) family, URAT1 encoded by the SLC22A12 gene and Glut9, are responsible for urate balance. In the luminal membrane of the proximal renal tubular epithelial cells urate/organic anion exchanger (URAT1) is present. The function of this transporter is independent of direct sodium—urate cotransport and is not driven by membrane potential. Inhibition of URAT1 is mediated by the following metabolites and drugs: probenecid, losartan, nonsteroidal anti-inflammatory agents, lactate, nicotinate, acetoacetate, hydroxybutyrate and succinate. To drive the entry of uric acid into the cell via the organic anion transporter (OAT) 1, alpha-ketoglutarate, a citric acid intermediate, can enter the cell by cotransport with sodium across the basolateral membrane (via the sodium-dicarboxylate symporter [NaDC-3]). This accumulation of alpha-ketoglutarate creates a favorable outward gradient for this compound and the entry of uric acid into the cell. Glucose transporter 9 (GLUT9), a voltage-driven urate efflux transporter, mediates urate reabsorption from the tubular cell to the circulation. GLUT9 is inhibited also by the uricosuric agents probenecid and benzbromarone. Overall energy for transport is provided by the Na^+/K^+ ATPase pump by maintaining a low cell Na^+ concentration and a concentration gradient is created favoring sodium to enter the cell.

The net effect is the excretion of 6—12% of the amount filtered. Alterations in excretion according to urate homeostasis are thought to be mediated primarily by changes in the rate of tubular secretion. Net urate reabsorption also varies directly with proximal Na^+ transport and, in the presence of volume depletion, both Na^+ and urate excretion are reduced. In the setting of diuretic therapy there is increased sodium loss and therefore increased sodium and uric acid reabsorption in the proximal tubule leading to hyperuricemia which is common with diuretic therapy.

Acute uric acid nephropathy (UAN) is a result of undissociated uric acid precipitation in renal tubules and crystals of monosodium urate in the renal interstitium, leading to acute oliguric renal failure. This is most often due to overproduction and overexcretion of uric acid in patients with lymphoma, leukemia, or a myeloproliferative disease (such as polycythemia vera), especially after chemotherapy or radiation has induced rapid cell lysis. Plasma uric acid concentration generally above 15 mg/dL and many uric acid crystals can be seen on urinanalysis. Chronic exposure to high levels of uric acid may lead to chronic renal disease. It has been shown in rats that experimental hyperuricemia induced by oxonic acid (uricase inhibitor) induced systemic hypertension, glomerular hypertrophy/hypertension, afferent arteriolar sclerosis, macrophage infiltration in normal rat kidney, tubulointerstitial fibrosis and eventually glomerulosclerosis [39]. Uric acid may have a key role in initiating renal arteriolar lesions in high-risk patients such as the elderly, obese black population, subjects with gout or hyperuricemia, chronic lead ingestion, metabolic syndrome and chronic diuretic use, therefore increasing their risk for early renal disease progression [40]. There is also evidence that an elevated uric acid may potentiate the effects of angiotensin II to induce renal vasoconstriction which could possibly be mediated by its effect to upregulate angiotensin type I receptors on vascular smooth muscle cells and lead to hypertension [41]. In cyclosporine nephropathy, which is a progressive renal disease, it has been shown in remnant kidney that there is glomerular hypertension and cortical vasoconstriction. Also, it has been shown that an increase in uric acid exacerbates cyclosporine nephropathy in the rat. Concomitant treatment with allopurinol or benzbromarone reduced the severity of renal disease [42]. In addition, uric acid stimulated inflammatory mediators in the vascular [43]. A study published in 2008 examined the association between uric acid and progression of renal disease. Data from 21,475 healthy volunteers who were followed prospectively for a median of 7 years were analyzed. The data indicated that the risk for incident kidney disease increased roughly linearly with uric acid level to a level of approximately 6 to 7 mg/dl in women and 7 to 8 mg/dl

in men; above these levels, the associated risk increased rapidly [44].

In the setting of cancer, acute kidney injury (AKI) associated with tumor lysis syndrome (TLS) may both have a crystal-dependent and a crystallin-dependent mechanism of renal injury. Uric acid has antiangiogenic effects such as inhibition of endothelial cell proliferation and migration, and stimulation of endothelial cell apoptosis. It also stimulates pro-inflammatory mechanisms such as MCP-1 and CRP, and activation of NF-κB and p38 MAPK [41]. Uric acid has been shown even with absence of crystal formation to have pro-oxidative properties (stimulation of oxidants and peroxynitrite-associated radicals) that may perpetuate renal injury. In the presence of crystal formation there is of course mechanical obstructive nephropathy which results during TLS [45].

Rasburicase is highly effective for prevention and management of hyperuricemia in adults at risk for tumor lysis syndrome (TLS). In a recent study published in *Annals of Oncology* (2011), a single-dose rasburicase was effective in the management of a patient with hyperuricemia secondary to TLS; only a subset of high-risk patients required a second dose {Vadhan-Raj, 2011 #143}.

PHOSPHATE

Serum phosphate is present in two forms: organic and inorganic. Organic phosphorus is composed entirely of phospholipid-bound proteins. Inorganic phosphorus is the form that is measured and used. Ninety percent of inorganic phosphorus is ultrafilterable of which 53% is dissociated in a 1:4 ratio of H_2PO_4- to H_2PO_4-2 and the rest are in salts form sodium, magnesium and calcium. When phosphorus reaches levels >8 mg/dl it complexes with calcium and is removed from the circulation. Phosphorus decreases during hyperventilation and alkalosis and increases during acidosis. Insulin, glucose and epinephrine cause decreases in serum phosphorus. Most of the phosphorus is absorbed in the jejunum and is an active process coupled to sodium via the NaPiIIb cotransporter. 1,25-Dihydroxyvitamin D3 increases stimulation of this pump and therefore absorption of phosphorus. This is maintained by the Na^+/K^+ ATPase pump in the basolateral membrane.

In the kidney 85% of serum inorganic phosphorus is filtered and the ratio of H_2PO_4- to H_2PO_4-2 depends on the PH. Seventy percent of phosphorus is reabsorbed in the proximal tubule via the NaPi cotransporter (70—80% of the filtered load) against electrochemical gradient which is maintained by the basolateral sodium pump. Increased dietary content of phosphorus is an important stimulus for urinary excretion of phosphorus. The remaining 20—30% is reabsorbed in the distal tubule. Metabolic acidosis, TSH, insulin and insulin-like growth factor increase phosphorus reabsorption and upregulation of the NaPi cotransporter. Increased ECF increases urinary excretion of phosphorus while depletion decreases. High calcium intake decreases urinary excretion of phosphorus. There are three types of NaPi cotransporter: type I, II and III. Type I and II are predominantly expressed in the kidneys. Type II cotransporter is the main site of most of the phosphorus reabsorption and a major target for regulation by PTH, fibrioblast growth factor 23 (FGF23), vitamin D and dietary phosphates. Urinary phosphorus excretion is directly related to dietary intake of phosphorus. Hypophosphatemia stimulates 1alpha-hydroxylase to convert calcidiol to calcitriol and increases phosphorus reabsorption in the intestine and kidney. Hyperphosphatemia can lead to increased excretion of phosphorus mediated by increased phosphorus, PTH and FGF23 [46].

Cytotoxic agents given for malignancy can lead to hyperphosphatemia, phosphaturia and hypocalcemia. Also, rapidly growing malignancies can lead to hypophosphatemia by incorporating phosphorus into new cells. In denervated kidneys such as kidney transplants there is an increased phosphorus excretion; this is believed to be due to increased dopamine production and decreased alpha/beta-adrenergic renal receptor activity. Hyperphosphatemia can also occur in the use of enemas and laxatives containing phosphorus. Cow's milk to infants can lead to tetany since there are higher phosphorus levels that lead to hypocalcemia, as observed when infusing phosphate can lead to hypocalcemia. This may be as a result of increased deposition in the bone, organs and soft tissues. Also in cancer patients, when treating tumors hyperphosphatemia may develop as a result of cytolysis. Tumor lysis from large tumor burdens can also lead to hyperphosphatemia and hypocalcemia.

CALCIUM

Forty percent of serum calcium is bound to serum proteins with 80—90% bound to albumin. An increase in serum albumin by 1 g/dl causes an increase in serum calcium by 0.8 mg/dl. Also, hyponatremia can lead to an increase in calcium-bound albumin, and hypernatremia can cause a decrease in calcium binding. The active form of calcium is ionized calcium, which is 47% of total serum calcium. Calcium can also be found in a complexed form — it complexes with bicarbonate, phosphate and acetate. As an example, complexed calcium is increased two-fold in uremic patients. A normal adult may ingest 1000 mg of Ca^{2+} per day, of which roughly 400 to 500 mg may be absorbed. Three hundred milligrams of calcium from digestive secretions are lost in the stool, resulting in a net absorption of only 100 to 200 mg. Calcium and phosphorus are regulated in the intestine, kidney and bone via PTH and vitamin D.

PTH controls calcium via increasing bone demineralization therefore resulting in phosphorus and calcium since the major form of calcium is in hydroxyapatite, $Ca_{10}(PO_4)_6(OH)_2$, the

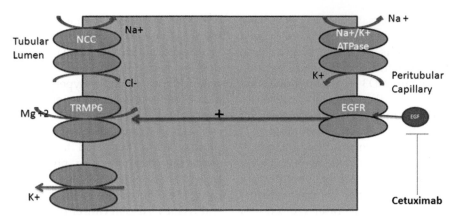

FIGURE 11.3 **EGFR pathway.** The epidermal growth factor (EGF) was discovered as the first hormone to regulate active magnesium reabsorption through TRPM6. Reabsorption of magnesium is primarily driven by the luminal membrane potential established by the voltage-gated potassium channel. Cetuximab targets EGFR and leads to decreased TRMP6-mediated magnesium reabsorption. This figure is reproduced in color in the color plate section.

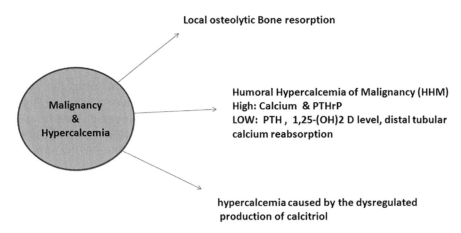

FIGURE 11.4 **Mechanisms of hypercalcemia in cancer patients.**

main mineral component of bone (Figure 11.4). Also, increasing renal reabsorption of calcium and excretion of phosphorus will result in enhancing GI absorption of both calcium and phosphorus mediated by activated vitamin D $(1,25(OH)_2D3)$ or calcitriol. PTH secretion is a result of hypocalcemia, hyperphosphatemia and calcitriol deficiency. Calcium-sensing receptors are present in both the thyroid C cells

and the kidney in the thick ascending loop of Henle and are responsible for sensing calcium levels; in hypocalcemia they cause increased secretion of PTH. PTH affects the kidney by activation of specific adenylyl cyclase systems in the proximal tubule and the early cortical distal nephron, including the cortical thick ascending limb, the distal tubule and the connecting segments. PTH diminishes the proximal reabsorption of phosphate by decreasing the activity of the type II Na^+-phosphate cotransporter in the luminal membrane [47].

An acidic environment will cause an increase in PTH and therefore net phosphorus excretion to act as a buffer for the excess hydrogen load. It also promotes bone buffering in the presence of acidosis. Vitamin D is manufactured in the skin via conversion of 7-dehydrocholestrol to vitamin D3 in response to sunlight. Vitamin D2 from plants or vitamin D3 cholecalciferol from fish is also carried in the blood while bound to vitamin D-binding proteins and in the liver is converted to 25(OH)D, also called calcidiol. In the kidney calcidiol is converted to calcitriol via 1alpha-hydroxylase CYP27B. This enzyme is affected by PTH, estrogen, calcitonin, prolactin, growth hormone low serum calcium and low serum phosphorus, and is inhibited by calcitriol. The formation of calcitriol is primarily stimulated by PTH and hypophosphatemia in an attempt to maintain Ca^{2+} and phosphate balance.

Calcium is absorbed more in the small intestine in the duodenum and proximal jejunum than in the ileum. It is absorbed trancellularly and paracellularly. The epithelial calcium channels TRPV5 (ECaC) are regulated by vitamin D. ECaC1 are channels in the kidney and ECaC2 are the channels in the intestine.

RENAL

Only ultrafilterable calcium crosses the glomerlular capillary walls and is absorbed by the tubular cells. Ninety-seven to ninety-nine percent of filterable calcium is reabsorbed more in the ionized form. Most of urinary calcium is chelated to citrate. Urinary excretion of calcium is linked to urinary excretion of sodium. Seventy percent is absorbed in the proximal tubule with the last 10% in the distal tubule. Eighty to ninety percent of reabsorbed calcium is via paracellular gradient created in the proximal and thick ascending loop of Henle. In the distal tubule and the connecting tubule the transport is via the epithelial calcium channels TRVP5 (ECaC1).

Extracellular calcium-sensing receptors (CaSR) are important in calcium and magnesium reabsorption in (thick ascending loop) TAL via altering the permeability of calcium in the paracellular pathway and changing the apical transport which generates the TAL luminal electropositivity, and is the driving force for calcium reabsorption. PTH and 1,25-dihydroxycholecalciferol are the major regulators of TRVP5 in the distal nephron. High extracellular PH stimulates activity of TRVP5 (ECaC1) and low PH decreases its activity. Acute or chronic load of phosphorus also leads to a decrease in calcium excretion secondary to likely deposition of calcium/phosphorus in the bones and other tissues. Medullary carcinoma of the thyroid is a tumor derived from parafolicular cells and as a result has high levels of calcitonin. Hyperuricemia may also develop in association with osteoblastic metastases such as osteoblastic disease in carcinoma of breast and prostate as a result of rapidly developing matrix and deposition of minerals.

CAUSES OF HYPOCALCEMIA

Citrate and sodium ethylenediaminetetra-acetate (Na-EDTA) when given intravenously can bind to calcium and lead to hypocalcemia. Also, ethylene glycol toxicity can lead to hypocalcemia by binding to the oxalate crystals. Excessive chloride can lead to hypocalcemia. Foscarnet can lead to hypocalcemia by causing chelation of calcium and hypomagnesemia. Also ketoconazole and pentamidine can lead to hypocalcemia. Mithramycin potent inhibitor of RNA synthesis decreases serum calcium and phosphorus and urinary hydroxyproline excretion. In malignancy, in order to correct hypercalcemia, mithramycin has been used where it has been shown to inhibit the rate of osteo-clastic resorption induced by PTH [48]. In cancer patients that are critically ill and ICU patients there is a notable presence of hypocal-cemia. This also correlates with septic patients. Circulating levels of calcitonin precursors appear to be elevated in such patients [49].

Malignancy-associated hypercalcemia is most commonly associated with breast, lung, kidney, ovary and hematological malignancies. In malignant cells there is an excess of intra-cellular organic and inorganic phosphate, up to four times as much compared to non-malignant cells. There is an increase in phos-phorus which is beyond the kidney's capacity to reabsorb and is worsened in uric acid nephropathy. Twenty-four to forty-eight hours after initiation of chemotherapy there is an increase of phosphorus. A large amount of ste-roids can also increase the circulating phosphate [4]. Hypocalcemia is also related to hyperphosphatemia where, due to the excess phosphorus, it precipitates in the soft tissues and tubular system which further leads to wors-ening hypocalcemia [4].

Hypercalcemia is a poor prognostic indicator with survival of 3 months thereafter. It is useful to divide malignancy-associated hypercalcemia into humoral hypercalcemia of malignancy (HHM) usually mediated by PTHrP, which will be discussed further below, local osteolytic hypercalcemia and hypercalcemia caused by the dysregulated production of calcitriol, the active metabolite of vitamin D. Humoral hyper-calcemia is a result of circulating factors from the malignant cells. In HHM this is induced by PTHrP. This peptide has effects of PTH and as a result will cause reduced phosphate reabsorp-tion in the kidney, increase calcium reabsorption in the kidney, increase osteoclast activity in the bone and increase excretion of cAMP. The pres-ence of hypercalcemia with normal PTH but increased urinary cAMP would confirm the diagnosis of HHM mediated by PTHrP. HHM patients not as primary hyperparathyroid

patients have elevated calcitriol instead due to FGF23 that are released from the tumors and cause suppression of 25(OH) 1alpha(OH)ase and inhibit production of $1,25(OH)_2D3$ from the precursor 25(OH)D3 [50]. In HHM bone formation and reabsorption are not matched as in hyperparathyroidism. Calcium-sensing receptor CaSR is expressed in many cells and hypercalcemia leads to activation and increased secretion of PTHrP leading to increased osteoly-sis, growth and tumor spread [51]. In Hodgkin and non-Hodgkin lymphoma there is develop-ment of hypercalcemia from the increased $1,25(OH)_2D3$ levels that are believed to be a result of the tumor's ability to produce calcitriol and lead to hypercalcemia. Successful treatment with chemotherapy will lead to normalization of calcium. Overall, PTHrP and tumor-produced calcitriol act synergistically in malignancy-related hypercalcemia.

Tumors also have the ability to release fac-tors called osteoclast activating cytokines known as IL-1, IL-6, tumor necrosis factor-alpha (TNF-alpha), TNF-beta, lymphotoxin, transforming growth factor-alpha (TGF-alpha) and arachadonic acid metabolites. Malignant cells also produce mediators such as granulo-cyte macrophage colony-stimulating factors (M-CSF) that induce immune cells to produce TNF and IL-1 [52]. Patients with hematologic malignancies complicated by hypercalcemia do not have elevated systemic levels of PTHrP but increased calcitriol production. On the con-trary solid tumors have suppressed levels of cacitriols. Hodgkin disease, NHL and HTLV-1-related ATLL, where hypercalcemia has been reported to occur in 5% and 15% of pa-tients, respectively, are directly related to increased calcitriol levels [53]. However, some patients have been triggered to develop hyper-calcemia only after significant sun exposure presumably secondary to enhanced production of 25(OH)D and vitamin D supplementation. The following are the associated changes: an increased osteoclastic bone resorption and excessive gastrointestinal calcium absorption; lab abnormalities such as a normal or suppressed PTH concentration; a normal or slightly elevated serum phosphate; and normal levels of the inactive precursor 25(OH)D, with an elevated calcitriol level, or a calcitriol level that is inadequately suppressed for the degree of hypercalcemia. If measured, the tubular reabsorption of phosphate is normal or increased. This is all in contrast to PTHrP--mediated HHM. Many patients had bulky or advanced-stage disease, none had bone lesions identified clinically or radiographically, which helps in implicating mostly the high calcitonin levels and not humoral osteolysis as a major contributor to hypercalcemia. The most effective treatment initially is steroids. The third major category of malignancy-associated hypercalcemia acts locally as osteolytic factors. In multiple myeloma the cells produce osteoclastic activating factors such as TGF-beta, IL-1 and IL-6; there is also increased bone resorption and decreased osteoblastic bone formation. Patients with multiple myeloma and lytic lesion are secondary to the presence of high levels of Wnt-signaling antagonist Dickkopf1 (DKK1). Wnt (wingles/int) is an important gene and its products promote growth, maturation and differentiation of osteoblasts. In the presence of an antagonist DKK1 there is a block on proliferation and differentiation of osteoblasts [54].

References

[1] George JM, Capen CC, et al. Biosynthesis of vasopressin in vitro and ultrastructure of a bronchogenic carcinoma. Patient with the syndrome of inappropriate secretion of antidiuretic hormone. J Clin Invest 1972;51(1):141–8.

[2] Bartter FC. The syndrome of inappropriate secretion of antidiuretic hormone (SIADH). Dis Mon 1973;1–47.

[3] Doshi SM, Shah P, et al. Hyponatremia in hospitalized cancer patients and its impact on clinical outcomes. Am J Kidney Dis 2012;59(2):222–8.

[4] Howard SC, Jones DP, et al. The tumor lysis syndrome. N Engl J Med 2011;364(19):1844–54.

[5] Stewart AF. Clinical practice. Hypercalcemia associated with cancer. N Engl J Med 2005;352(4):373–9.

[6] Fakih M. Management of anti-EGFR-targeting monoclonal antibody-induced hypomagnesemia. Oncology (Williston Park) 2008;22(1):74–6.

[7] Adrogue HJ, Madias NE. Hyponatremia. N Engl J Med 2000;342(21):1581–9.

[8] Schrier RW. Water and sodium retention in edematous disorders: role of vasopressin and aldosterone. Am J Med 2006;119(7 Suppl. 1):S47–53.

[9] Mayinger B, Hensen J. Nonpeptide vasopressin antagonists: a new group of hormone blockers entering the scene. Exp Clin Endocrinol Diabetes 1999;107(3): 157–65.

[10] Berghmans T. Hyponatremia related to medical anticancer treatment. Support Care Cancer 1996;4(5):341–50.

[11] Bennett CL, Vogelzang NJ, et al. Hyponatremia and other toxic effects during a phase I trial of recombinant human gamma interferon and vinblastine. Cancer Treat Rep 1986;70(9):1081–4.

[12] Lei KI, WickhamNW, et al. Severe hyponatremia due to syndrome of inappropriate secretion of antidiuretic hormone in a patient receiving interferon-alpha for chronic myeloid leukemia. Am J Hematol 1995; 49(1):100.

[13] Jeppesen AN, JensenHK, et al. Hyponatremia as a prognostic and predictive factor in metastatic renal cell carcinoma. Br J Cancer 2010;102(5):867–72.

[14] Garrett CA, Simpson Jr TA. Syndrome of inappropriate antidiuretic hormone associated with vinorelbine therapy. Ann Pharmacother 1998;32(12):1306–9.

[15] Bode U, Seif SM, et al. Studies on the antidiuretic effect of cyclophosphamide: vasopressin release and sodium excretion. Med Pediatr Oncol 1980;8(3):295–303.

[16] List AF, Hainsworth JD, et al. The syndrome of inappropriate secretion of antidiuretic hormone (SIADH) in small-cell lung cancer. J Clin Oncol 1986;4(8):1191–8.

[17] Berghmans T, Paesmans M, et al. A prospective study on hyponatraemia in medical cancer patients: epidemiology, aetiology and differential diagnosis. Support Care Cancer 2000;8(3):192–7.

[18] Korinek AM, Languille M, et al. Effect of postoperative extradural morphine on ADH secretion. Br J Anaesth 1985;57(4):407–11.

[19] Bell C, Anderson D. SSRI-induced hyponatraemia. Int J Geriatr Psychiatry 1998;13(2):128.

[20] Johnson BE, Chute JP, et al. A prospective study of patients with lung cancer and hyponatremia of malignancy. Am J Respir Crit Care Med 1997;156(5): 1669–78.

[21] Chute JP, Taylor E, et al. A metabolic study of patients with lung cancer and hyponatremia of malignancy. Clin Cancer Res 2006;12(3 Pt 1):888–96.

[22] Ellison DH, Berl T. Clinical practice. The syndrome of inappropriate antidiuresis. N Engl J Med 2007;356(20): 2064—72.

[23] Berl T, Anderson RJ, et al. Clinical disorders of water metabolism. Kidney Int 1976;10(1):117—32.

[24] Schrier RW. Treatment of hyponatremia. N Engl J Med 1985;312(17):1121—3.

[25] Verbalis JG. Hyponatremia: epidemiology, pathophysiology, and therapy. Curr Opin Oncol 1993;2(4): 636—52.

[26] Upadhyay A, Jaber BL, et al. Incidence and prevalence of hyponatremia. Am J Med 2006;119(7 Suppl. 1): S30—5.

[27] Waikar SS, Mount DB, et al. Mortality after hospitalization with mild, moderate, and severe hyponatremia. Am J Med 2009;122(9):857—65.

[28] Zilberberg MD, Exuzides A, et al. Epidemiology, clinical and economic outcomes of admission hyponatremia among hospitalized patients. Curr Med Res Opin 2008;24(6):1601—8.

[29] Upadhyay A, Jaber BL, et al. Epidemiology of hyponatremia. Semin Nephrol 2009;29(3):227—38.

[30] Khuri RN, Strieder WN, et al. Effects of flow rate and potassium intake on distal tubular potassium transfer. Am J Physiol 1975;228(4):1249—61.

[31] Satlin LM, Carattino MD, et al. Regulation of cation transport in the distal nephron by mechanical forces. Am J Physiol Renal Physiol 2006;291(5):F923—31.

[32] Lazrak A, Liu Z, et al. Antagonistic regulation of ROMK by long and kidney-specific WNK1 isoforms. Proc Natl Acad Sci U S A 2006;103(5):1615—20.

[33] Zeidel ML, Kikeri D, et al. Atrial natriuretic peptides inhibit conductive sodium uptake by rabbit inner medullary collecting duct cells. J Clin Invest 1988; 82(3):1067—74.

[34] Will A, Tholouli E. The clinical management of tumour lysis syndrome in haematological malignancies. Br J Haematol 2011;154(1):3—13.

[35] Hoorn EJ, Zietse R. Combined renal tubular acidosis and diabetes insipidus in hematological disease. Nat Clin Pract Nephrol 2007;3(3):171—5.

[36] Quamme GA. Renal magnesium handling: new insights in understanding old problems. Kidney Int 1997;52(5):1180—95.

[37] Fakih MG, Wilding G, et al. Cetuximab-induced hypomagnesemia in patients with colorectal cancer. Clin Colorectal Cancer 2006;6(2):152—6.

[38] Freitag JJ, Martin KJ, et al. Evidence for skeletal resistance to parathyroid hormone in magnesium deficiency. Studies in isolated perfused bone. J Clin Invest 1979;64(5):1238—44.

[39] Nakagawa T, Mazzali M, et al. Uric acid — a uremic toxin? Blood Purif 2006;24(1):67—70.

[40] Heinig M, Johnson RJ. Role of uric acid in hypertension, renal disease, and metabolic syndrome. Cleve Clin J Med 2006;73(12):1059—64.

[41] Kang DH, Johnson RJ. Vascular endothelial growth factor: a new player in the pathogenesis of renal fibrosis. Curr Opin Nephrol Hypertens 2003;12(1): 43—9.

[42] Mazali FC, Johnson RJ, et al. Use of uric acid-lowering agents limits experimental cyclosporine nephropathy. Nephron Exp Nephrol 2012;120(1):e12—9.

[43] Sanchez-Lozada LG, Nakagawa T, et al. Hormonal and cytokine effects of uric acid. Curr Opin Nephrol Hypertens 2006;15(1):30—3.

[44] Johnson RJ, Segal MS, et al. Essential hypertension, progressive renal disease, and uric acid: a pathogenetic link? J Am Soc Nephrol 2005;16(7):1909—19.

[45] Lapsia V, Johnson RJ, et al. Elevated uric acid increases the risk for acute kidney injury. Am J Med 2012;125(3): 302. e309—17.

[46] Quarles LD. Endocrine functions of bone in mineral metabolism regulation. J Clin Invest 2008;118(12): 3820—8.

[47] Green J, Goldberg R, et al. PTH ameliorates acidosis-induced adverse effects in skeletal growth centers: the PTH-IGF-I axis. Kidney Int 2003;63(2):487—500.

[48] Perlia CP, Gubisch NJ, et al. Mithramycin treatment of hypercalcemia. Cancer 1970;25(2):389—94.

[49] Zivin JR, Gooley T, et al. Hypocalcemia: a pervasive metabolic abnormality in the critically ill. Am J Kidney Dis 2001;37(4):689—98.

[50] Wysolmerski JJ, Broadus AE. Hypercalcemia of malignancy: the central role of parathyroid hormone-related protein. Annu Rev Med 1994;45:189—200.

[51] Chattopadhyay N. Effects of calcium-sensing receptor on the secretion of parathyroid hormone-related peptide and its impact on humoral hypercalcemia of malignancy. Am J Physiol Endocrinol Metab 2006;290(5):E761—70.

[52] Dranoff G. Cytokines in cancer pathogenesis and cancer therapy. Nat Rev Cancer 2004;4(1):11—22.

[53] Seymour JF, Gagel RF. Calcitriol: the major humoral mediator of hypercalcemia in Hodgkin's disease and non-Hodgkin's lymphomas. Blood 1993;82(5): 1383—94.

[54] Heath DJ, Chantry AD, et al. Inhibiting Dickkopf-1 (Dkk1) removes suppression of bone formation and prevents the development of osteolytic bone disease in multiple myeloma. J Bone Miner Res 2009;24(3): 425—36.

12

Infections of the Kidney in Cancer Patients

Brett Stephens

University of Texas Medical School at Houston, Houston, TX, USA

INTRODUCTION

Patients with cancer are at increased risk of infections due to multiple mechanisms including alterations in innate and adaptive immunity from the malignancy itself as well as from aggressive cancer therapies. The first line of defense in the host includes phagocytic cells such as neutrophils, monocytes and macrophages. These cells are able to mount a response against organisms through phagocytosis, release of oxidative and non-oxidative mediators, complement activation and release of B- and T-cell stimulating cytokines. This immune response can be disrupted by chemotherapeutic or neoplastic induction of neutropenia, as well as qualitative dysfunction via therapies such as glucocorticoids or radiation. Humoral and cell-mediated responses can also be affected. Leukemias, lymphomas, multiple myeloma and hematopoietic stem-cell transplantation (HSCT) can all induce lymphopenias. Furthermore, chemotherapeutic agents can magnify these deficits, and agents such as calcineurin inhibitors used following HSCT can alter T-cell function (Figure 12.1). Thus, even organisms with low virulence can cause significant morbidity in these susceptible patients [1–3]. This chapter deals specifically with kidney-related infections and their subsequent complications in this population (Table 12.1). Bacterial, fungal and parasitic infections will be reviewed in brief, followed by a more in-depth review of viral infections, particularly after HSCT.

EPIDEMIOLOGY

Cancer patients have an increased risk of developing an infection and are 10 times more likely to develop sepsis compared to the general population [2]. Large database reports have shown that up to 20% of intensive care unit (ICU) admissions are patients with malignancies, sepsis being the leading reason for admission. These complications contribute significantly to length of stay and overall

Renal Disease in Cancer Patients
http://dx.doi.org/10.1016/B978-0-12-415948-8.00012-X

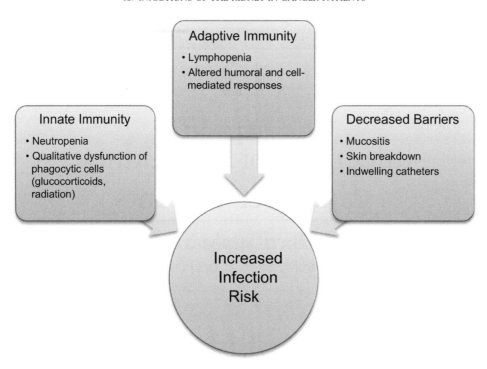

FIGURE 12.1 Infection risk in cancer patients is related to multiple alterations in host responses due to the malignancy itself or toxicities of therapy.

costs [3–4]. Furthermore, there has been a decline in the cancer-related death rate in the United States and Western Europe, as well as an increasing and aging population. These have all contributed to increasing health care expenditures. In the United States, approximately 16% of the gross domestic product is spent on health care annually ($2 trillion), with expectations to reach 20% by the year 2017. The National Institutes of Health reported that in 2007 nearly $89 billion was spent on cancer care, with future estimates predicting a continued rise [5]. In 2006 an estimated $3 billion and 2.3 million hospital bed days were attributed to infections in cancer patients in the USA; and by the year 2025 these numbers are projected to increase to $4.5 billion and 3.4 million hospital bed days [6]. No data exist specifically on the proportion of kidney-related infections or their direct cost.

BACTERIAL INFECTIONS

Bacterial Pyelonephritis

In addition to the immunologic dysfunction in cancer patients, other risk factors for bacterial infections in the urinary tract include: therapy-induced damage to the urothelium, obstruction from mechanical blockage or neurogenic bladder, chronic in-dwelling urinary catheters and ureteral stents. While most infections occur in an ascending manner, hematogenous spread does occasionally occur. Common pathogens include *Esherichia coli*, *Klebsiella* and *Staphylococcus saprophyticus* [1]. Pyelonephritis is more likely in patients with functional or structural urinary abnormalities, and complications can range from renal abscess and xanthogranulomas, to renal functional impairment, to severe sepsis [8–10].

TABLE 12.1   Infections of the Kidney in Cancer Patients with Related Risk Factors and Renal Complications

Infections	Risk factors	Renal involvement
BACTERIAL		
— Pyelonephritis — multiple organisms, including *Esherichia coli*, *Klebsiella*, and *Staphylococcus saprophyticus* — Tuberculosis	— Damaged urothelium — Mechanical obstruction — Functional abnormality — Indwelling catheters — Ureteral stents	— Acute renal failure — Interstitial nephritis — Obstructive nephropathy
FUNGAL		
— *Candida* species — *Candida albicans*, *glabrata*, *tropicalis*, and *parapsilosis* — *Aspergillus* — Zygomycoses — mucormycosis	— Prior use of steroids — Prior antibiotics — Advanced age — Intensity of chemotherapy — Indwelling catheters	— Microabscesses — Obstructive nephropathy — Infarction — Acute renal failure
PARASITIC		
— Schistosomiasis	— Corticosteroids — Hematologic malignancies	— Obstructive nephropathy — Reflux nephropathy — Nephrolithiasis
VIRAL		
— Adenovirus — BK virus — Cytomegalovirus — Epstein—Barr virus	— Level of immunosuppression — HLA mismatch — Graft-versus-host disease — T-cell depletion	— Acute tubular necrosis — Interstitial nephritis — Obstructive nephropathy — Vasculitis — Glomerulonephritis

Complicated pyelonephritis is defined as pyelonephritis in the setting of structural or functional urinary tract abnormalities, or in patients with significant co-morbidities and immunocompromised states. The 2010 Infectious Disease Society of America Guidelines recommend a urine culture and susceptibility testing in all cases, with therapy consisting of at least 7 days (in uncomplicated cases) to 2 weeks (in complicated cases) with quinolones or trimethoprim-sulfamethoxazole, depending on local resistance patterns. Parenteral antibiotics may be needed, and predictors of trimethoprim-sulfamethoxazole resistance include prior treatment with trimethoprim within the previous 6 months or travel outside of the United States [7]. A recent study comparing the efficacy of carbapenems versus third-generation cephalosporins in febrile, complicated pyelonephritis showed equal efficacy between the two groups at 2 weeks of therapy, with 97.3 and 96% success rates, respectively [9]. Possible indications for hospitalization include persistent vomiting, progression of symptoms despite therapy, obstruction and suspected sepsis, with obstruction being the most important risk factor for overall prognosis. Nevertheless, no good prospective trials currently exist regarding oral versus parenteral therapy, or inpatient versus outpatient management [8].

One recent retrospective trial evaluated the risk of acute pyelonephritis in patients with ureteral stents due to malignant obstruction in the setting of systemic chemotherapy. A total of 74 patients with ureteral stents were analyzed with a median follow-up time of 10.5 months. No difference in fever or acute pyelonephritis was found in patients who received chemotherapy versus those who did not ($p = .651$). A total of 6.8% of patients were diagnosed with acute pyelonephritis, but chemotherapy did not appear to further increase the risk in a relatively short term follow-up [10]. Tuberculosis rarely affects the kidney, but contributes to renal disease mainly through actions on the lower urinary tract with subsequent obstruction. Only about 20–30% of patients with genitourinary tuberculosis have a history of pulmonary infection [11]. In one retrospective review of 40 patients diagnosed with renal granulomatoses, tuberculosis accounted for 7.5% of the cases [12]. Tuberculosis of the kidney in the association with underlying malignancies has been reported in rare cases [13–14].

FUNGAL INFECTIONS

Risk factors for fungal infections in cancer patients include prior use of steroids and antibiotics, advanced age, intensity of chemotherapy and the presence of indwelling catheters. In neutropenic patients, *Candida* species remain the most common fungal infections, including *Candida albicans, glabrata, tropicalis* and *parapsilosis*. *Aspergillus* is also a significant cause of invasive disease, especially in HSCT recipients with delayed engraftment [1]. In one report of patients with acute myeloid leukemia, the rate of mold infections reached 7.9%, and invasive, fatal fungal infections have been detected in up to 30% of cancer patients at autopsy [15,16].

Candida Species

In large surveys, candidemia has been associated with overall mortality rates of 38%, with rates reaching 45% in hematological malignancies and 49% in patients with solid tumors. Response rate appears to be directly correlated to neutrophil count or recovery [16].

Candidal infections are rarely isolated to the kidney, and when the kidney is involved, it likely represents disseminated infection. While candida does have a predilection for the collecting system, it can invade the papilla, medulla and occasionally the cortex causing microabscesses. Obstruction from fungal bezoars does occur and often necessitates endoscopic or surgical removal [17–19]. Additionally, one case report described a patient with a renal infarction from invasion and occlusion of the hilar vessels in disseminated candidiasis [20]. With the routine use of fluconazole prophylaxis in patients undergoing HSCT, invasive candidal infections have declined, but fluconazole resistance is subsequently on the rise [16].

Aspergillus and Zygomycosis

Filamentous fungal infections predominantly affect patients with acute myeloid leukemia, with mortality rates from 38 to 66%. *Aspergillus* occurs mainly in patients with severe and protracted neutropenia, with primary locations including the lung and sinuses, although isolated renal involvement and ureteral obstruction have been reported. Voriconazole has been shown to be superior to therapy with amphotericin B in invasive aspergillosis, yet the number of cases of infection continues to rise [1,16,21].

Isolated renal zygomycosis (particularly mucormycosis) has been reported as early as 1960, with most of the reports occurring in the last two decades. In one series of 26 patients with zygomycosis in the setting of hematologic malignancies, 21 were found to have involvement of the lungs, with none of the 26 patients surviving. The survival rate of patients with isolated renal zygomycosis, however, appears to be more favorable, with survival rates in one series of 76%, although only one patient in this group had a known malignancy [22]. The hallmark findings in these infections include vascular invasion and tissue necrosis. Oral antifungal prophylaxis with triazoles and nystatin has proven to be ineffective. Thus, early recognition and therapy with amphotericin B, reduction in immunosuppression and surgical debridement are essential to the overall prognosis, with the most important factor being the outcome of the underlying malignancy [23].

PARASITE INFECTIONS

Little data exist on the number and association of parasite infections in cancer patients; however, in one series of 151 corticosteroid-treated patients with strongyloidiasis, 34 patients had hematological malignancies and 32 had renal transplants. In all these patients, the mean daily dose of prednisone was 40 mg with a cumulative prednisone-equivalent dose of greater than 1000 mg. None of these patients had direct involvement of the kidney [24].

Schistosomiasis is one of the most widespread parasitic infections caused by blood-dwelling trematodes, and it is endemic in approximately 74 tropical and subtropical countries, affecting 200 million people. Schistosomiasis causes kidney disease through ova-induced urothelial damage, granuloma formation, calcification and fibrosis, which can lead to obstruction, reflux and stone formation. It has also been associated more commonly with squamous cell carcinoma of the bladder through chronic inflammation, oxidative damage to DNA and subsequent malignant transformation [25,26].

VIRAL INFECTIONS

Adenovirus

Adenovirus is a non-enveloped, double-stranded DNA virus that is transmitted through aerosolized droplets and fecal–oral routes. Immunocompromised patients are at significant risk of serious and potentially lethal infections, either through newly acquired virus or reactivation of latent disease. Symptoms of renal involvement include fever, hematuria and flank pain [27]. While the virus has an affinity for tubular epithelial cells and ATN is a common finding, glomerulonephritis, interstitial inflammation and obstruction have all been described [28]. In one case series of 21 patients who underwent HSCT, 90% of patients with adenovirus infections demonstrated acute renal failure, with graft-versus-host disease being a significant risk factor [29]. While no standardized therapy exists, cidofovir appears to be safe and effective [30].

BK Virus

BK virus is a non-enveloped, icosahedral encapsulated DNA virus that belongs to the Polyomaviridae family, a family that also includes simian virus 40 and human JC virus. BK virus is widespread, and the majority of primary infections occur in childhood, with 50% of the population affected by 3 years of age. Eighty percent of the population is seropositive by adulthood, and most primary infections in immunocompetent hosts are asymptomatic [27]. It is believed that the virus is disseminated during the primary infection to the renal tubular epithelial cells and urinary tract epithelial cells where it remains dormant until states of immunosuppression and reactivation occur [31]. BK viral infection was first described in 1971 after it was isolated in the urine of a 39-year-old man with ureteric stenosis 4 months after renal transplantation. The virus was named after the initials of the Sudanese patient (also true of the JC virus) [32].

Asymptomatic viruria occurs in a number of settings, including up to 0.3% of non-immunosuppressed patients, 3% of pregnant women, 10–45% of renal transplant patients and 50% of bone marrow transplant recipients. BK virus has been isolated in other tissues, including leukocytes, liver, lung and brain. Demonstration of the virus in the tissue and asymptomatic shedding of the virus in the urine do not always correlate with functional impairment. Viral replication is a highly regulated process involving multiple cellular processes which have recently been described, detailing genome delivery to the nucleus, DNA replication, protein expression and viron assembly. These specific processes are likely the sites of future targeted therapies [27,31,32].

Involvement of the urinary tract can range from hemorrhagic cystitis to urethral and ureteral stenosis with subsequent hydronephrosis to nephropathy and renal impairment. Suspicion of infection can be enhanced by detection of "decoy cells" in the urine. These epithelial cells have large nuclei with basophilic intranuclear inclusions, but they can also be found in JC and adenovirus infections. Definitive diagnosis of BK nephropathy requires renal biopsy demonstrating tubulointerstitial nephritis, inflammatory infiltrates and epithelial cells with viral inclusions, which help differentiate it from acute rejection in transplant patients. Electron microscopy will show epithelial intranuclear viral particles 45–55 nm in size. Confirmation of the virus type is accomplished with immunohistochemical staining, *in situ* hybridization, or *in situ* polymerase chain reaction (PCR). Although biopsy is the definitive test in diagnosing nephropathy, serologic and urine tests are often used when less invasive measures are needed. Urine BK virus PCR has a 100% sensitivity, 95% specificity and when combined with urine cytology has a 100% negative predictive value. Plasma BK virus PCR has a 100% sensitivity and 88% specificity, but care must be taken when using these tests in children, as primary infection may be different from reactivation (Table 12.2). Additionally, as stated earlier, viruria and viremia are not necessarily associated with nephropathy or dysfunction [27,32,33].

In renal transplant recipients, there is a bimodal distribution of infection. The first peak occurs within 4–8 weeks after transplantation, with the second peak not occurring until many months to years later. There exists a high

TABLE 12.2 Diagnostic Tests for BK Virus Infection [27,32,33]. Note that Infection does not always Equate with Dysfunction

Test	Sensitivity	Specificity	Positive predictive value	Negative predictive value
Decoy cells			25–30%	99%
Urine BK PCR	100%	95%	40%	100% (when combined with urine cytology)
Plasma BK PCR	100%	88%	60%	100%
BK DNA on biopsy			70%	100%

association with BK nephropathy and acute rejection, but it is uncertain if the infection precipitates the rejection, or if rejection and subsequent therapy predisposes patients to infection [32]. Emphasis has been placed on identifying those patients at risk of infection. In one study of 880 renal transplant patients using over 3000 renal biopsies and over 8100 urine samples, Prince and colleagues demonstrated that induction therapy with anti-thymocyte globulin, maintenance therapy with tacrolimus and mycophenolate, and a higher number of transplant rejection episodes were correlated with the risk of BK nephropathy [34]. While some studies show that successful therapy often consists of lowering of the immunosuppression dose as well as switching from tacrolimus to cyclosporine and from mycophenolate to imuran, one newer study has shown benefit with lower doses of tacrolimus compared to cyclosporine [35].

In patients with cancer, cases of BK infection are often seen in those undergoing HSCT. As mentioned earlier, viruria is present in up to half of all of these patients, with hemorrhagic cystitis and obstruction commonly occurring [36]. In fact, patients with persistent viruria are four times more likely to develop hematuria and hemorrhagic cystitis than those without viruria [32]. It has been hypothesized that BK nephropathy occurs with immune reconstitution after HSCT. Viral antigens exposed to emerging and functioning lymphocytes are thought to trigger an enhanced inflammatory response [27].

One large prospective study looked at the association of BK infection in patients after HSCT. One hundred and twenty-four patients diagnosed with mostly acute myeloid leukemia and non-Hodgkin lymphoma were monitored for BK viruria, viremia and nephropathy after HSCT. Viruria occurred in 64.8% of the patients with a mean onset at 24 days after transplantation, while viremia was found in 16.9% of the patients at a mean onset 128 days after transplantation. Only two patients developed nephropathy, but this study supports other evidence that viruria often precedes viremia which precedes nephropathy. Graft-versus-host disease and HLA mismatched transplants were identified as risk factors for development of nephropathy [37]. Given such results, there has been a growing interest in routine screening and early intervention. In one study of 66 renal transplant patients, a monthly screening protocol was initiated over a 1-year period. Eleven patients were identified as having a positive plasma BK PCR test and underwent prompt reduction of immunosuppression with either a 50% reduction in baseline dosage or complete discontinuation of mycophenolate mofetil. Ten of the patients became negative for BK virus at 6 months, with no evidence of nephropathy and only one episode of cellular rejection [38]. Further studies for screening and intervention are needed to elucidate best practice guidelines.

No definitive therapy exists for BK nephropathy, but minimization of immune suppression along with antiviral therapies has been used with success. Cidofovir is often used but does have nephrotoxic effects, especially at doses normally used for CMV infection. In one study of 18 patients with BK viruria and viremia after allogeneic HSCT, low-dose cidofovir proved effective in three-quarters of the patients with only three patients demonstrating transient renal dysfunction [39]. Leflunomide, a pyrimidine synthesis inhibitor, has also been used with good results. A recent review included five case reports, two retrospective cohort studies and three prospective observational trials, showing a target blood concentration of 40 mg/L in addition to immunosuppression reduction reduced BK viruria/viremia and graft failure with few adverse events [40].

BK virus remains a significant and increasingly recognized problem in all immunocompromised patients, even with reports of nephropathy occurring in patients after systemic chemotherapy [41,42]. Continued efforts will be needed to minimize risk and improve therapeutic outcomes.

Cytomegalovirus

Cytomegalovirus (CMV) is a beta-herpes virus, a large virus that includes over 200 proteins. CMV has been demonstrated in varied cell types, including endothelial cells, epithelial cells, neutrophils and smooth muscle cells. Similar to the other herpes viruses, CMV after primary infection remains in the human body for life, mostly in a dormant state. However, little is known about the site and mechanism of latency and persistence. In immunosuppressed patients and particularly HSCT patients, CMV can cause multiorgan disease, including: pneumonia, hepatitis, gastroenteritis, retinitis and rarely encephalitis. Both T-cell-mediated immunity and natural killer cells are important in controlling replication, with data showing that deficiency of natural killer cells is associated with severe CMV infection [43].

Risk factors in HSCT patients include serologic status of the donor and recipient, high-dose corticosteroids, T-cell depletion, graft-versus-host disease and HLA mismatch. Approximately 30% of seronegative recipients transplanted from seropositive donors will develop primary CMV infection, and approximately 40% of seropositive patients will develop disease after autologous HSCT [43,44].

Diagnosis has traditionally relied on the characteristic "owl's eye" appearance in histopathological specimens with immunohistochemical confirmation; however, a positive CMV pp65 antigen in peripheral blood leukocytes is a rapid and semiquantitative method for diagnosis. PCR is the most sensitive method for detecting CMV in the bloodstream, but its specificity and positive predictive values in bronchoalveolar lavage fluid is not known [43].

No universal guideline exists on prevention of disease and timing of intervention, with risks and benefits existing for both prophylaxis and preemptive therapy. There may be some enhanced benefit with prophylaxis in HSCT patients within the first 100 days after transplant, but there appears to be no difference between prophylaxis and preemptive therapy in regards to mortality after day 180 [44,45]. Therapy with immune globulin has not been proven to reduce CMV disease, but it has been associated with increased risk of veno-occlusive disease. Ganciclovir is currently the first line therapeutic agent, although uncontrolled studies have shown that oral valganciclovir is comparable to intravenous ganciclovir in terms of efficacy and safety in preemptive therapy [43].

Most of the injury to the kidney in CMV-infected patients comes from concurrent infections, sepsis, CMV-specific medications (particularly cidofovir) and other nephrotoxic agents during the course of therapy [46]. However, CMV has been demonstrated in epithelial cells of the proximal tubules in renal transplant patients [47]. One case series analyzed 62 biopsies in 30 renal transplant patients who showed signs of clinical rejection to look for evidence of CMV infection. CMV DNA was demonstrated in 70% of the patients and 52% of the biopsies, with 90% of patients with systemic CMV disease having viral DNA in the renal biopsy. Patients who demonstrated CMV had significantly higher creatinine levels even at 5 years of follow-up [48]. Other reports of CMV-mediated renal disease include type II cryoglobulinemic vasculitis as well as ARF from interstitial nephritis [49,50].

Epstein—Barr Virus

Epstein—Barr virus (EBV) is a ubiquitous latent gamma-herpes virus infecting more than 90% of the world's population, with memory B-cells becoming infected during the primary phase of exposure. It is speculated that these B-cells travel from the circulation to the lymphoid tissue of the oropharynx where periodic reactivation causes lysis and continued reinfection of more B-cells. The cellular T-cell-mediated response controls both primary and latent infections. The virus was first isolated in 1964 from Burkitt's lymphoma specimens and has since been associated with a wide range of malignancies, including lymphoproliferative disease after solid organ and HSCT. After HSCT, lymphoproliferative disease has an incidence of 2—40%, depending on the transplant regimen, with most of the cases occurring in the first year. Risk factors include T-cell depletion in the donor cells, HLA mismatch, intensive immunosuppression and primary immunodeficiency. Early detection is key to overall prognosis, with the most successful therapies consisting of B-cell monoclonal antibodies and the adoptive transfer of donor-derived T-cells [51,52].

In the kidney EBV is associated with acute tubulointerstitial nephritis and renal failure in both immunocompetent and immunocompromised patients [53,54]. Other renal lesions associated with EBV and infectious mononucleosis include acute glomerulonephritis, hemolytic—uremic syndrome and rhabdomyolysis-induced acute renal failure [55].

SUMMARY

Patients with cancer are at risk for infections, including those with normally low virulence, due to alterations in the immune system and toxicities related to therapies. While disseminated infection and sepsis contribute significantly to the overall morbidity and mortality as well as health care-related expenditures in this population, kidney-specific infections and nephrotoxicity related to treatment in cancer patients remain a substantial burden. Bacterial and fungal infections are common and often associated with disruption in the architecture or normal function of the urinary tract as well as with chronic indwelling catheters. These organisms can often disseminate, and thus require early and accurate diagnosis along with aggressive therapy. Primary viral infections and reactivation of latent disease are fundamental concerns in immunosuppressed patients, particularly after HSCT. Risk factors for these infections include HLA mismatch, donor and recipient serologic status, level of immunosuppression and T-cell function, and graft-versus-host disease. Multiple targeted therapies exist but often bring about other serious toxicities. Therefore, screening, prophylaxis and early intervention have been areas of focus and will continue to be the subjects of future studies.

References

[1] Thirumala R, Ramaswamy M, Chawla S. Diagnosis and management of infectious complications in critically ill patients with cancer. Crit Care Clin 2010; 26:59—91.

[2] Danai PA. The epidemiology of sepsis in patients with malignancy. Chest 2006;129:1432—40.

[3] Rosolem MM, Rabello L, Lisboa T, et al. Critically ill patients with cancer and sepsis: clinical course and prognostic factors. J Crit Care 2011:1—7.

[4] Vincent JL, Rello J, Marshall J, et al. International study of the prevalence and outcomes of infection in intensive care units. JAMA 2009;302:2323—9.

[5] Meropol N, Schrag D, Smith TJ, et al. American Society of Clinical Oncology guidance statement: the cost of cancer care. J Clin Oncol 2009;23:3868—74.

[6] Cooksley CD, Avritscher EB, Rolston KV, et al. Hospitalizations for infection in cancer patients: impact of an aging population. Support Care Cancer 2009; 17:547—54.

[7] Gupta K, Hooton TM, Naber KG, et al. International clinical practice guidelines for the treatment of acute uncomplicated cystitis and pyelonephritis in women: a 2010 update by the Infectious Diseases Society of America and the European Society for Microbiology and Infectious Diseases. Clin Infec Dis 2011; 52:103—20.

[8] Neumann I, Rojas MF, Moore P. Pyelonephritis in non-pregnant women. Clin Evid 2008;2:807.

[9] Takashashi S, Kurimura Y, Takeyama K, et al. Efficacy of treatment with carbapenems and third-generation cephalosporins for patients with febrile complicated pyelonephritis. J Infect Chemother 2009;15:390—5.

[10] Oh SJ, Ku JH, Lee SW, et al. Systemic chemotherapy in patients with indwelling ureteral stenting. Int J Urol 2005;12:548—51.

[11] Wise GJ, Shteynshlyuger A. An update on lower urinary tract tuberculosis. Curr Urol Rep 2008;9:305−13.

[12] Javaud N, Belenfant X, Stirnemann J, et al. Renal granulomatoses: a retrospective study of 40 cases and review of the literature. Medicine (Baltimore) 2007;86:170−80.

[13] Makni SK, Chaari C, Ellouze S, et al. Mucinous tubular and spindle cell carcinoma of the kidney associated with tuberculosis. Saudi J Kidney Dis Transpl 2011;22:335−6.

[14] Ballesteros JJ, Munne A, Rivalta T, et al. Association of renal xanthogranuloma and urological neoplasia. Eur Urol 1988;15:306−10.

[15] Pagano L, Caira M, Candoni A, et al. The epidemiology of fungal infections in patients with hematologic malignancies: the SEIFEM 2004 study. Haematologica 2006;91:1068−75.

[16] Maschmeyer G, Haas A. The epidemiology and treatment of infections in cancer patients. Int J Antimicrob Agents 2008;31:193−7.

[17] Modi P, Goel R. Synchronous endoscopic management of bilateral kidney and ureter fungal bezoar. Urol Int 2007;78:374−6.

[18] Raghavan R, Date A, Bhaktaviziam A. Fungal and nocardial infections of the kidney. Histopathology 1987;11:9−20.

[19] Morris BS, Chudgar PD, Manejwaia O. Primary renal candidiasis: fungal mycetomas in the kidney. Australas Radiol 2002;46:57−9.

[20] McGee SM, Thompson CA, Granberg CF, et al. Acute renal infarction due to fungal vascular invasion in disseminated candidiasis. Urology 2009;73:535−7.

[21] Simaldone MC, Cannon GM, Benoit RM. Case report: bilateral ureteral obstruction secondary to Aspergillus bezoar. J Endourol 2006;20:318−20.

[22] Weng DE, Wilson WH, Little R, et al. Successful medical management of isolated renal zygomycosis: case report and review. Clin Infec Dis 1998;26:601−5.

[23] Lee DG, Choi JH, Choi SM, et al. Two cases of disseminated mucormycosis in patients following allogeneic bone marrow transplantation. J Korean Med Sci 2002;17:403−6.

[24] Fardet L, Genereau T, Poirot JL, et al. Severe strongyloidiasis in corticosteroid-treated patients: case series and literature review. J Infect 2007;54:18−27.

[25] Vennervald BJ, Polman K. Helminths and malignancy. Parasite Immunol 2009;31:686−96.

[26] Barsoum RS. Schistosomiasis and the kidney. Semin Nephrol 2003;23:34−41.

[27] Waldman M, Marshall V, Whitby D, et al. Viruses and kidney disease: beyond HIV. Semin Nephrol 2008;28:595−607.

[28] Teague MW, Glick AD, Fogo AB. Adenovirus infection of the kidney: mass formation in a patient with Hodgkin's disease. Am J Kidney Dis 1991;18: 499−502.

[29] Bruno B, Zager RA, Gooley TA, et al. Adenovirus nephritis in hematopoietic stem-cell transplantation. Transplantation 2004;15:1049−57.

[30] Yusuf U, Hale GA, Carr J, et al. Cidofovir for the treatment of adenoviral infection in pediatric hematopoietic stem cell transplant patients. Transplantation 2006;27:1398−404.

[31] Jiang M, Abend JR, Tsai B, et al. Early events during BK virus entry and disassembly. J Virol 2009;83:1350−8.

[32] Pahar A, Rees L. BK virus-associated renal problems − clinical implications. Pediatr Nephrol 2003;18: 743−8.

[33] Wong W, Chandraker A. BK virus nephropathy: a challenging complication in kidney transplant recipients. Nephrol Rounds 2009;7:1−6.

[34] Prince O, Savic S, Dickenmann M, et al. Risk factors for polyoma virus nephropathy. Nephrol Dial Transplant 2009;24:1024−33.

[35] Geddes CC, Gunson R, Mazonakis E, et al. BK viremia surveillance after kidney transplant: single-center experience during a change from cyclosporine to lower dose tacrolimus-based primary immunosuppression regimen. Transpl Infec Dis 2011;13: 109−16.

[36] Khan H, Oberoi S, Mahvash A, et al. Reversible ureteral obstruction due to polyomavirus infection after percutaneous nephrostomy catheter placement. Biol Blood Marrow Transplant 2011;17:1551−5.

[37] O'Donnell PH, Swanson K, Josephson MA, et al. BK virus infection is associated with hematuria and renal impairment in recipients of allogeneic hematopoietic stem cell transplants. Biol Blood Marrow Transplant 2009;15:1038−48.

[38] Petrov R, Elbahloul O, Gallichio MH, et al. Monthly screening for polyomavirus eliminates BK nephropathy and preserves renal function. Surg Infec 2009;10:85−90.

[39] Ganguly N, Clough LA, Dubois LK, et al. Low-dose cidofovir in the treatment of symptomatic BK virus infection in patients undergoing allogeneic hematopoietic stem cell transplantation: a retrospective analysis of an algorithmic approach. Transpl Infec Dis 2010;12:406−11.

[40] Wu JK, Harris MT. Use of leflunomide in the treatment of polyomavirus BK-associated nephropathy. Ann Pharmacother 2008;42:1679−85.

[41] Van der Bij A, Betjes M, Weening J, et al. BK virus nephropathy in an immunodeficient patient with

chronic lymphocytic leukemia. J Clin Virol 2009; 45:341—4.

[42] Aoki K, Kotani S, Ichinohe T, et al. Acute renal failure associated with systemic polyoma BK virus activation in a patient with peripheral T-cell lymphoma. Int J Hematol 2010;92:638—41.

[43] Ljungman P, Hakki M, Boeckh M. Cytomegalovirus in hematopoietic stem cell transplant recipients. Infect Dis Clin N Am 2010;24:319—37.

[44] Mori T, Kato J. Cytomegalovirus infection/disease after hematopoietic stem cell transplantation. Int J Hematol 2010;91:588—95.

[45] Boeckh M, Ljungman P. How we treat cytomegalovirus in hematopoietic cell transplant recipients. Blood 2009;113:5711—9.

[46] Jacobsen T, Sifontis N. Drug interactions and toxicities associated with the antiviral management of cytomegalovirus infection. Am J Health Syst Pharm 2010;67:1417—25.

[47] Hsieh CL, Lin SY, Huang CC, et al. Cytomegalovirus in the kidney allograft. Inter Med 2010;49:2185.

[48] Li YT, Emery VC, Surah S, et al. Extensive human cytomegalovirus (HCMV) genomic DNA in the renal tubular epithelium early after renal transplantation: relationship with HCMV DNAemia and long-term graft function. J Med Virol 2010;82:85—93.

[49] Suneja M, Nair R. Cytomegalovirus glomerulopathy in a kidney allograft with response to oral valganciclovir. Am J Kidney Dis 2008;52:e1—4.

[50] Kramer J, Hennig H, Lensing C, et al. Multi-organ affecting CMV-associated cryoglobulinemic vasculitis. Clin Nephrol 2006;66:284—90.

[51] Shaffer DR, Rooney CM, Gottschalk S. Immunotherapeutic options for Epstein—Barr virus-associated lymphoproliferative disease following transplantation. Immunotherapy 2010;2:663—71.

[52] Cohen JM, Cooper N, Chakrabarti S, et al. EBV-related disease following haematopoietic stem cell transplantation with reduced intensity conditioning. Leuk Lymphoma 2007;48:256—69.

[53] Becker JL, Miller F, Nuovo GJ, et al. Epstein—Barr virus infection of renal proximal tubule cells: possible role in chronic interstitial nephritis. J Clin Invest 1999;104:1673—81.

[54] Frazao JM, Elangovan L, Felsenfeld AJ, et al. Epstein—Barr-virus-induced interstitial nephritis in an HIV-positive patient with progressive renal failure. Nephrol Dial Transplant 1998;13:1849—52.

[55] Mayer HB, Wanke CA, Williams M, et al. Epstein—Barr virus-induced infectious mononucleosis complicated by acute renal failure: case report and review. Clin Infect Dis 1996;22:1009—18.

Drug Nephropathies

Ilya G. Glezerman

Memorial Sloan-Kettering Cancer Center, New York, NY, USA
and Weill-Cornell Medical College, New York, NY, USA

INTRODUCTION

Despite the fact that cancer incidence declined 0.6% between 1999 and 2008, lifelong risk of developing cancer was a staggering 41.21% based on data from 2006 to 2008. On the other hand, with significant advances in anti-cancer therapies the 5-year survival has increased from 35.0% in 1950–1954 to 68.6% in 2001–2007 [1]. These data indicate that a significant portion of the population is likely to be exposed to chemotherapy and suffer various short-term and long-term side-effects of the treatment, affecting the health and quality of life of cancer survivors.

Kidneys are vulnerable to the development of drug toxicity due to the role they play in metabolism and excretion of toxic agents. The kidneys receive close to 25% of cardiac output resulting in high rate of delivery of potentially toxic drugs. Renal tubules and proximal segment in particular have significant capacity for the uptake of drugs either via endocytosis at the apical membrane or via transporter proteins at the basilar membrane. A high rate of delivery and uptake results in high intracellular concentration of medications and other substances which then undergo extensive metabolism via renal enzymes such as CYP 450 and flavin-containing monoxygenases leading to formation of potentially toxic metabolites and reactive oxygen species (ROS) [2]. Although adverse drug reaction probability scales may be necessary to establish the causal relationship between the drug and toxic reaction [3], numerous chemotherapy agents have been associated with various renal toxicities including tubulo-interstitial damage, glomerular disease, electrolyte abnormalities, hypertension and proteinuria. This chapter reviews renal side-effects of the most commonly used anti-cancer drugs.

AGENTS WITH PREDOMINANTLY TUBULAR TOXICITY

Cisplatin

Clinical Case

The patient was a 63-year-old male with a past medical history significant for benign prostatic hypertrophy, gastroesophageal reflux and recently

Renal Disease in Cancer Patients
http://dx.doi.org/10.1016/B978-0-12-415948-8.00013-1

diagnosed locally advanced squamous cell carcinoma of the larynx. Baseline serum creatinine (SCr) was 1.0 (06.1.3) mg/dL. The patient received three doses of cisplatin at 50 mg/m². Post-treatment he was noted to have an elevated SCr of 2.0 mg/dl but bland urinalysis and a random urinary protein to creatinine ratio of 0.06. The patient's magnesium level was 0.8 (1.4–2.2) mEq/L; he was normotensive and his physical exam was unremarkable. Nine months after the treatment the SCr remained elevated at a new baseline of 1.9 mg/dL.

The cisplatin (cis-dichlorodiammineplatinum)— platinum coordination complex is an effective chemotherapy against a wide spectrum of tumors including testicular, head and neck, ovarian, lung, cervix and bladder. Nephrotoxicity is one of the dose-limiting toxicities of cisplatin. Several mechanisms have been invoked to explain renal toxicity. Cisplatin induces production of ROS and inhibits antioxidant enzymes leading to oxidative stress injury. Exposure to cisplatin also leads to increased renal expression of tumor necrosis factor-α (TNF-α) which plays a pivotal role in the development of renal injury through increased tubular cell apoptosis and production of ROS [4]. Inflammation has also been recognized as an important pathophysiologic mechanism of cisplatin toxicity. Cisplatin-induced injury results in increased levels of a number of cytokines and chemokines including TNF-α, which in turn activate inflammatory response by attracting inflammatory cells such as neutrophils and T-cells to the area of injury [5].

Cisplatin is excreted and concentrated in the kidneys with concentration in proximal tubules five times higher than in plasma. It enters renal cells via organic cation transporter 2 which is kidney specific [4]. Cisplatin is highly protein bound with 90% of the drug bound 2 hr after infusion [6]. Excretion of cisplatin is biphasic with initial rapid phase with a half-life ($t_{1/2}$) of 23–49 min, which correlates with glomerular filtration rate (GFR) and reflects excretion of unbound platinum, and a slow phase with a $t_{1/2}$ of 58–73 hr, which represents the degradation of plasma proteins bearing bound platinum [7].

Renal toxicity manifests as a decrease in renal blood flow leading to a decline in GFR within 3 hr of cisplatin administration. These changes are probably due to increased vascular resistance secondary to tubulo-glomerular feedback and increased sodium chloride delivery to macula densa. The decline in GFR appears to be dose dependent. In a group of patients who received four cycles of 100 mg/m² the ^{51}Cr-EDTA-measured GFR declined by 11.7% whereas in patients who received three cycles of 200 mg/m² the mean decline was 35.7%. This effect was noted to be lasting as GFR was still 30% below baseline at 2 years [6]. Acute tubular toxicity of cisplatin causes mitochondrial dysfunction, decreased ATPase activity, impaired solute transport and altered cation balance. As a result, sodium and water reabsorption is decreased and salt and water excretion is increased leading to polyuria [4]. Cisplatin also causes dose-dependent renal magnesium wasting.

Tubulo-interstitial injury is a predominant finding on pathologic examination of human kidneys affected by cisplatin toxicity with glomeruli relatively spared. Both proximal and distal tubules have been affected and in patients with acute kidney injury (AKI) there is evidence of acute tubular necrosis. Long-term cisplatin exposure may cause cyst formation and interstitial fibrosis [4].

Clinical presentation is typical of the case report presented earlier. Patients develop azotemia in setting of bland urine and minimal proteinuria. Although renal function improves in most patients, a significant minority develop permanent renal impairment. Hypomagnesemia is common and may be present in 42–100% of patients depending on total cisplatin dose and length of exposure. Hypomagnesemia and renal magnesium wasting may persist for up to 6 years after initial dose

[8]. Renal salt wasting syndrome has been reported in up to 10% of patients manifesting as hyponatremia and severe orthostatic hypotension in setting of high urinary sodium concentration. This syndrome may present 2–4 months after initiation of cisplatin therapy [9]. Rare cases of thrombotic microangiopathy have been reported in patients who were also receiving bleomycin [6]. The syndrome of inappropriate antidiuretic hormone secretion has also been documented in patients receiving vigorous hydration [10] but appears less common now as cisplatin-associated nausea is treated successfully with new generation antiemetics diminishing the stimulus for antidiuretic hormone secretion.

Vigorous hydration with saline has significantly reduced the incidence of AKI in patients receiving cisplatin. Both mannitol and loop diuretics have been used to increase urine flow to ameliorate toxicity; however, randomized studies have not shown a clear cut benefit of diuresis in this setting [11]. Numerous compounds have been studied to prevent cisplatin nephrotoxicity. The efforts to prevent nephrotoxicity had focused on four preventive strategies including interference with cisplatin renal cell entry and activation via inhibition of OTC2 and activating enzymes; antioxidant compounds to counteract ROS produced by exposure to cisplatin; anti-apoptotic agents and anti-inflammatory drugs. The goal of the research is to develop renal protective strategies without compromising anti-tumor effect [5]. Despite ongoing efforts only amifostine has been FDA approved for protection against cumulative nephrotoxicity from cisplatin therapy. Amifostine offers protection via binding of free radicals by the thiol group. Side-effects, cost and concerns that it also diminishes the anti-tumor effect of chemotherapy have limited the use of this drug in clinical practice [4]. Recently, liposomal formulation of cisplatin has been tested in non-small cell lung cancer, pancreatic, head and neck and breast cancers. It showed similar efficacy but reduced nephrotoxicity as compared to unmodified cisplatin [12].

Other Platinum Agents

Carboplatin is another platinum-based agent but its potential for nephrotoxicity is significantly lower than cisplatin. It is safe at doses <400 mg/m^2 [13] and acute renal toxicity appears to occur only at myeloablative doses of >800–1200 mg/m^2 [14]. However, statistically but not clinically significant reduction in GFR of 22 ml/min/1.73 m^2 has been reported in a group of pediatric patients who received a median cumulative dose of 2590 (1364–7133) mg/m^2 with weekly doses ranging between 124 and 282 mg/m^2. The reduction in GFR persisted 2 years after the last dose [15].

Oxaliplatin is a third generation platinum compound which has virtually no nephrotoxic potential and is widely used in the treatment of colorectal cancers [16].

Ifosfamide

Case Report

The patient was a 28-year-old male with unresectable retroperitoneal seminoma pretreated with cisplatin 6 months ago with baseline SCr of 1.3 mg/dL and bland urine presented with AKI after receiving three doses of ifosfamide (one dose of daily 2.0 g/m^2 for 3 days and two doses of 3.3 g/m^2 for 2 days). The patient also received two concomitant doses of carboplatin (AUC of 7). Post-treatment the patient developed rising SCr, glucosuria, proteinuria, hypokalemia, metabolic acidosis and hypophosphatemia. Despite discontinuation of ifosfamide the patient progressed to ESRD and required initiation of HD 10 months after last dose of ifosfamide. He remained in complete remission from seminoma 26 months after treatment.

Ifosfamide is an alkylating agent used in the treatment of a variety of childhood and adult malignancies. It has significant potential for nephrotoxicity. Ifosfamide is metabolized in the liver into active ifosfamide mustard form and in the liver and kidneys into urotoxic acrolein and chloroacetaldehyde (CAA) which has presumed nephrotoxic activity. CAA purportedly causes renal tubular damage via production of ROS, ATP depletion, decrease in Na^+/K^+ ATPase activity and increase in intracellular Ca^{2+}. Ifosfamide toxicity is also associated with an increase in inflammatory cytokines including TNF-α which has been linked to an increase in oxidative stress via depletion of glutathione [17]. Ifosfamide is excreted in the urine as inactive metabolites, acrolein and in unchanged form, which represent 20% of administered dose [18].

Most of the data pertaining to nephrotoxicity of ifosfamide was obtained in children. In one study GFR was noted to decrease below 90 ml/min/1.73 m² in 50% of the patients and below 60 ml/min/1.73 m² in 11% with median follow-up of 6 (1−47) months and median dose of 62 (6.1−165) g/m². Overall the drop in GFR was 35.1 ml/min/1.73 m² [19]. Fanconi syndrome characterized by proximal tubular dysfunction with glucosuria in setting of normoglycemia, renal phosphate and potassium wasting, proximal tubular acidosis, hypouricemia and aminoaciduria were reported in 5% of patients treated with ifosfamide [20]. Patients who receive a cumulative dose <60 g/m² are at lower risk of renal toxicity while patients receiving >100 g/m² are at the highest. Cisplatin and high-dose carboplatin combination therapy, renal irradiation, nephrectomy and hydronephrosis were other risk factors [21,22]. Renal disease may progress even after ifosfamide is discontinued and may lead to ESRD [23].

Ifosfamide urotoxicity manifesting as hemorrhagic cystitis has been successfully treated with sodium 2-mercaptoethane sulfonate (MESNA). However, it has not been shown to prevent renal toxicity of CAA in experimental data [24,25] and in clinical practice severe toxicity has occurred despite concurrent administration of MESNA [21]. Several other substances with antioxidative properties including N-acetylcysteine, agmatine, melatonin, taurine and glycine have been shown to attenuate renal toxicity *in vitro* and in experimental animals [17,25].

Methotrexate

Methotrexate (MTX) is an anti-folate agent which inhibits dihydrofolate reductase (DHFR), an important step in DNA synthesis. Fifty to seventy percent of the drug is bound to plasma proteins. In subjects with normal renal function 95% of the drug is found in the urine 30 hr after administration [26]. MTX is both filtered and secreted by the kidneys. It is a weak organic acid and is poorly soluble in acidic urine [27].

Although it is administered over a large therapeutic range only a high-dose methotrexate (HDMTX) therapy of 1−33 g/m² has potential for nephrotoxicity. MTX renal toxicity is presumed to be due to direct precipitation of the drug as well as due to the toxic effect on renal tubules. Renal dysfunction developed in 1.8% of 3887 patients treated with HDMTX in clinical trials. The mortality was 4.4% in this group [28]. Patients develop nonoliguric and in more severe cases oliguric acute kidney injury shortly after administration of MTX. The urinalysis is generally bland and there is no proteinuria. Since MTX is excreted in the urine renal impairment affects the clearance of the drug. Prolonged exposure to toxic levels of MTX (10 μmol/L>at 24 hr; >1 μmol/L at 48 hr and >0.1 μmol at 72 hr) may lead to life-threatening non-renal toxicities such as prolonged cytopenias, mucositis, neurotoxicity and hepatic dysfunction.

MTX solubility is 10-fold higher in urine with pH 7.5 than in acidic urine (pH of 5.5). Urinary alkalinization and aggressive hydration (2.5−3.5 L/m² per 24 hr starting 12 hr prior to chemotherapy administration) is important to establish brisk diuresis and prevent methotrexate precipitation in the tubules. Probenecid, penicillins, salicylates, sulfisoxazole and non-steroid anti-inflammatory drugs may increase the risk of nephrotoxicity as they interfere with renal tubular secretion of MTX and delay excretion.

Leucovorin rescue is used in patients who develop nephrotoxicity and toxic MTX levels due to inadequate hydration. Leucovorin acts as an antidote by bypassing the blocked DHFR pathway. It is used at a standard rescue dose of $10 \, mg/m^2$ with HDMTX but in patients who have toxic levels of MTX the leucovorin rescue dose is escalated according to established nomograms [26]. Doses of $100-1000 \, mg/m^2$ every 6 hr are given depending on the MTX level. Lower rescue doses of leucovorin of $20-50$ mg every 6 hr have been used in patients with 24-hr HDMTX levels of $10-50 \, \mu mol/l$ resulting in low rates of hematologic toxicities [29].

Leucovorin rescue is an effective sole therapy in patients with MTX toxicity [30]; however, other modalities have also been employed. Thymine can also act as an antidote by bypassing the DHFR step in DNA synthesis but this agent is not currently available [27]. HD and hemoperfusion have been used in an attempt to remove MTX from circulation. While both modalities result in lower MTX plasma levels immediately after treatment there is significant rebound effect with levels reaching $90-100\%$ of pre-procedure MTX concentrations [28].

Glucarpidase (carboxypeptidase-G_2) is a recombinant bacterial enzyme which rapidly metabolizes MTX to inactive compounds and has been used successfully to treat HDMTX toxicity. It is able to decrease MTX plasma level $>98\%$ within 15 min after administration and may protect against the development of grade 4 nonrenal toxicity if administered <96 hr after an HDMTX dose [31]. Leucovorin is also a substrate for this enzyme and should be held during administration of carboxypeptidase.

Because of MTX redistribution from the intracellular compartment the second dose of glucarpidase may be required 48 hr later. Since MTX immunoassays cross react with inactive metabolites produced by carboxypeptidase reaction, only high-performance chromatography should be used to measure MTX levels after administration of glucarpidase [27].

In patients who have recovered renal function additional doses of HDMTX may be given without untoward side-effects [30,32].

Pemetrexed

Pemetrexed is an anti-folate agent which inhibits several enzymes involved in DNA synthesis. The drug is not metabolized significantly. It enters cells via reduced folate carrier (RFC) and folate receptor-α (FR-α) and is polyglutamated intracellularly. Polyglutamation results in significant increase in affinity of pemetrexed to the enzymes involved in folate metabolism and decreased affinity to RFC and FR-α leading to prolonged intracellular life [33]. Up to 80% of the drug is bound to plasma proteins and 70 to 90% of an unchanged drug is excreted in the urine within the first 24 hr. The half-life of pemetrexed is 3.5 hr in patients with normal renal function. In patients with renal insufficiency the half-life is prolonged and exposure to the drug is increased [34]. It has not been studied in patients with creatinine clearance (CrCl) $<45 \, ml/min$ but there was a report of a fatality related to treatment when pemetrexed was given to a patient with a CrCl of $19 \, ml/min$ [35].

Mild renal toxicity was reported in patients who received high-dose therapy ($\geq 600 \, mg/m^2$), but it was reversible and not progressive. Recently, several cases of pemetrexed-induced tubular injury were reported [36–39]. All patients received at least three cycles of therapy. Five patients underwent renal biopsies which revealed acute tubular injury, interstitial inflammation and fibrosis. Two patients had clinically significant diabetes insipidus. After discontinuation of pemetrexed the renal function stabilized but did not return to pre-treatment baseline.

Both FR-α and RFC are expressed by kidney tubular cells [40]. It has been suggested that renal toxicity is a result of pemetrexed uptake by tubular cells and intracellular polyglutamation of pemetrexed resulting in "trapping" of pemetrexed in the tubular cells, impairment of RNA and DNA synthesis and ultimately tubular injury [36,39].

Pentostatin

Pentostatin is an inhibitor of adenosine deaminase and has been used in hairy cell leukemia and T-cell lymphomas. The renal toxicity is both dose and schedule dependent. The toxicity usually develops when the pentostatin dose exceeds $4 \, mg/m^2/d$ and with regimens of $4 \, mg/m^2$ every other day the toxicity is uncommon. Nephrotoxicity of pentostatin is manifested by elevated SCr levels and fluid retention. Renal abnormalities may be delayed by a median of 14 days. The etiology of renal dysfunction is unknown but presumed to be due to acute tubular necrosis. Hydration with at least 1.5 L of fluids per day is a cornerstone in prevention of pentostatin renal toxicity [41].

AGENTS WITH PREDOMINANTLY GLOMERULAR TOXICITY

Gemcitabine

Gemcitabine is a pyrimidine analog and is used in the treatment of a variety of solid tumors. Nephrotoxicity of this agent manifests as thrombotic microangiopathy (TMA). During early clinical experience TMA was reported at a low rate of 0.015% [42]. However, as the drug became more widely used the incidence of TMA was noted to increase to as high as 0.4% [43] and possibly even 2.2% [44]. TMA

presents as new onset renal insufficiency, microangiopathic hemolytic anemia (MAHA) and new or worsening hypertension (HTN). The etiology of renal toxicity is unclear but endothelial injury and clotting cascade activation appears to be crucial in the pathogenesis of gemcitabine-induced TMA [43].

The largest case series to date reported 29 patients who developed TMA with gemcitabine [45]. All patients developed renal dysfunction *de novo* or had worsening of pre-existing CKD. Active sediment and proteinuria was present in most patients. Kidney biopsy was performed in four cases and showed microthrombi, mesangiolysis and widening of the subendothelial space with detachment of endothelial cells from the glomerular basement membrane. MAHA was characterized by anemia, thrombocytopenia, elevated lactate dehydrogenase (LDH), low serum haptoglobin levels and peripheral schistocytes. Development of TMA appears to be independent of the total dose as the cumulative dose prior to the diagnosis of TMA ranged from 4 to 81 g/m^2. After TMA was recognized, gemcitabine was promptly discontinued and patients were treated with supportive therapy. Nine patients required hemodialysis. Overall, 28% of patients experience full renal recovery and 48% had partial recovery or stable renal function. Two patients were able to discontinue hemodialysis. Although patients in this study did not undergo plasmapheresis some authors advocate this treatment for patients with TMA due to gemcitabine. In the literature review of 10 cases of patients treated with this modality four progressed to ESRD, three developed CKD, two had partial recovery and one died of progression of malignancy [45]. These outcomes appear compatible to those in patients treated conservatively.

Mitomycin

Mitomycin is an anti-tumor antibiotic isolated from *Streptomyces caespitosus* and used for treatment of gastrointestinal and other solid tumors. It has been associated with life-threatening TMA with renal failure and MAHA. Unlike gemcitabine, mitomycin nephrotoxicity is dose dependent. The risk of TMA is 1.6% with cumulative doses ≤ 49 mg/m^2 and as high as 30% at doses exceeding 70 mg/m^2 [46]. Therefore doses exceeding 40 mg/m^2 are not recommended.

Antiangiogenic Agents

Clinical Case

The patient was a 59-year-old male with glioblastoma but no other significant medical history treated with temozolomide and bevacizumab (10 mg/kg biweekly). The patient's baseline SCr was 1.0 mg/dL. Four months after initiation of chemotherapy the patient developed HTN, AKI (SCr 1.9 mg/dl), severe thrombocytopenia and anemia, high LDH and undetectable haptoglobin. Urinalysis was bland and U_{prot}/U_{creat} was <0.1. Kidney biopsy showed TMA with mesangiolysis and microthrombi. Despite discontinuation of bevacizumab the patient progressed to ESRD.

In the past decade a group of agents called antiangiogenic therapies have been utilized in the treatment of a variety of solid tumors. Angiogenesis, the formation of new blood vessels, is seminal to the growth of tumors and development of metastases making it an attractive target for therapeutic intervention. Angiogenesis is a complex process regulated by a variety of proangiogenic and antiangiogenic factors. Vascular endothelial growth factor (VEGF) is a proangiogenic factor that binds to a family of VEGF receptors (VEGFR), a group of tyrosine kinase receptors (TKR). The receptor binding triggers intracytoplasmic signaling pathways leading to proliferation of endothelial cells and pericytes, recruitment of endothelial cell precursors and growth of capillaries [47]. In the kidneys, VEGF is expressed in podocytes and signals glomerular endothelial cells as well as regulates survival of podocytes via an autocrine mechanism. VEGF maintains podocyte cytosolic calcium concentration and selective barrier to macromolecules [48]. VEGF influences blood pressure (BP) via upregulation of synthesis of nitric oxide in vascular beds and increased production of prostacycline resulting in vasodilatation and relaxation [49].

Two classes of antiangiogenic therapies targeting the VEGF pathway are now available. The first, bevacizumab, is a function blocking humanized monoclonal antibody directed against VEGF. The second is represented by a group of drugs known as small molecule multi-target tyrosine kinase inhibitors (mTKI). These agents inhibit VEGFR as well as a number of other TKRs and include sunitinib, sorafenib, axitinib and several other drugs in development.

The renal effects of VEGF inhibition have been studied in murine models. The VEGF gene was deleted only from the podocytes in mice at 3,12 and 24 weeks of age. All mice developed proteinuria and hypertension 4—5 weeks after induction. Pathologic findings in the kidneys revealed typical features of TMA with intracapillary thrombi, endotheliosis and obliterated capillary loops [50]. In humans, a similar spectrum of disorders has been associated with VEGF inhibition. HTN, proteinuria and TMA have all been reported either during initial trials or in clinical case reports.

The effects of anti-VEGF antibody therapy on blood pressure were reviewed in the meta-analysis of seven randomized clinical trials which included 1850 patients treated with bevacizumab. In patients who received a low dose (3—7.5 mg/kg/dose) of the drug the relative risk (RR) of developing HTN was 3.0 (95% confidence interval (CI), 2.2—4.2; $p < 0.001$). In a high-dose group (10—15 mg/kg/dose) the RR was 7.5 (95% CI, 4.2—13.4; $p < 0.001$). Grade III HTN (requiring therapy or more intense therapy) was observed in 8.7% of patients in the low-dose group and 16.0% in the high-dose group. Proteinuria was also more common in treated patients. In the low-dose group RR for proteinuria was 1.4 (95% CI, 1.1–1.7, $p < 0.003$) and in the high-dose group the RR was 2.2 (95% CI, 1.6–2.9, $p < 0.001$). Grade III (>3.5 gm/24 hr) proteinuria was noted in 1.8% of patients in the high-dose group vs. only 0.1% of controls [51].

TMA is a predominant glomerular lesion associated with anti-VEGF antibody therapy. It has been reported after intravenous [50,52,53] as well as intraocular administration [54]. Two patients also had concurrent mesangial IgA deposits. Other lesions reported with anti-VEGF antibody therapy are cryoglobulinemic glomerulonephritis [55] and immune complex-mediated focal proliferative glomerulonephritis [56]. In patients with kidney biopsy findings of TMA the clinical course varied from sub-nephrotic range proteinuria to more fulminant disease with worsening renal function, hypertension and microangiopathic anemia as is also illustrated by our case report.

HTN is also a major side-effect of mTKI therapy. In the meta-analysis of 13 clinical trials of 4999 patients with renal cell carcinoma (RCC) and other malignancies treated with sunitinib the incidence of all-grade HTN was 21.6% and high grade was 6.8%. However, RR was only statistically significant for patients with high-grade HTN at 22.72 (95% CI: 4.48–115.3). Furthermore, when patients were analyzed by the type of malignancy, only those with RCC had statistically significant RR of developing both all-grade and high-grade HTN. More pronounced effects of mTKI in RCC may be due to higher VEGF levels in patients with RCC resulting in a more marked anti-VEGF effect. The majority of patients with RCC also undergo nephrectomies resulting in reduction in renal function which probably leads to decreased excretion of sunitinib and prolonged exposure to the drug [57].

Proteinuria has not been reported in clinical trials of mTKI agents except for phase II trials of axitinib in which the incidence of all-grade proteinuria was 18–36% and grade ≥ 3 was 0–5% [58]. Proteinuria and nephrotic syndrome due to sunitinib or sorafenib have been described in a number of case reports and one case series [59–63]. Proteinuria of up to 20 g/24 hr was reported and the majority of patients also had new or worsening HTN. The proteinuria generally resolved after discontinuation of mTKI. Two patients had a kidney biopsy which showed features of TMA in one patient and TMA as well as podocyte effacement in another. MAHA was not present in either case [61,63]. Several fulminant cases of TMA with worsening renal function, severe hypertension and MAHA with low haptoglobin, high LDH levels and schistocytosis have also been reported [52,64–66].

Because the putative mechanism of HTN in patients treated with anti-VEGF therapies is intricately related to the anti-tumor action of these drugs it has been proposed that development of HTN can be used as a biomarker of response [67]. Two small retrospective studies showed that development of hypertension was associated with improved oncologic outcomes in patients with RCC treated with axitinib and sunitinib [68,69]. In a retrospective analysis of more than 500 patients treated with sunitinib in the setting of RCC, overall survival (OS) and progression-free survival (PFS) were more than four-fold higher in a group of patients who developed sunitinib-induced HTN which was defined as a maximum systolic blood pressure of at least 140. However, hypertensive patients had more renal adverse events (5% vs. 3%, $p = 0.013$) [70]. OS and PFS were also improved in patients with advanced non-small cell lung cancer treated with bevacizumab who developed treatment-related HTN. In this study HTN was defined as BP >150/100 or a ≥ 20 mm Hg rise in diastolic blood pressure (DBP) [71].

Nephrologists should be aware of these data as recommendations to discontinue anti-VEGF therapy due to the development of HTN and proteinuria should be weighed against the possible enhanced anti-tumor effect in this setting. An expert panel from the National Institute of Cancer has proposed guidelines for the management of anti-VEGF therapy-induced HTN. It recommends careful assessment of the patients prior to the initiation of therapy to identify those with cardiovascular risk factors, addressing pre-existing HTN prior to initiation of anti-VEGF therapy and monitoring BP on a regular basis, particularly during the first cycle. The patients should be treated if they develop BP >140/90 or DBP ≥20 mm Hg higher than baseline. The panel did not make any specific recommendations about anti-hypertensive regimen due to lack of data and stated that treatment should be individualized to fit the patient's co-morbid conditions and minimize drug interaction [72]. Other considerations include concurrent development of proteinuria as a complication of anti-VEGF therapy. In this setting it may be appropriate to use angiotensin converting enzyme inhibitors or angiotensin receptor blockers for their anti-proteinuric effect. In summary, although long-term effects of anti-VEGF therapy-induced HTN and proteinuria are unknown it is probably prudent to continue the anti-cancer therapy if HTN and proteinuria are controlled with medical therapy. However, if complications such as nephrotic syndrome, HTN with end-organ damage, renal insufficiency or evidence of MAHA develop, discontinuation of antiangiogenic therapy should be considered promptly.

In addition to HTN, proteinuria and TMA, both mTKI and anti-VEGF antibody agents have been reported to cause acute interstitial nephritis (AIN) [62,73–76]. While some cases were confirmed by renal biopsy, in others the diagnosis was made on clinical grounds since biopsy was precluded by thrombocytopenia or the presence of solitary kidney. Patients had eosinophilia, eosinophiluria and kidney dysfunction. Renal function either improved or stabilized after discontinuation of antiangiogenic therapy. In two cases mTKI were administered intermittently (4 weeks on and 2 weeks off) and patients exhibited "saw tooth" fluctuations in eosinophilia and SCr levels with both parameters improving just before the initiation of the next cycle [62].

AGENTS ASSOCIATED WITH ELECTROLYTE ABNORMALITIES

Case Report

The patient was an 81-year-old male with a history of metastatic colorectal cancer who presented to the renal clinic for evaluation of hypomagnesemia. Three months prior to presentation he was started on panitumumab (6 mg/kg) and irinotecan. The patient's serum magnesium (Mg^{2+}) level was 1.4 (1.4–2.2) mEq/L. One month after initiation of chemotherapy he developed hypomagnesemia (Mg^{2+}-level of 1.2–1.0 mEq/L). Urinary fractional excretion of Mg^{2+} was 10.86. Despite intravenous (IV) Mg^{2+} supplementation and panitumumab dose reduction, the Mg^{2+} level was 0.8 mEq/L 6 months after initiation of panitumumab. The patient continued to require 6 g of IV $MgSO_4$ weekly in addition to oral Mg^{2+} supplementation.

Hypomagnesemia as a common complication of cisplatin therapy and Fanconi syndrome due to ifosfamide treatment has been addressed by this review already. However, recently a number of targeted biological agents have been associated with electrolyte imbalance.

Cetuximab

Cetuximab is a chimeric monoclonal antibody directed against the epithelial growth factor receptor (EGFR). The EGFR is overexpressed in several tumors of epithelial origin and cetuximab is used in combination with chemotherapy for treatment of these malignancies. Although in initial clinical trials hypomagnesemia was not reported [77], numerous published reports have established a link between low serum

Mg^{2+} and use of cetuximab. Active Mg^{2+} transport in the kidney occurs predominantly in the distal convoluted tubule (DCT). TRPM 6 (transient receptor potential cation channel, subfamily M, member 6) has been demonstrated to play a role in this process. EGFR is also expressed on DCT. Experiments show that epithelial growth factor (EGF) markedly increases the activity of TRMP 6 leading to the hypothesis that EGFR activation is necessary for reabsorption of Mg^{2+} and that blockage of EGFR leads to renal Mg^{2+} wasting [78]. In one of the earlier reports 34 patients on cetuximab had the Mg^{2+} level measured at least once. Of these patients, 23% had grade 3 (<0.9—0.7 mg/dL) and 6% grade 4 (<0.7 mg/dL) hypomagnesemia [79]. In another report the incidence of grade 3 or 4 hypomagnesemia was 27% [80]. The severity of hypomagnesemia appears to correlate with duration of exposure and is difficult to manage. Daily infusions of up to 6—10 g of $MgSO_4$ were required to correct the deficit in one cohort [80]. The hypomagnesemia resolved in all cases ≥4 weeks after discontinuation of cetuximab. Patients who developed clinically significant hypomagnesemia also had hypocalcemia due to parathyroid hormone resistance which is seen in patients with low Mg^{2+} levels. Hypocalcemia resolved after Mg^{2+} levels normalized [79,80].

In more recent randomized trials the incidence of grade 3/4 hypomagnesemia ranged between 5.8 and 0.8% in the cetuximab arm versus 0.4 and 0% in the chemotherapy or best supportive care (BSC) arms. However, in these studies the Mg^{2+} level was not routinely measured accounting for lower incidence of hypomagnesemia [81].

Panitumumab

Panitumumab is a fully human antibody directed at EGFR and is used in the treatment of metastatic colorectal cancer. In randomized trials it was also shown to cause low serum Mg^{2+} level with incidence of grade 3/4 hypomagnesemia ranging between 5 and 3% in the panitumumab arm versus 0 and <1% in the chemotherapy or BSC arms [82,83].

Imatinib

Imatinib is a small molecule mTKI with specificity for BCR-Abl, C-kit and platelet-derived growth factor receptor (PDGFR). Imatinib showed activity against tumors characterized by dysregulation of function of these enzymes. Imatinib has been shown to cause hypophosphatemia. In the initial report, hypophosphatemia developed in 25 (51%) of 49 patients who had at least one measurement of serum phosphorus. Patients with both low and normal serum phosphate levels were found to have high urine fractional excretion of phosphate as compared to controls but only hypophosphatemic patients had elevated parathyroid hormone (PTH) levels [84]. In another study 14 (39%) of 36 patients treated with imatinib developed hypophosphatemia and high PTH levels [85]. Additionally, serum phosphate levels were measured routinely in two clinical trials of 403 patients with chronic myeloid leukemia receiving imatinib. Hypophosphatemia was observed in 50% of the patients but hypophosphatemia as an adverse event was only reported in 3% of the patients [86]. The exact mechanism by which imatinib causes hypophosphatemia is unknown but it may inhibit bone resorption via inhibition of PDGFR and lead to decreased calcium and phosphate efflux from the bone. Lower calcium egress from bone has been postulated to cause mild secondary hyperparathyroidism which in turn leads to increased renal phosphate losses [84].

CONCLUSIONS

Despite advances in diagnosis, treatment and prevention of chemotherapy-induced kidney injury significant challenges still remain. In many cases the only therapeutic intervention available is the discontinuation of the offending agent. Future research may be directed towards development of antidote agents that protect normal cells and allow continuation of chemotherapy without compromising anti-tumor effects. In addition to traditional cytotoxic agents, new targeted biological therapies have been associated with renal disease due to interference with signaling pathways in non-malignant cells. Since development of HTN may be a biomarker for anti-tumor activity for targeted therapies, further investigations into long-term effects of treatment-induced HTN on morbidity and mortality are needed.

References

[1] http://seer.cancer.gov/. Accessed 2012.
[2] Perazella MA. Renal vulnerability to drug toxicity. Clin J Am Soc Nephrol 2009;4(7):1275–83.
[3] Naranjo CA, Busto U, Sellers EM, Sandor P, Ruiz I, Roberts EA, et al. A method for estimating the probability of adverse drug reactions. Clin Pharmacol Ther 1981;30(2):239–45.
[4] Yao X, Panichpisal K, Kurtzman N, Nugent K. Cisplatin nephrotoxicity: a review. Am J Med Sci 2007;334(2):115–24.
[5] Miller RP, Tadagavadi RK, Ramesh G, Reeves WB. Mechanisms of cisplatin nephrotoxicity. Toxins 2010; 2(11):2490–518.
[6] Meyer KB, Madias NE. Cisplatin nephrotoxicity. Miner Electrolyte Metab 1994;20(4):201–13.
[7] Gormley PE, Bull JM, LeRoy AF, Cysyk R. Kinetics of cis-dichlorodiammineplatinum. Clin Pharmacol Ther 1979;25(3):351–7.
[8] Lajer H, Daugaard G. Cisplatin and hypomagnesemia. Cancer Treat Rev 1999;25(1):47–58.
[9] Hutchison FN, Perez EA, Gandara DR, Lawrence HJ, Kaysen GA. Renal salt wasting in patients treated with cisplatin. Ann Intern Med 1988;108(1):21–5.
[10] Littlewood TJ, Smith AP. Syndrome of inappropriate antidiuretic hormone secretion due to treatment of lung cancer with cisplatin. Thorax 1984;39(8):636–7.
[11] Launay-Vacher V, Rey JB, Isnard-Bagnis C, Deray G, Daouphars M. Prevention of cisplatin nephrotoxicity: state of the art and recommendations from the European Society of Clinical Pharmacy Special Interest Group on Cancer Care. Cancer Chemother Pharmacol 2008;61(6):903–9.
[12] Stathopoulos GP, Boulikas T. Lipoplatin formulation review article. J Drug Deliv 2012;2012:581363.
[13] Cornelison TL, Reed E. Nephrotoxicity and hydration management for cisplatin, carboplatin, and ormaplatin. Gynecol Oncol 1993;50(2):147–58.
[14] Isnard-Bagnis C, Launay-Vacher V, Karie S, Deray G. Anticancer drugs. In: De Broe M, Porter G, Bennett W, Deray G, editors. Clinical Nephrotoxins Renal Injury from Drug and Chemicals. 3rd ed. New York: Springer Scientific; 2008.
[15] English MW, Skinner R, Pearson AD, Price L, Wyllie R, Craft AW. Dose-related nephrotoxicity of carboplatin in children. Br J Cancer 1999;81(2):336–41.
[16] Extra JM, Marty M, Brienza S, Misset JL. Pharmacokinetics and safety profile of oxaliplatin. Semin Oncol 1998;25(2 Suppl. 5):13–22.
[17] Hanly L, Chen N, Rieder M, Koren G. Ifosfamide nephrotoxicity in children: a mechanistic base for pharmacological prevention. Expert Opin Drug Saf 2009;8(2):155–68.
[18] Li YF, Fu S, Hu W, Liu JH, Finkel KW, Gershenson DM, et al. Systemic anticancer therapy in gynecological cancer patients with renal dysfunction. Int J Gynecol Cancer 2007;17(4):739–63.
[19] Skinner R, Cotterill SJ, Stevens MC. Risk factors for nephrotoxicity after ifosfamide treatment in children: a UKCCSG Late Effects Group study. United Kingdom Children's Cancer Study Group. Br J Cancer 2000;82(10):1636–45.
[20] Suarez A, McDowell H, Niaudet P, Comoy E, Flamant F. Long-term follow-up of ifosfamide renal toxicity in children treated for malignant mesenchymal tumors: an International Society of Pediatric Oncology report. J Clin Oncol 1991;9(12): 2177–82.
[21] Skinner R, Sharkey IM, Pearson AD, Craft AW. Ifosfamide, mesna, and nephrotoxicity in children. J Clin Oncol 1993;11(1):173–90.
[22] Jones DP, Spunt SL, Green D, Springate JE. Renal late effects in patients treated for cancer in childhood: a report from the Children's Oncology Group. Pediatr Blood Cancer 2008;51(6):724–31.
[23] Berns JS, Haghighat A, Staddon A, Cohen RM, Schmidt R, Fisher S, et al. Severe, irreversible renal failure after ifosfamide treatment. A clinicopathologic report of two patients. Cancer 1995;76(3):497–500.
[24] Yaseen Z, Michoudet C, Baverel G, Dubourg L. In vivo mesna and amifostine do not prevent chloroacetaldehyde nephrotoxicity in vitro. Pediatr Nephrol 2008;23(4):611–8.

[25] Nissim I, Horyn O, Daikhin Y, Luhovyy B, Phillips PC, Yudkoff M. Ifosfamide-induced nephrotoxicity: mechanism and prevention. Cancer Res 2006;66(15):7824–31.

[26] Bleyer WA. The clinical pharmacology of methotrexate: new applications of an old drug. Cancer 1978;41(1):36–51.

[27] Smith SW, Nelson LS. Case files of the New York City Poison Control Center: antidotal strategies for the management of methotrexate toxicity. J Med Toxicol 2008;4(2):132–40.

[28] Widemann BC, Adamson PC. Understanding and managing methotrexate nephrotoxicity. Oncologist 2006;11(6):694–703.

[29] Zelcer S, Kellick M, Wexler LH, Gorlick R, Meyers PA. The Memorial Sloan Kettering Cancer Center experience with outpatient administration of high dose methotrexate with leucovorin rescue. Pediatr Blood Cancer 2008;50(6):1176–80.

[30] Flombaum CD, Meyers PA. High-dose leucovorin as sole therapy for methotrexate toxicity. J Clin Oncol 1999;17(5):1589–94.

[31] Widemann BC, Balis FM, Kim A, Boron M, Jayaprakash N, Shalabi A, et al. Glucarpidase, leucovorin, and thymidine for high-dose methotrexate-induced renal dysfunction: clinical and pharmacologic factors affecting outcome. J Clin Oncol 2010;28(25):3979–86.

[32] Christensen AM, Pauley JL, Molinelli AR, Panetta JC, Ward DA, Stewart CF, et al. Resumption of high-dose methotrexate after acute kidney injury and glucarpidase use in pediatric oncology patients. Cancer 2012;118(17):4321–30.

[33] Adjei AA. Pharmacology and mechanism of action of pemetrexed. Clin Lung Cancer 2004;5(Suppl. 2):S51–5.

[34] Villela LR, Stanford BL, Shah SR. Pemetrexed, a novel antifolate therapeutic alternative for cancer chemotherapy. Pharmacotherapy 2006;26(5):641–54.

[35] Mita AC, Sweeney CJ, Baker SD, Goetz A, Hammond LA, Patnaik A, et al. Phase I and pharmacokinetic study of pemetrexed administered every 3 weeks to advanced cancer patients with normal and impaired renal function [see comment]. J Clin Oncol 2006;24(4):552–62.

[36] Stavroulopoulos A, Nakopoulou L, Xydakis AM, Aresti V, Nikolakopoulou A, Klouvas G. Interstitial nephritis and nephrogenic diabetes insipidus in a patient treated with pemetrexed. Ren Fail 2010;32(8):1000–4.

[37] Michels J, Spano JP, Brocheriou I, Deray G, Khayat D, Izzdine H. Acute tubular necrosis and interstitial nephritits during pemetrexed therapy. Case Rep Oncol 2009;2:53–6.

[38] Vootukuru V, Liew YP, Nally Jr JV. Pemetrexed-induced acute renal failure, nephrogenic diabetes insipidus, and renal tubular acidosis in a patient with non-small cell lung cancer. Med Oncol 2006;23(3):419–22.

[39] Glezerman IG, Pietanza MC, Miller V, Seshan SV. Kidney tubular toxicity of maintenance pemetrexed therapy. Am J Kidney Dis 2011;58(5):817–20.

[40] Birn H. The kidney in vitamin B12 and folate homeostasis: characterization of receptors for tubular uptake of vitamins and carrier proteins. Am J Physiol Renal Physiol 2006;291(1):F22–36.

[41] Margolis J, Grever MR. Pentostatin (Nipent): a review of potential toxicity and its management. Semin Oncol 2000;27(2 Suppl. 5):9–14.

[42] Fung MC, Storniolo AM, Nguyen B, Arning M, Brookfield W, Vigil J. A review of hemolytic uremic syndrome in patients treated with gemcitabine therapy. Cancer 1999;85(9):2023–32.

[43] Izzedine H, Isnard-Bagnis C, Launay-Vacher V, Mercadal L, Tostivint I, Rixe O, et al. Gemcitabine-induced thrombotic microangiopathy: a systematic review. Nephrol Dial Transplant 2006;21(11):3038–45.

[44] Desrame J, Duvic C, Bredin C, Bechade D, Artru P, Brezault C, et al. [Hemolytic uremic syndrome as a complication of gemcitabine treatment: report of six cases and review of the literature]. La Revue de medecine interne/fondee par la Societe Nationale Francaise de Medecine Interne 2005;26(3):179–88.

[45] Glezerman I, Kris MG, Miller V, Seshan S, Flombaum CD. Gemcitabine nephrotoxicity and hemolytic uremic syndrome: report of 29 cases from a single institution. Clin Nephrol 2009;71(2):130–9.

[46] Valavaara R, Nordman E. Renal complications of mitomycin C therapy with special reference to the total dose. Cancer 1985;55(1):47–50.

[47] Mena AC, Pulido EG, Guillen-Ponce C. Understanding the molecular-based mechanism of action of the tyrosine kinase inhibitor: sunitinib. Anticancer Drugs 2010;21(Suppl. 1):S3–11.

[48] Breen EC. VEGF in biological control. J Cell Biochem 2007;102(6):1358–67.

[49] Yogi A, O'Connor SE, Callera GE, Tostes RC, Touyz RM. Receptor and nonreceptor tyrosine kinases in vascular biology of hypertension. Curr Opin Nephrol Hypertens 2010;19(2):169–76.

[50] Eremina V, Jefferson JA, Kowalewska J, Hochster H, Haas M, Weisstuch J, et al. VEGF inhibition and renal thrombotic microangiopathy. N Engl J Med 2008;358(11):1129–36.

[51] Zhu X, Wu S, Dahut WL, Parikh CR. Risks of proteinuria and hypertension with bevacizumab, an antibody against vascular endothelial growth factor:

systematic review and meta-analysis. Am J Kidney Dis 2007;49(2):186–93.

[52] Frangie C, Lefaucheur C, Medioni J, Jacquot C, Hill GS, Nochy D. Renal thrombotic microangiopathy caused by anti-VEGF-antibody treatment for metastatic renal-cell carcinoma. Lancet Oncol 2007;8(2): 177–8.

[53] Roncone D, Satoskar A, Nadasdy T, Monk JP, Rovin BH. Proteinuria in a patient receiving anti-VEGF therapy for metastatic renal cell carcinoma. Nat Clin Pract Nephrol 2007;3(5):287–93.

[54] Pelle G, Shweke N, Van Huyen JP, Tricot L, Hessaine S, Fremeaux-Bacchi V, et al. Systemic and kidney toxicity of intraocular administration of vascular endothelial growth factor inhibitors. Am J Kidney Dis 2011;57(5):756–9.

[55] Johnson DH, Fehrenbacher L, Novotny WF, Herbst RS, Nemunaitis JJ, Jablons DM, et al. Randomized phase II trial comparing bevacizumab plus carboplatin and paclitaxel with carboplatin and paclitaxel alone in previously untreated locally advanced or metastatic non-small-cell lung cancer. J Clin Oncol 2004;22(11):2184–91.

[56] George BA, Zhou XJ, Toto R. Nephrotic syndrome after bevacizumab: case report and literature review. Am J Kidney Dis 2007;49(2):e23–9.

[57] Zhu X, Stergiopoulos K, Wu S. Risk of hypertension and renal dysfunction with an angiogenesis inhibitor sunitinib: systematic review and meta-analysis. Acta Oncol 2009;48(1):9–17.

[58] Izzedine H, Massard C, Spano JP, Goldwasser F, Khayat D, Soria JC. VEGF signalling inhibition-induced proteinuria: mechanisms, significance and management. Eur J Cancer 2010;46(2):439–48.

[59] Patel TV, Morgan JA, Demetri GD, George S, Maki RG, Quigley M, et al. A preeclampsia-like syndrome characterized by reversible hypertension and proteinuria induced by the multitargeted kinase inhibitors sunitinib and sorafenib. J Natl Cancer Inst 2008;100(4):282–4.

[60] Obhrai JS, Patel TV, Humphreys BD. The case/progressive hypertension and proteinuria on anti-angiogenic therapy. Kidney Int 2008;74(5):685–6.

[61] Overkleeft EN, Goldschmeding R, van Reekum F, Voest EE, Verheul HM. Nephrotic syndrome caused by the angiogenesis inhibitor sorafenib. Ann Oncol 2010;21(1):184–5.

[62] Jhaveri KD, Flombaum CD, Kroog G, Glezerman IG. Nephrotoxicities associated with the use of tyrosine kinase inhibitors: a single-center experience and review of the literature. Nephron Clin Pract 2011;117(4):c312–9.

[63] Bollee G, Patey N, Cazajous G, Robert C, Goujon JM, Fakhouri F, et al. Thrombotic microangiopathy secondary to VEGF pathway inhibition by sunitinib. Nephrol Dial Transplant 2009;24(2):682–5.

[64] Kapiteijn E, Brand A, Kroep J, Gelderblom H. Sunitinib induced hypertension, thrombotic microangiopathy and reversible posterior leukencephalopathy syndrome. Ann Oncol 2007;18(10):1745–7.

[65] Choi MK, Hong JY, Jang JH, Lim HY. TTP-HUS associated with sunitinib. Cancer Res Treat 2008;40(4):211–3.

[66] Levey SA, Bajwa RS, Picken MM, Clark JI, Baron K, Leehey DJ. Thrombotic microangiopathy associated with sunutinib, a VEGF inhibitor, in a patient with factor V Leiden mutation. Nephrol Dial Transplant Plus 2008;3:154–6.

[67] van Heeckeren WJ, Ortiz J, Cooney MM, Remick SC. Hypertension, proteinuria, and antagonism of vascular endothelial growth factor signaling: clinical toxicity, therapeutic target, or novel biomarker? J Clin Oncol 2007;25(21):2993–5.

[68] Rixe O, Billemont B, Izzedine H. Hypertension as a predictive factor of sunitinib activity. Ann Oncol 2007;18(6):1117.

[69] Rixe O, Dutcher JP, Motzer RJ, Wilding G, Stadler WM, Kim S, et al. Association between diastolic blood pressure (DBP) ≥90 mm Hg and efficacy in patients (pts) with metastatic renal cell carcinoma (MRCC) receiving axitinib (AG-013736; AG). Ann Oncol 2008;19(Suppl. 8): viii, 189.

[70] Rini BI, Cohen DP, Lu DR, Chen I, Hariharan S, Gore ME, et al. Hypertension as a biomarker of efficacy in patients with metastatic renal cell carcinoma treated with sunitinib. J Natl Cancer Inst 2011;103(9): 763–73.

[71] Dahlberg SE, Sandler AB, Brahmer JR, Schiller JH, Johnson DH. Clinical course of advanced non-small-cell lung cancer patients experiencing hypertension during treatment with bevacizumab in combination with carboplatin and paclitaxel on ECOG 4599. J Clin Oncol 2010;28(6):949–54.

[72] Maitland ML, Bakris GL, Black HR, Chen HX, Durand JB, Elliott WJ, et al. Initial assessment, surveillance, and management of blood pressure in patients receiving vascular endothelial growth factor signaling pathway inhibitors. J Natl Cancer Inst 2010;102(9):596–604.

[73] Winn SK, Ellis S, Savage P, Sampson S, Marsh JE. Biopsy-proven acute interstitial nephritis associated with the tyrosine kinase inhibitor sunitinib: a class effect? Nephrol Dial Transplant 2009;24(2): 673–5.

[74] Izzedine H, Brocheriou I, Rixe O, Deray G. Interstitial nephritis in a patient taking sorafenib. Nephrol Dial Transplant 2007;22(8):2411.

[75] Khurana A. Allergic interstitial nephritis possibly related to sunitinib use. Am J Geriatr Pharmacother 2007;5(4):341—4.

[76] Barakat RK, Singh N, Lal R, Verani RR, Finkel KW, Foringer JR. Interstitial nephritis secondary to bevacizumab treatment in metastatic leiomyosarcoma. Ann Pharmacother 2007;41(4):707—10.

[77] Cunningham D, Humblet Y, Siena S, Khayat D, Bleiberg H, Santoro A, et al. Cetuximab monotherapy and cetuximab plus irinotecan in irinotecan-refractory metastatic colorectal cancer. N Engl J Med 2004;351(4): 337—45.

[78] Izzedine H, Bahleda R, Khayat D, Massard C, Magne N, Spano JP, et al. Electrolyte disorders related to EGFR-targeting drugs. Crit Rev Oncol Hematol 2010;73(3):213—9.

[79] Schrag D, Chung KY, Flombaum C, Saltz L. Cetuximab therapy and symptomatic hypomagnesemia. J Natl Cancer Inst 2005;97(16):1221—4.

[80] Fakih MG, Wilding G, Lombardo J. Cetuximab-induced hypomagnesemia in patients with colorectal cancer. Clin Colorectal Cancer 2006;6(2):152—6.

[81] Fakih M. Management of anti-EGFR-targeting monoclonal antibody-induced hypomagnesemia. Oncology (Williston Park) 2008;22(1):74—6.

[82] Peeters M, Price TJ, Cervantes A, Sobrero AF, Ducreux M, Hotko Y, et al. Randomized phase III study of panitumumab with fluorouracil, leucovorin, and irinotecan (FOLFIRI) compared with FOLFIRI alone as second-line treatment in patients with metastatic colorectal cancer. J Clin Oncol 2010;28(31): 4706—13.

[83] Van Cutsem E, Peeters M, Siena S, Humblet Y, Hendlisz A, Neyns B, et al. Open-label phase III trial of panitumumab plus best supportive care compared with best supportive care alone in patients with chemotherapy-refractory metastatic colorectal cancer. J Clin Oncol 2007;25(13):1658—64.

[84] Berman E, Nicolaides M, Maki RG, Fleisher M, Chanel S, Scheu K, et al. Altered bone and mineral metabolism in patients receiving imatinib mesylate. N Engl J Med 2006;354(19):2006—13.

[85] Osorio S, Noblejas AG, Duran A, Steegmann JL. Imatinib mesylate induces hypophosphatemia in patients with chronic myeloid leukemia in late chronic phase, and this effect is associated with response. Am J Hematol 2007;82(5):394—5.

[86] Owen S, Hatfield A, Letvak L. Imatinib and altered bone and mineral metabolism. N Engl J Med 2006;355(6):627; author reply 8—9.

Paraneoplastic Glomerulopathy

Sheron Latcha[1], Surya V. Seshan[2]

[1]Memorial Sloan-Kettering Cancer Center, Weill-Cornell Medical College, New York, NY, USA
[2]Weill-Cornell Medical College and New York-Presbyterian Medical Center, New York, NY, USA

GENERAL FEATURES

Introduction

The most frequently cited characterization for paraneoplastic glomerulonephritis (PNGN) comes from Ronco, who stated that the "paraneoplastic syndrome refers to clinical manifestations that are not directly related to tumor burden, invasion, or metastasis, but are caused by the secretion of tumor cell products such as hormones, growth factors, cytokines, and tumor antigens" [1]. Bacchetta later elaborated on the concept, adding, "the diagnosis of paraneoplastic syndrome may be suspected in the presence of the following criteria: (i) no obvious alternative etiology for the associated syndrome; (ii) existence of a temporal relationship between the diagnosis of the syndrome and cancer; (iii) clinical (and histological) remission after complete surgical removal of the tumor or full remission achieved by chemotherapy; (iv) recurrence of the tumor associated with an increase of associated symptoms" [2]. A range of renal functional and structural abnormalities have been described in patients with neoplastic disease [1,3–5]. Renal parenchymal changes can occur in the glomeruli, tubulointerstitial compartment and vasculature.

A proposed link between neoplasia and glomerulonephritis (GN) dates back to the first published case report on cancer and the nephrotic syndrome in 1966 [6]. Since then, a spectrum of glomerular histopathology has been described in association with a variety of primary neoplasms. There remains some skepticism that paraneoplastic-associated glomerulonephritis (PNGN) actually exists. Table 14.1 [7] lists cancer incidence based on tumor type. The most common cancers overall are prostate and breast, in men and women, respectively. Lung cancer is followed, in descending order, by colorectal, melanoma, bladder, non-Hodgkin lymphoma (NHL), kidney, thyroid, pancreas and leukemia (all types). Table 14.2 [2,8] lists the total number of reported cases of PNGN reported in association with the most common tumor types. While breast and prostate cancer collectively account for 13% of these, lung carcinoma accounts for 27%. Nonetheless, less than 1% of adult cancer patients develop PNGN with overt renal disease [9]. Among the most common solid tumors, there have been fewer than 200 case reports of PNGN in the literature since 1966. On occasion, certain benign tumors, namely carotid body tumors and others, have

Renal Disease in Cancer Patients
http://dx.doi.org/10.1016/B978-0-12-415948-8.00014-3

TABLE 14.1 Estimated New Cases of Cancer for 2012

Cancer type	Estimated new cases
Prostate	241,740
Breast (female/male)	226,870/2,190
Lung	226,160
Colorectal	143,460
Melanoma	76,250
Bladder	73,510
Non-Hodgkin lymphoma	70,130
Renal	59,588
Endometrial	47,130
Pancreatic	43,920
Leukemia (all types)	47,150

Adapted from the American Cancer Society Facts and Figures database, 2012.

TABLE 14.2 Summary of Paraneoplastic Glomerulonephritis (PNGN) with Solid Tumors

PNGN	Solid tumor type	Number of cases
Membranous nephropathy		
	Gastrointestinal	26
	Lung	26
	Renal	12
	Prostate	9
	Breast	5
Rapidly proliferative glomerulonephritis		
	Renal	10
	Gastrointestinal	8
	Lung	4
	Prostate	3
	Breast	3

TABLE 14.2 Summary of Paraneoplastic Glomerulonephritis (PNGN) with Solid Tumors—(*cont'd*)

PNGN	Solid tumor type	Number of cases
Minimal change disease		
	Lung	10
	Gastrointestinal	9
	Renal	7
	Breast	2
IgA nephropathy		
	Renal	19
	Lung	2
	Gastrointestinal	1
Membranoproliferative glomerulonephritis		
	Lung	7
	Renal	4
	Gastrointestinal	2
	Breast	2
	Prostate	1
Focal segmental glomerulosclerosis		
	Renal	6
	Gastrointestinal	2
	Lung	1
	Breast	1
Total		182

also been linked to onset of nephrotic syndrome (NS) with remission after excision of the tumor [10].

Although the reported prevalence of PNGN does not coincide with the prevalence of primary neoplasia in the general population, data from retrospective studies with large cohorts support a higher incidence of glomerular disease in those with neoplastic disease, emphasizing a role of tumor-associated phenomena.

The prevalence of carcinoma in patients with IgA nephropathy (IgAN) has been reported to be as high as 23%; 22% for those with membranous glomerulopathy (MGN), and 13% for patients with nephrotic syndrome (NS) [1]. Conversely, when compared with the general population, the incidence of cancer in patients with MN has been observed to be 10-fold higher [11]. Additionally, in an age-matched control population, the relative risk of malignancy in any patient with ANCA-associated vasculitis is increased six-fold [12]. These retrospective studies and case series have their inherent biases and may overstate the prevalence of glomerular disease with malignancy. Population-based studies can avoid some of these biases. Using Danish Kidney Biopsy Registry data, when compared with the general population, an excess rate of GN was observed in individuals with colon, lung and skin cancer, Hodgkin disease, leukemia and non-Hodgkin lymphoma [13]. Despite reporting biases, the reported cases of PNGN represent something other than expected frequency of GN in the general population.

The objectives of this chapter are to (1) describe the histopathologic features of primary GNs; (2) report on the prevalence of PNGNs and their associated malignancies; (3) discuss the purported pathogenetic mechanisms for neoplasia-induced glomerular injury based on information obtained from case reports, clinical and experimental models of PNGN; and (4) offer suggestions for the screening and management of patients with suspected PNGN.

Pathogenetic Mechanisms

A number of clinical studies and experimental models have investigated the mechanistic relationship between neoplasia and glomerular disease. Thus far, a causal link between neoplasia and PNGN remains ill defined. To date, the proposed hypotheses include: (1) Deposition of tumor antigens or circulating tumor antigen antibody complexes in the glomeruli and subsequent activation of inflammatory pathways. The neoplasia could possibly express an otherwise privileged antigen or incite an immune response via molecular mimicry [9]. (2) Prior immunosuppressive therapy for primary GNs may activate tumorigenesis. (3) Intrinsic viral oncogenic activity. Alternatively, viral oncogenes could be shed into circulation as free antigens or circulating immune complexes (ICs) and could be qualified as biomarkers. (4) Elaboration of cytokines or permeability factors by the tumor which then initiate glomerular injury [2,14].

Some of the tumor-specific antigens also serve as circulating biomarkers of specific diseases and may indicate their existence, persistence or recurrence following treatment (e.g. carcinoembryonic antigen in colorectal and gastric cancer, prostatic-specific antigen in prostate cancer, alpha-feto protein in liver and germ cell tumors, monoclonal immunoglobulin proteins in B-lymphocyte or plasma cell-associated malignancies). A proportion of malignant tumors secrete a variety of hormonal substances which can have significant effects on distant organs and their function, often presenting with appropriate clinical manifestations. However, the vast majority of tumors associated with paraneoplastic syndrome or glomerular lesions have no documented evidence of specific markers. About 20% of patients develop NS, 6 or more months preceding the clinical manifestations of the underlying tumor [15]. Although the exact incidence of PNGN presenting commonly as nephrotic syndrome in occult malignancies is not known, a thorough examination and analysis of the renal tissue specimen using light microscopy (LM), immunofluorescence (IF) and electron microscopy (EM) with appropriate immunohistochemistry to identify specific markers in susceptible age groups of patients is helpful.

Studies have suggested that glomerular deposits in patients with tumors may or may not be composed of immunoglobulins and complement, and depending on their location (often mesangial or subendothelial), they may represent either non-specific trapping or *in-situ* formation of ICs following binding of tumor antigens to glomerular structural elements [16]. These have been termed as subclinical GN. Such deposits were found in 30% of patients with cancer in one study [17] by IF and EM of both renal biopsy and autopsy tissue, while these findings were rare in a control group. This observation can probably be ascribed to a defect in immunologic surveillance or immunoregulatory mechanisms in patients with malignant tumors, often expressing varied levels of foreign antigen [9,16,18]. Therefore, clinically manifest PNGN mediated by IC deposits is relatively uncommon [3].

A clinical, pathological and immunohistochemical analysis of autopsy kidney tissue in 21 patients with malignancy who died without cancer treatment revealed a range of glomerular alterations along with abnormal urinary sediment and renal function in all patients [19]. They included thickening of glomerular capillary basement membranes, two cases of IgA nephropathy, three with focal segmental glomerulosclerosis (FSGS) and one case of membranous GN. The authors were able to localize a specific tumor marker within the glomerular deposits of the latter case [19].

The various patterns of paraneoplastic glomerular disease in patients with malignancies are broadly dependent on (1) the duration of the neoplasm, (2) the state of differentiation of the tumor which could dictate the elaboration of specific or non-specific markers, (3) the type of tumor antigen or other products expressed, (4) the type and extent of host response to these antigens involving cell- or antibody-mediated mechanisms, and (5) the physico-chemical characteristics of circulating ICs that render them pathogenic or nephritogenic. Although there is a high prevalence of detectable ICs in cancer patients [20], and asymptomatic or nonpathogenic glomerular deposits are commonly found in these patients, the exact role of these ICs in initiating glomerular disease remains speculative [16].

In PNGN with clinical renal disease, apart from LM, IF and EM studies of the glomerular disease are essential in defining the composition of the immune deposits as well as their exact location in the glomerular structures to determine the pattern of the lesion. This in turn contributes towards appropriate management and predicts prognosis. Each of these modalities has the ability to point toward a more definitive diagnosis [17,18,21,22]. Moreover, several investigators have cited reports [1,10,15] that have gone further to confirm the association of tumor-related antigen as a principal component of the ICs in the causation of the glomerular injury by: (1) elution of the immunoglobulins from the glomerular deposits and documenting their reactivity towards specific antigens on the cell membrane of the respective tumor, (2) localization of tumor-specific circulating biomarkers as antigens in the glomeruli and immunohistochemical identification of their specificity, (3) isolation of tumor-specific antigens from glomerular deposits reacting to specific circulating antibodies or directly on tumor cells, and (4) identification of tumor-associated ICs that fix complement. Since there are only about 15–20 cases in the literature that have been studied in this manner, specific tests are needed to identify tumor antigens in the glomeruli at the molecular level, to implicate their participation in producing PNGN by a broad range of tumors [1]. This will be particularly useful in patients with suspected PNGN and to differentiate them from other coincidental, similar appearing glomerular lesions.

The pathogenetic mechanisms underlying other non-immune complex-mediated PNGN, such as minimal change disease (MCD), focal segmental glomerulosclerosis (FSGS), crescentic glomerulonephritis with or without vasculitis, thrombotic microangiopathy and AA amyloidosis, are diverse, and can involve tumor-associated cell-mediated mechanisms, or secondary auto-immune phenomena directed against glomer-ular cells or microvascular endothelial cells.

The occurrence of a wide range of glomerular lesions affecting the epithelial, mesangial and endothelial cells, with or without immune com-plexes, manifesting as non-proliferative and proliferative forms of glomerulonephritides, has prompted usage of the term "glomerulo-pathy" in the setting of a paraneoplastic syn-drome. However, in the interest of maintaining uniformity, the appropriate terminology cur-rently used for the primary and secondary glomerular diseases is recommended for the purpose of reporting with the associated malig-nancy, when it is known. This method would also reflect the different patterns of glomerular lesions that are linked to a specific histologic type of malignant tumor, as well as common forms of glomerular injury, that are associated with a number of different tumor phenotypes from the various organs.

Clinical Manifestations of PNGN

Though PNGN is often encountered in adults and the elderly with malignant tumors, similar mechanisms may cause glomerular disease in children and adolescents. This group is affected by a variety of tumors, most frequently second-ary to hematological malignancies [2,23].

Since the earliest reports of the association of cancer with PNGN [6], NS has been by far the most common clinical presentation. A smaller proportion presents with a nephritic picture characterized by hematuria, hypertension and varying degrees of renal insufficiency or failure, often related to the type of GN noted, such as proliferative or crescentic forms. Lee et al. [6] have raised an important issue regarding the application of the full criteria of nephrotic syn-drome when estimating the prevalence in this patient population, as there may be consider-able variability in the manifestations of the

clinical and laboratory features of PNGN. While the classic definition of nephrotic syndrome, which includes massive proteinuria, hypoalbu-minemia, hyperlipidemia and edema, is not al-ways encountered in patients with cancer, the cause of proteinuria or hematuria requires further testing, including renal biopsy examina-tion, to define the glomerular lesion. In addition, appropriate serologic testing for viral and other infections, auto-immune disorders, monoclonal proteins and complement levels, urinalysis (with examination of the urinary sediment) should be routinely performed to identify related or concomitant unrelated renal disease in cancer patients. Complications secondary to chemotherapeutic agents or radiotherapy are not uncommon and may require monitoring of renal function and a kidney biopsy, if necessary.

GLOMERULAR LESIONS IN SOLID TUMORS

Membranous Glomerulonephritis (MGN)

Idiopathic MGN accounts for the majority of MGN cases in the developed countries and in the adult Caucasian population. Worldwide, chronic infections (hepatitis B, hepatitis C, syph-ilis, malaria and schistosomiasis) account for most cases of secondary forms of MGN. Other secondary etiologies for MGN include autoim-mune disease (SLE, rheumatoid arthritis, mixed connective tissue disease), drugs/toxins (D penicillamine, mercury, NSAIDs, COX-2 inhibi-tors) and malignancy. Ronco [1] pointed out the significantly higher annual incidence of neoplastic disease (>1000 per 100,000 popula-tion) than the annual incidence of MGN (2.8 per 100,000 population) in adults over 60 years of age. Furthermore, Brueggemeyer and Ramirez [24] found a 10-fold increase in the inci-dence of cancer in their cohort of 128 MGN pa-tients than in age-matched controls, suggesting that MGN occurred with an occult malignancy at the time of renal presentation. A similar incidence was also found in another study, where in 24 out of 240 patients with MGN, a cancer was diagnosed at the time or within a year after renal biopsy [11]. Burstein et al. reported nine out of 87 (10.3%) patients presumed to have idiopathic MGN had or developed a malignancy associated with their renal disease, involving various solid tumors and hematologic malignancies [25]. The relative paucity of subepithelial deposits in biopsy and autopsy series in asymptomatic cases [16,19], the low number of cases reported with clinical disease, as well as fewer cases in our own practice, does not support this view.

Epidemiology of PN MGN

The available clinical information, which is based on case series, reports a temporal relationship between neoplasia and MGN in 6–22% of patients with NS. In approximately 80% of reported cases of PN MGN, the neoplastic condition was diagnosed before or at the time of renal disease. When MGN was diagnosed first, the malignancy was generally discovered within 12 months [14]. Solid malignancies of epithelial origin, particularly lung, renal, breast and gastrointestinal, are most frequently diagnosed with PN MGN [2,8,26–29]. Prostate cancer is increasingly being reported with PN MGN (Table 14.3) [2,8]. This may reflect increased use of the prostate-specific antigen (PSA) as a screening test. Patients with PN MGN tend to be older (>50 years), with a male preponderance, and may have a history of heavy smoking [1,14].

Histopathology

On histopathology, as the IC deposits localize to the subepithelial space, the glomerular basement membrane (GBM) appears thickened on LM. This thickening represents immune deposits, basement membrane spikes and the additional matrix material that is laid down by the injured podocytes as the disease progresses, best seen on silver methenamine stain (Figure 14.1A). This is generally not accompanied by significant intraglomerular inflammatory cell infiltrate or proliferation in idiopathic MGN. However, Lefaucher and colleagues also found an increased number of infiltrating inflammatory cells in the glomeruli (>8 cells/glomerulus) in PN MGN [11]. Mild mesangial expansion with increased matrix or cellularity may be observed, suggesting a secondary form of MGN. Immunofluorescence demonstrates primarily polyclonal IgG (positive for both kappa and lambda light chain), complement component C3 and, rarely, lower intensity of IgM or IgA, along the glomerular capillary walls in a diffuse, segmental or relatively global granular pattern (Figure 14.1B). Whereas IgG4 is the predominant subclass found in idiopathic MGN along with IgG1, IgG2 and IgG3 are characteristically found in secondary MGN [14]. Depending on the duration, extent of deposits and natural history of the lesion, there are amorphous/granular electron dense deposits in the subepithelial and intramembranous spaces, evidence of foot process effacement and signs of podocyte injury by EM (Figure 14.1C). On occasion, the pattern of glomerular basement membrane involvement in secondary forms may be heterogeneous in distribution, characterized by variation in size and distribution of deposits and varied stage of resolution. Secondary MGN can often have mesangial and subendothelial deposits.

Clinical Reports and Experimental Animal Models

Heymann nephritis is an experimental rat model for active and passive immune-mediated nephritis. When rats were immunized with homogenates of homologous renal cortex and an immunopotentiator, Freund's adjuvant, they developed massive proteinuria, and granular immune deposits of IgG and C3 developed in the subepithelial space of the GBM [30]. Megalin, the target antigen, localized to the podocyte

TABLE 14.3 Prevalence of Membranous Nephropathy According to Cancer Subtypes

Solid tumors			Hematologic malignancies		
Site	**Tumor type**	**# cases**	**Lineage**	**Tumor type**	**# cases**
Gastrointestinal tumors			Lymphoid tumors		
	Gastric carcinoma	16		Chronic lymphocytic leukemia	10
	Colorectal carcinoma	5		Non-Hodgkin lymphoma	5
	Pancreatic carcinoma	3		Hodgkin lymphoma	5
	Esophageal carcinoma	2		Acute lymphocytic leukemia	1
	Liver/Hepatocellular carcinoma	2		Cutaneous T-cell lymphoma	1
Respiratory system tumors			Myeloid tumors		
	Lung/Bronchus carcinoma	14		Myelodysplastic syndrome	3
	Small cell carcinoma	6		Chronic myelomonocytic leukemia	1
	Bronchial carcinoid	2		Acute myeloid leukemia	1
	Mesothelioma	2		Primary myelofibrosis	1
	Laryngeal carcinoma	2	Total		28
Renal tumors		11			
Genitourinary tumors					
	Prostate carcinoma	9			
	Bladder carcinoma	2			
	Cervical carcinoma	2			
	Endometrial carcinoma	1			
	Seminoma	1			
	Choriocarcinoma	1			
Head and neck tumors					
	Thymoma	7			
	Adrenal ganglioneuroma	1			
	Parotid adenolymphoma	1			
	Mandible squamous cell carcinoma	1			
	Carotid body tumor	1			
	Brain tumor	1			

(*Continued*)

TABLE 14.3 Prevalence of Membranous Nephropathy According to Cancer Subtypes—(cont'd)

Solid tumors		
Site	**Tumor type**	**# cases**
Others		
	Unspecified	57
	Breast carcinoma	5
	Sarcoma	3
	Melanoma	1
	Sacro-coccygeal chordoma	1
	Spinal schwannoma	1
	Pulmonary lympho-epithelioma	1
Total		162

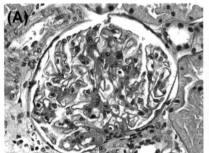 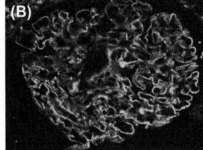 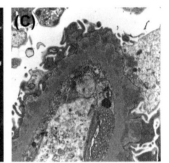

FIGURE 14.1 Paraneoplastic membranous glomerulonephritis. (A) A 69-year-old woman with breast cancer developed nephrotic syndrome. The glomerulus shows global, moderate thickening of the capillary walls. PAS × 400. This figure is reproduced in color in the color plate section. (B) Immunofluorescence demonstrates global, granular, polyclonal IgG and C3 along the capillary walls. FITC IgG × 400. This figure is reproduced in color in the color plate section. (C) Electron microscopy of a capillary loop with numerous subepithelial, finely granular deposits and basement membrane spikes. The overlying foot processes are effaced. × 20,000.

foot process. Megalin is not present in human glomeruli, so investigators have sought to identify the epithelial antigen in human idiopathic MGN and PN MGN.

In the majority of cases of idiopathic MGN, circulating autoantibodies react with the transmembrane glycoprotein M type phospholipase A2 receptor (PLA2R), a protein that is expressed by the human podocyte [31]. PLA2R is highly specific for idiopathic MGN and is not found in patients with other etiologies for NS, or in

normal controls. PLA2R antigen co-localizes with IgG4 in subepithelial deposits on renal biopsies of patients with idiopathic MGN, and that IgG reactive with PLA2R can be eluted from these tissue specimens. Additionally, circulating levels of PLA2R antibodies match the course of the clinical disease in MGN [14]. Since the clinicopathological findings are indistinguishable between idiopathic and PN MGN, testing for PLA2R antibody titers may be helpful in differentiating the two entities.

Tumor-derived antigens have been detected in the subepithelial deposits in biopsy specimens of PN MGN. Antigens, such as carcinoembryonic antigen (CEA), a reexpressed fetal protein, have been suggested as the targets of T- and B-cell immune responses in gastrointestinal or colonic carcinoma patients with PN MGN. There are several clinical case reports on various solid tumors presenting with MGN in which typical subepithelial deposits were found on EM [32–34]. By immunohistochemical techniques using fluorescein or peroxidase labeling techniques, these deposits stained positively for CEA or other specific tumor antigens. Prior digestion of immune complexes *in situ* to remove blocking immunoglobulins was performed in some cases. Circulating immune complexes or immunoglobulins eluted from the glomeruli of some patients have been shown to react with surface plasma membranes of the tumor cells from the same patient by radioimmunodiffusion [32,35].

Investigators using experimental rat models have attempted to elucidate the role of tumor cells in the pathogenesis of PNGN. Tumor antigen antibody complexes have been observed in several mouse models, suggesting that the deposition of antigen–antibody complexes in the glomeruli mediated by the host immune response to antigens is an essential factor in the pathogenesis of renal disease [36–38]. Whether these immune complexes are directly pathogenic remains to be proven, and may be determined by the local milieu as well as their physico-chemical properties. The possible mechanisms include (1) that the antigen and/or antibody could have been passively deposited, (2) that low affinity antigen–antibody complexes can initially be trapped in the subendothelial space and later disassociate and relocate to the subepithelial space, and (3) that cationic antigens can lodge in the GBM and that freely circulating antibody can then target these antigens to form *in situ* immune complexes, often with participation of the alternate pathway of complement activation and C3 fixation. Consistent with the Heymann model for nephritis, antigen and antibodies alone do not appear to be adequate to produce glomerular pathology. In an experimental rat model, rats injected with colon cancer cells developed PN MGN with no evidence of tumor involvement in the kidney. T-cell-deficient rats that were similarly injected had none of these findings, suggesting a role for T-cell immune response in the development of cancer-induced proteinuria and glomerulopathy [39].

Minimal Change Disease (MCD)

MCD is classically defined by the pentad of proteinuria greater than >3.5 g/d; serum albumin lower than 3 g/dL; cholesterol greater than 300 mg/dL; lipiduria; and pitting edema. MCD is the most common cause of childhood NS, and accounts for NS in 90% of cases in children <10 years old and for 50% of cases >10 years old. In adults with NS, MCD is the underlying diagnosis in 10–15% of cases [40]. Most cases of adult MCD are idiopathic, but this lesion has been linked with medications (NSAIDs, COX2 inhibitors, lithium, D penicillamine, pamidronate), neoplastic disease (commonly, lymphoid malignancies), infection (syphilis, tuberculosis, HIV) and atopy.

Epidemiology of PN MCD

As seen in Table 14.4 [2,8], PN MCD is most often associated with the lymphoid malignancies, specifically Hodgkin lymphoma [41]. Solid tumors are only less commonly associated with PN MCD. When PN MCD has been reported with solid tumors, thymoma accounts for about 40% of cases, and is followed by gastrointestinal, respiratory and renal tumors.

Histopathology

A moniker for MCD is Nil disease, **N**othing **I**n **L**ight microscopy, and is characterized by normal appearing glomeruli on LM with abundant proximal tubular protein reabsorption

TABLE 14.4 Prevalence of Minimal Change Disease According to Cancer Subtypes

Solid tumors			Hematologic malignancies		
Site	Tumor type	# cases	Lineage	Tumor type	# cases
Thymoma		26	Lymphoid tumors		
Gastrointestinal carcinoma				Hodgkin lymphoma	61
	Colorectal carcinoma	6		Non-Hodgkin lymphoma	6
	Pancreatic carcinoma	2		Chromic lymphocytic leukemia	2
	Esophageal carcinoma	1	Myeloid tumors		
Respiratory system carcinoma				Chronic myelogenous leukemia	2
	Lung/Bronchus carcinoma	8	Total		71
	Mesothelioma	1			
	Small cell carcinoma	1			
Renal carcinoma		7			
Genitourinary carcinoma					
	Urothelial carcinoma	2			
	Bladder carcinoma	1			
Others					
	Breast	2			
	Ovarian	1			
	Melanoma	1			
	Sarcoma	1			
	Angiomyolipoma	1			
	Neurilemminoma	1			
	Undifferentiated carcinoma	1			
	Vaginale testis mesothelioma	1			
Total		64			

droplets (Figure 14.2A), absence of complement or immunoglobulins on IF, and no immune deposits on EM. The distinctive histologic finding is diffuse foot process effacement on EM (Figure 14.2B). MCD and FSGS are often discussed together. Both glomerular diseases are considered to be podocytopathies since the primary lesion involves podocyte, or the visceral glomerular epithelial cell. The glomerular filtration barrier consists of three layers, the fenestrated endothelium, the GBM and the podocyte and their foot processes. The tertiary cytoplasmic foot processes of the podocytes are connected to one another by the slit diaphragm and adhere to

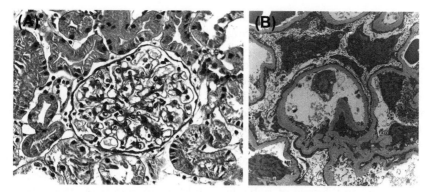

FIGURE 14.2 **Paraneoplastic minimal change disease.** (A) A 63-year-old man with renal cell carcinoma. Glomerulus showing preserved capillary architecture without significant changes. PAS × 600. This figure is reproduced in color in the color plate section. (B) Electron microscopy shows diffuse, global, epithelial foot process effacement with microvillous transformation in the urinary space. × 20,000.

the GBM via several intrinsic podocyte proteins including dystroglycans, adhesion proteins (integrins) and extracellular matrix constituents of the GBM. Inherited or acquired defects of any of these components have been shown to play a role in the pathogenesis of proteinuria.

Clinical Reports and Experimental Animal Models

For the acquired podocytopathies, it has long been postulated that MCD and FSGS are the consequence of immune factors, specifically a disorder in T-cell regulation. From the very early reports of NS, there was evocative data suggesting a link between NS and T-cell-mediated immunity. NS was observed in patients with atopy and could be precipitated by an allergic reaction to bee stings or poison ivy. Increased serum levels of IgE were noted in patients with NS, in the absence of identifiable allergies. Also, infection with measles, a virus known to suppress cell-mediated immunity, could induce remission in patients with MCD. Lastly, there is a rapid response and decrease in proteinuria when patients with MCD are treated with corticosteroids (CCS). CCS are especially effective at blocking cell-mediated immune responses [42,43].

Table 14.4 [2,8] lists the prevalence of MCD according to tumor types. Notably, there is an increased prevalence of thymoma associated with PN MCD. Thymoma, a relatively rare malignancy, is associated with multiple autoimmune disorders (myasthenia gravis, pure red cell aplasia, pemphigus vulgaris, SLE). The reported prevalence of all paraneoplastic glomerular lesions (MCD, FSGS, MGN) in patients with thymoma is a conspicuously high rate of 2% [8]. In light of these associations, a proposed mechanism for PN MCD is dysregulated thymic T-cell production. Normally, T-cells mature and go through positive and negative selection through the thymus. Autoimmune diseases can arise when autoreactive T-cells are not eliminated; when there is an imbalance between autoreactive T-cells and immunoregulatory mechanisms; or when immunoregulatory mechanisms are not effectively controlled. PN MCD is often diagnosed after the thymoma is removed, and responds to CCS. If the thymic tissue was suppressing an immunoregulatory population of cells, this would explain the development of PN MCD after thymectomy [44]. Alternatively, PN MCD could be the result of persistent T-cell dysfunction after thymectomy.

A number of investigators have tested this hypothesis that T-cell dysregulation plays a role in corrupting the integrity of the glomerular filtration barrier. Whether there is a triggering factor (cytokines, oncogenic virus) for T-cell dysregulation has been the subject of several studies. In a gross oversimplification of T-cell immunity, one can divide the system into Th1 and Th2 subdivisions. The two subdivisions have different cytokine profiles and functional effects. Gamma interferon is the dominant cytokine in Th1 immune responses, and IL-4 and IL-13 dominate Th2 responses. IL-13 levels are increased in the serum and T-cells of patients with MCD. It has been demonstrated that there are IL-13 receptors in podocyte cell culture and glomeruli of humans and rats [45]. Studies done on Wistar rats transfected with a vector-cloned IL-13 gene showed that the transfected rats developed proteinuria, hypoalbuminemia and hypercholesterolemia. When the transfected rats were compared to control rats, their LM studies were histologically unremarkable, and the EM revealed 80% foot process fusion. Reverse transcription and quantitative PCR with hybridization probes and IF staining used to examine glomerular gene expression of nephrin, podocin, dystroglycan and IL-13 receptor subunits demonstrated that gene expression and IF staining intensity for these moieties was diminished in the transfected rats when compared with controls. Glomerular gene expression of IL-13 receptors, IL-13R alpha 1 and IL-13R alpha 2, were significantly upregulated, as was IF staining intensity for these proteins [45].

Another lymphokine candidate for PN MCD is IL-8. IL-8 is produced by macrophages and some subsets of T-cells. Levels of IL-8 are increased in sera and peripheral blood mononuclear cell supernatants from patients with MCD. IL-8 infusion into the renal artery of rats produces proteinuria, which can then be blocked by anti-IL-8 antibodies [46,47]. It remains speculative whether the cytokine milieu of malignancy affects the immune system, particularly upregulation of the macrophage and Th lymphocytes, which then elaborate other putative factors, which in turn cause glomerular epithelial injury. An alternative explanation is the neutralization of the anion layer of the GBM by the cationic cytokines.

Vascular endothelial growth factor (VEGF) has also been proposed as a mediator of MCD lesions. Measured serum levels and mRNA expression of VEGF are higher in children with NS and plasma VEGF and mRNA were higher in patients with active NS compared to children in remission from their disease [48]. In a case report of a female with advanced rectal cancer with 1.8 gm proteinuria, hypoalbuminemia and a renal biopsy showing MCD, serum VEGF levels were markedly elevated (1880 pg/ml) and immunohistochemical analysis of the rectal tumor using monoclonal antibody-specific VEGF showed strong expression of VEGF. Three months after tumor resection, the proteinuria resolved, serum VEGF levels decreased and serum albumin level was restored [49]. Additional information that VEGF may have a role in PN MCD comes from the von Hippel—Lindau tumor suppressor gene. A mutation of the von Hippel—Lindau tumor suppressor gene is identified in most cases of sporadic clear cell renal cancer. This mutation results in overproduction of VEGF. Whether overexpression of VEGF due to mutation of the von Hippel—Lindau tumor suppressor gene explains the relatively high prevalence of renal cell cancer (RCCa) in association with PN MCD and paraneoplastic focal segmental glomerulosclerosis (PN FSGS) is a matter of speculation. On the other hand, it is becoming increasingly apparent that VEGF biology is very complex, and the kidney is a prime target for its physiologic as well as pathologic action.

When bevacizumab, a humanized monoclonal antibody to VEGF, was used to treat RCCa, 54% of patients given bevacizumab developed grade 2 or 3 proteinuria [50]. A systematic literature review and meta-analysis of published RCCa with bevacizumab therapy in cancer patients demonstrated that, regardless of tumor type, bevacizumab treatment was associated with a higher risk for proteinuria. When compared with chemotherapy alone, when bevacizumab was added to the treatment, the relative risk of high-grade proteinuria was 4.79; and the relative risk for NS was 7.78 [51]. The biology of VEGF is complex and proteinuria induced by inhibitory monoclonal VEGF antibodies may involve manifold pathways. There are likely many polymorphisms in the VEGF gene which may explain the myriad clinical sequelae of overexpression, underexpression, or inhibition of this protein.

Focal Segmental Glomerulosclerosis (FSGS)

FSGS and MCD are discussed in proximity to one another since they are generally considered to be at different parts of the spectrum of podocytopathies and are believed to share some pathogenetic pathways. FSGS accounts for 40% of cases of NS in adults and is the most common cause of primary glomerular disease causing ESRD in the USA. Approximately 80% of FSGS cases overall are idiopathic in nature [52].

Epidemiology of PN FSGS

Table 14.5 [2,8,53] lists the prevalence of PN FSGS according to their associated cancer types. As is the case with PN MCD, more than half of the reports of PN FSGS are linked to hematologic malignancies, being slightly more common with the lymphoid malignancies. Thymoma and RCCa are the most frequently reported solid malignancies in association with PN FSGS.

Histopathology

Histologically, the lesion is characterized by segmental obliteration of the glomerular capillary with solidification on LM leading to sclerosis, frequently capsular adhesion and hyaline deposition (Figure 14.3). Usually a cuff of hyperplastic epithelial cells overlays this area

of the glomerulus. Increased proximal tubular reabsorption droplets can also be observed, indicating significant proteinuria. On EM, there is extensive effacement of the epithelial cell foot processes and electron dense immune deposits are not present. Evidence of podocyte injury such as swelling, discrete and confluent cytoplasmic vacuolization, protein droplets and reactive nuclear changes may be observed. IF typically reveals coarsely granular staining for IgM and C3 in the mesangial areas, which are generally due to non-specific trapping, particularly in the areas of sclerosis.

FSGS is considered a common endpoint for podocyte injury from diverse clinical entities. Some of the insults which lead to foot process effacement and loss of the integrity of the GBM barrier include viruses (HIV), drugs (heroin, interferon, pamidronate) and mechanical stress (hyperfiltration, hypertension). Podocytes or glomerular visceral epithelial cells are terminally differentiated cells which cannot repair themselves via cell division. Consequently, podocyte depletion, detachment, apoptosis and necrosis will all result in glomerulosclerosis [52].

Clinical Reports and Experimental Animal Models

Idiopathic FSGS has been attributed to a circulating permeability factor (PF). Evidence cited to support this hypothesis includes that a kidney taken from a donor with nephrosis will no longer show proteinuria when transplanted into a patient without nephrosis. Conversely, FSGS can recur in a patient with FSGS who has received a transplanted kidney. Furthermore, when FSGS recurs in the transplanted kidney, plasmapheresis, presumably by removal of soluble factors responsible for the proteinuria, can cause reversal of NS. Recently, the identity of one such factor has been elucidated by Wei et al. as soluble urokinase receptor (suPAR) [54]. When discussing potential permeability factors, it bears keeping in mind that podocyte function is mediated by autocrine pathways as well as via

TABLE 14.5   Prevalence of Focal Segmental Glomerulosclerosis According to Cancer Subtypes

Solid tumors			Hematologic malignancies		
Site	Tumor type	# cases	Lineage	Tumor type	# cases
Renal carcinomas		6	Lymphoid malignancies		
Thymoma		4		Hodgkin lymphoma	7
Gastrointestinal carcinoma		2		Chronic lymphocytic leukemia	6
Respiratory system carcinoma				Non-Hodgkin lymphoma	3
	Lung/bronchus carcinoma	1		Cutaneous T-cell lymphoma	2
	Mesothelioma	1		Acute lymphocytic leukemia	1
Others			Myeloid malignancies		
	Breast carcinoma	1		Polycythemia vera	6
	Melanoma	1		Essential thrombocythemia	3
	Sarcoma	1		Primary myelofibrosis	2
	Pheochromocytoma	1		Myelodysplastic syndrome	1
	Hydaditiform mole	1		Acute myeloid leukemia	1
Total		19	Total		32

receptor-mediated interaction with exogenous mediators. The possible link between T-cell and podocyte regulatory pathways remains a topic of ongoing inquiry, as discussed to some extent in the subsection on PN MCD.

A potential paraneoplastic link between thymoma and podocyte dysfunction in FSGS was studied in Buffalo/Mna rats because of their association with spontaneous thymoma. Data showed that the thymic disease did not cause the proteinuria, as thymectomy had no effect on proteinuria [55]. Two autosomal recessive genes located on chromosome 13 (which is also known to carry one out of four genes for thymic enlargement), seem to confer susceptibility to glomerulosclerosis. Of note, the localization of this chromosome corresponds to human chromosome 1, where the NEPHS2 gene coding for podocin, a protein integral to the glomerular filtration barrier, has been located. This gene co-localization suggests that perhaps there is a genetic predisposition to PN FSGS [56].

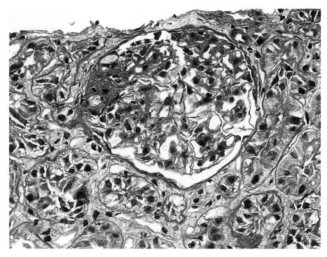

FIGURE 14.3 **Paraneoplastic focal segmental glomerulosclerosis.** A 40-year-old man presented with nephrotic syndrome and subsequently diagnosed with thymoma. The figure shows a normal appearing glomerulus showing segmental collapse and sclerosis containing a trapped foam cell at the periphery with adhesion to the Bowman capsule. This figure is reproduced in color in the color plate section.

Additional investigations in the Buffalo/Mna rats, which spontaneously develop FSGS, suggest that the cytokine milieu of malignancy creates a number of potential PFs. Serial testing and the kinetics of renal immune cell populations and various cytokines were tested (lymphocytes, macrophages, T-, B- and natural killer [NK] cells, transforming growth factor beta [TGFb], tumor necrosis factor alfa [TNFa], interferon [IFN], interleukins [IL-1, IL-2, IL-4, IL-6, IL-10, IL-12 and IL-13], regulated on activation, normal T expressed and secreted [RANTES] cytokines and monocyte chemo-attractant protein 1 [MCP1], and T-cell receptor chain transcripts). It was observed that, prior to the onset of overt proteinuria and ultrastructural podocyte changes, there was increased production of macrophage-associated cytokines, particularly TNFa. Also, cytokines associated with Th2 increased while there was downregulation of Th1 cytokines [57]. The cytokine milieu of malignancy and its effects on the immune system, particularly the macrophage and Th lymphocytes, may induce other factors which, in turn, cause glomerular epithelial injury.

IgA Nephropathy

IgA nephropathy (IgAN) is the most common form of primary GN worldwide, accounting for up to 10% of patients reaching end stage renal disease in some countries. There is geographic variation in the frequency of the disease, where in Europe, Asia and Australia, IgAN accounts for 20—40% of patients with primary GN. Japan has the highest frequency and the USA and Canada the lowest. The clinical presentation ranges from recurrent gross hematuria at the time of an upper respiratory tract infection, isolated persistent microhematuria and varying degrees of proteinuria, only rarely reaching nephrotic range proteinuria. Hypertension often is a presenting symptom in young or middle-aged adults.

Epidemiology of PN IgAN

When it has been reported, it is most often associated with solid tumors, specifically RCCa and lung carcinomas (Table 14.6) [2,8,58]. Secondary forms of IgAN have been described with autoimmune diseases (rheumatoid arthritis, Behcet's disease, ankylosing spondylitis, etc.), alcoholic

TABLE 14.6 Prevalence of IgA Nephropathy According to Cancer Types

Solid tumors		Hematologic malignancies		
Site	# cases	Lineage	Tumor type	# cases
Renal carcinomas	17	Lymphoid malignancies		
Gastrointestinal carcinoma	1		Cutaneous T-cell lymphoma	6
Respiratory system carcinoma	7	Myeloid malignancies		
Total	25		Polycythemia vera	3
			Myelodysplastic syndrome	2
			Chronic myelogenous leukemia	1
			Total	12

cirrhosis, dermatitis herpetiformis, inflammatory bowel disease, celiac disease and carcinoma. IgAN has a tendency to recur in renal transplants with little impact on graft outcome.

Histopathology

The characteristic finding on LM is glomerular mesangial expansion with cell proliferation and increased mesangial matrix. Other variants of LM appearance are segmental endocapillary proliferation with or without crescents, segmental sclerosis and rarely global endocapillary proliferation (Figure 14.4A). The former two findings along with mesangial proliferation have prognostic significance [59]. IF study is required for the diagnosis of IgAN. On IF, IgA is the principal or sole immunoglobulin in the glomerular mesangium, even in those glomeruli that are optically normal on LM (Figure 14.4B). IgA1 is the exclusive subtype in these deposits along with C3 staining. The question remains whether IgA in the deposits acts as an antigen or an antibody that fixes C3 complement. EM reveals granular electron dense deposits in the mesangial and

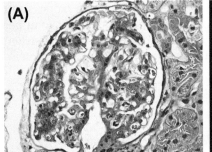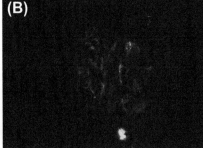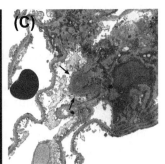

FIGURE 14.4 Paraneoplastic IgA nephropathy. A 72-year-old man presented with hematuria and flank pain, diagnosed with renal cell carcinoma, followed by total nephrectomy. The non-neoplastic portion of kidney examined. (A) Glomerulus shows global, mild mesangial hypercellularity and increased matrix. PAS × 400. This figure is reproduced in color in the color plate section. (B) Immunofluorescence microscopy localized IgA deposits, mainly in the mesangial areas. FITC IgA × 300. This figure is reproduced in color in the color plate section. (C) Electron microscopy of the glomerular mesangial area shows electron dense deposits (arrows). The peripheral capillary basement membranes are unremarkable. × 15,000.

paramesangial areas corresponding to the immune deposits (Figure 14.4C).

Clinical Reports and Experimental Animal Models

Although IgA nephropathy is a common primary form of GN, the exact pathogenesis is not known. IgA deposits have been found in the mesangium of patients without any clinical evidence of renal disease. Autopsy data on non-selected patients and allograft biopsies taken at zero hour have shown glomerular IgA deposits in up to 20% of cases. IgA nephropathy was found in 1.6% of supposedly normal kidney donors. These data would suggest that the clinical presentation and severity of IgAN may depend on modifying environmental or genetic factors [60]. The most current data show that there are increased levels of abnormally galactosylated IgA1 subtype in patients with active IgAN and proliferative mesangial changes. The basis for overproduction of the polymeric, abnormal IgA1 subtype with galactose-deficient O-glycans in the hinge region remains elusive. The most current pathogenetic pathway is the four-hit hypothesis: (1) increased circulating levels of IgA1 with galactose-deficient O-glycans in the hinge region; (2) antibodies are directed against the galactose-deficient O-glycans in the hinge region; (3) immune complexes form and accumulate in the glomeruli and mesangium; (4) the immune complexes induce mesangial cells to secrete proliferative and profibrotic cytokines and chemokines [61]. Details of the proposed pathogenetic pathway still need to be elucidated. It is not clear whether paraneoplastic IgAN (PN IgAN) results from derangements at any or none of the above steps.

The lack of good animal models for IgAN may be attributed to the existence of major differences between mice and human IgA systems. In studies of PN IgAN associated with RCCa, the same IgA subtype was found on the tumor and in the glomerular immune deposits in the majority of cases [58,62]. It is possible that "molecular mimicry" could explain PN IgAN. Tumor antigens could stimulate secretion of abnormal IgA1-like particles, which would then induce an IgG response, or induce an IgA immune response in the host. The production of interleukin-6 and IgA by the tumor infiltrating lymphocytes and plasma cells respectively have been implicated in three cases of PN IgAN with RCCa in elderly patients [58]. However, any mechanistic pathway for PN IgAN remains speculative at this time.

Although an idiopathic form of IgAN can occur at any age, a new onset IgAN in older patients begs further testing for an underlying malignancy, particularly originating from the respiratory tract, buccal cavity or nasopharynx [63]. In one series, 6/26 patients (23%) with IgAN who were 60 years or older had a malignancy while none of the patients under 60 (158) were found to have a neoplasm. Beaufils et al. also found asymptomatic IgA deposits in autopsy kidney tissue in patients who died due to gastro-intestinal cancers [18]. This is thought to be due to increased circulating IgA secondary to invasion of the intestinal mucosa by tumor [63].

While nearly 40% of patients with RCCa manifest some form of paraneoplastic syndrome, a strong association also exists between RCCa and PN IgAN [58,62]. In one clinicopathologic study of 60 nephrectomy cases with RCCa, 11/60 (18%) of them had PN IgAN. Von Hippel—Lindau protein, a product of the VHL gene co-localized with the IgA deposits in the glomerular mesangial areas of several cases, confirms the paraneoplastic nature of the renal lesion [62]. About 55% of these patients (6/11) showed recovery from proteinuria and hematuria following removal of the tumor.

Henoch—Schonlein purpura (HSP) is a form of systemic small vessel vasculitis which involves multiple organs, including skin, gastrointestinal tract, joints and the kidney. HSP nephritis displays a proliferative GN with crescents and deposits of IgA containing immune complexes. Additionally, an increased risk of malignancy was reported in HSP patients rather than their age-matched controls [12]. There are 20 reported cases of HSP nephritis associated with solid tumors and hematologic malignancies. The patients were mostly male with a median age of 59 [64,65].

Rapidly Progressive Glomerulonephritis (RPGN)

RPGN is characterized by acute renal failure, azotemia, hypertension, proteinuria and hematuria. The urine sediment is indicative of glomerular disease and consists of RBC and WBC casts,

cellular debris and pigmented casts. If the renal failure is severe, uremic symptoms (nausea, vomiting, pericarditis, encephalopathy), and clinically significant volume overload can be present. The other moniker for RPGN is crescentic GN.

Epidemiology of Paraneoplastic ANCA-associated Pauci-immune Crescentic GN (PN CrGN)

Table 14.7 [2,8,66] indicates that PN CrGN with ANCA-positive serology are common with solid tumors, particularly RCC, gastric

TABLE 14.7 Prevalence of Crescentic Glomerulonephritis According to Cancer Types

Solid tumors			Hematologic malignancies			
Site	**Tumor type**	**# cases**	**Lineage**	**Tumor type**		**# cases**
Renal cell carcinoma		10	Myeloid malignancies			
Gastrointestinal carcinoma				Polycythemia vera		1
	Gastric carcinoma	6		Myelodysplastic syndrome		1
	Esophageal carcinoma	1		Chronic myelogenous leukemia		1
	Hepatic carcinoma	1	Total			3
	Colorectal carcinoma	1				
Respiratory system carcinoma						
	Larynx/pharynx carcinoma	2				
	Lung/bronchus carcinoma	4				
Genitourinary carcinoma						
	Prostate carcinoma	3				
	Bladder carcinoma	1				
Breast carcinoma		3				
Others						
	Solid without details	10				
	Skin squamous cell carcinoma	1				
	Kaposi sarcoma	1				
	Thyroid carcinoma	1				
	Ovarian carcinoma	1				
	Total	46				

and lung carcinomas. Lymphoid tumors have not been reported with PN RPGN.

Histopathology

RPGN is a strictly clinical scenario and, based on the immunopathological findings on renal biopsy, it is generally classified into three groups (1) antiglomerular basement disease (antiGBM disease); (2) immune complex vasculitis and (3) antineutrophil cytoplasmic antibody-mediated (ANCA) vasculitis. All three forms of glomerular lesions display segmental necrotizing features with crescents or extracapillary epithelial proliferation, suggesting a severe form of glomerular injury (Figure 14.5). ANCA-associated GN, or pauci-immune crescentic GN, is the most common form of RPGN, accounting for 80% of cases. This entity lacks tissue immune deposits though the glomerular disease is mediated by an immunologic mechanism. IF staining shows a lack of immunoglobulin deposits except for fibrin staining in the necrotizing lesions. However, in one series, 54% of patients were found to have some glomerular immune deposits on EM study [67]. A mild to severe interstitial inflammatory infiltrate, composed primarily of mononuclear cells, is frequently present.

Clinical Reports and Experimental Animal Models

Immunologically mediated injury and inflammation of the small blood vessels and capillaries appears to be a fundamental component to the pathogenesis on ANCA-mediated crescentic GN [68]. ANCA in the serum is reactive to either proteinase 3 (PR3-ANCA) or myeloperoxidase (MPO-ANCA), which are components of azurophilic neutrophil granules and monocyte lysosomes. After ANCA binds to the PR3 or MPO antigen expressed on the cell membranes of cytokine primed neutrophils and monocytes, there is a release of oxygen radicals, lytic enzymes and inflammatory cytokines. ANCA also promotes inflammation by disrupting the normal process of phagocytic clearance of apoptotic neutrophils [69].

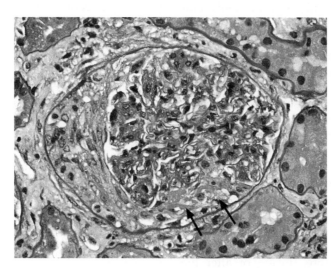

FIGURE 14.5 **Paraneoplastic crescentic glomerulonephritis.** A 59-year-old woman diagnosed with squamous cell carcinoma of the lung has hematuria, mild proteinuria and renal insufficiency. Serology for ANCA was negative. The figure shows the glomerulus showing a cellular crescent in the Bowman space partly compressing the underlying glomerulus. An area of fibrinoid material due to necrosis is visible (arrows). PAS × 400. This figure is reproduced in color in the color plate section.

As previously mentioned, there may be a higher prevalence of malignancy in patients with ANCA-associated vasculitis. In one retrospective analysis, the odds ratio for neoplasia in patients with Wegener's granulomatosis, now known as granulomatosis with polyangiitis (GPA) [70], was 1.79. RCCa was the most frequent malignancy observed overall, with an odds ratio for RCCa in the GPA (Wegener) group of 8.73. PR3 was not detected on any of the tumor samples [71]. In another series, the relative risk of malignancy for ANCA GN was 6.02, but the presence of ANCA was not predictive of malignancy [12]. Of course, all of this data are retrospective and may be prejudiced by referral bias and detection bias. Using registry data from Sweden, which followed a cohort of patients with GPA (Wegener) for 25 years, the relative risk (RR) of cancer was measured using a standard incidence ratio (SIR) between the observed and expected numbers of cancers. Overall, the RR of cancer was increased two-fold. For bladder cancer, the SIR was 4.8; for squamous cell cancer 7.3; for malignant lymphoma 4.2; and for leukemias 5.7 [72]. This study may also reflect the risks of malignancy related to prior exposure to cyclophosphamide as treatment for GPA (Wegener). Unfortunately, these studies do not shed any new insights into the actual relationship of ANCA serology, onset of paraneoplastic crescentic glomerulonephritis (PN CrGN) and concurrent existence of a malignancy. The underlying mechanism of PN CrGN remains largely undefined.

Anecdotal case reports have been cited [1,2,8] which suggest that there may be some direct or indirect link between ANCA-associated crescentic GN (the older cases lack serologic data) and the concurrent malignancy that was diagnosed shortly before, during or after the detection of the small vessel vasculitis process. They are: (1) improvement of renal function after treatment of underlying malignancy only by surgery and radiation, (2) granular or linear immunoglobulin or immune complex deposits are localized in the glomeruli (one case with prostate cancer showed prostate-specific antigen and prostate-specific acid phosphatase in glomerular deposits), and (3) carcinomas of the respiratory tract and urinary tract diagnosed soon after the clinical presentation of vasculitis and ANCA-associated crescentic GN, raising the possibility of tumor-associated trigger for the development of ANCA vasculitis. In most other cases, either the cancer was treated with chemotherapy or the PN CrGN was treated appropriately with steroids and cyclophosphamide to prevent further renal damage. Therefore, one could not confirm whether the renal disease regressed due to treatment of tumor alone, chemotherapy, or to a specific regimen for crescentic GN [73,74].

Membranoproliferative Glomerulonephritis (MPGN)

Membranoproliferative glomerulonephritis is a unique form of glomerular pattern of injury primarily affecting children and young adults in the second or early third decade of life. It can present with a nephritic or nephrotic clinical picture.

Epidemiology of PN MPGN

Idiopathic forms of MPGN seldom occur in older adults and are often secondary to infections (bacterial, viral, parasitic), autoimmune diseases, or, commonly, hematological malignancies. Close to 60% of all reported cases of PN MPGN are related to lymphoid malignancies (chronic lymphoid leukemia [CLL] and NHL). In a review of the literature, solid tumors of diverse organs have been implicated in the development of PN MPGN (Table 14.8) [2,8].

Histopathology

MPGN is a form of indolent, progressive chronic GN, where the pattern of glomerular injury is secondary to IC deposition in the

TABLE 14.8 Prevalence of Membranoproliferative Glomerulonephritis According to Cancer Types

Solid tumors			Hematologic malignancies		
Site	Tumor type	# cases	Lineage	Tumor type	# cases
Respiratory system carcinomas			Lymphoid malignancies		
	Lung/bronchial carcinoma	5		Chronic lymphocytic leukemia	20
	Pulmonary carcinoid	1		Non-Hodgkin lymphoma	13
Renal carcinomas		4		Hairy cell leukemia	5
Melanoma		3		Acute lymphocytic leukemia	2
Gastric carcinoma		2	Myeloid malignancies		
Breast carcinoma		2		Chronic myelogenous leukemia	2
Genitourinary carcinoma				Chronic myelomonocytic leukemia	1
	Prostate carcinoma	1		Polycythemia vera	1
	Bladder carcinoma	1	Total		44
	Ovarian germinal carcinoma	1			
Other					
	Carcinoma (type unknown)	4			
	Hydatidiform mole	1			
	Desmoplastic round cell tumor	1			
	Thymoma	1			
	Angiosarcoma	1			
Total		28			

subendothelial and/or mesangial space. On LM, there is marked mesangial cell proliferation and increased matrix, encroaching on the capillary lumina, giving a lobular glomerular architecture. The hypercellularity and activity of the lesion is contributed by infiltrating leukocytes (Figure 14.6A). The specific morphological feature is due to interposition of mesangial cells and matrix into the subendothelial space of the capillary wall with new basement membrane formation giving rise to double contours by silver staining. On IF, granular deposition of IgM, IgG and C3 can be seen in a segmental or global distribution (Figure 14.6B). On EM, mainly granular subendothelial and mesangial electron dense deposits, and cellular interposition within the capillary basement membranes, are evident (Figure 14.6C).

Clinical Reports

Since most of them are in the absence of HCV infection or cryoglobulins, it was suggested that PN MPGN may be induced by tumor antigen-mediated immune complexes and the failure of the host immune system to completely eliminate the circulating tumor antigens or complexes [75].

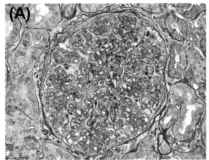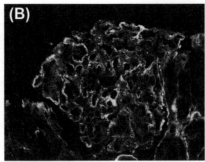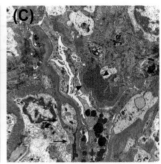

FIGURE 14.6 **Paraneoplastic membranoproliferative glomerulonephritis.** An elderly man with hematuria and nephrotic syndrome recently treated for lung cancer. (A) Glomerulus is enlarged and hypercellular with a lobulated configuration, infiltrated by mononuclear cells and cell proliferation as well as peripheral capillary wall thickening with double contours. PAS × 400. This figure is reproduced in color in the color plate section. (B) Immunofluorescence microscopy reveals segmental, granular, capillary wall and mesangial deposits of polyclonal IgG, C3 and lesser IgM with an irregular distribution. FITC IgG × 400. This figure is reproduced in color in the color plate section. (C) Electron microscopy shows thickened glomerular basement membranes with cellular interposition and new basement membrane formation (arrows) and subendothelial deposits (arrow heads). × 20,000.

On occasion, resection of the tumor was associated with remission of MPGN [75,76]. In other studies, MPGN developed after the primary tumor was resected [77], or MPGN had responded to corticosteroid (CCS) therapy without tumor ablation [78,79]. The paucity of cases, combined with the diverse renal responses to treatment of the primary neoplasia, makes it very difficult to discern any causal relationship or pathogenetic mechanism for PN MPGN.

Other Glomerular Lesions

A reactive type of amyloidosis with AA protein has been documented with several types of solid organ tumors [80], 25–33% of which are linked to RCCa [81]. Glomerular involvement is manifested by nephrotic syndrome with remission after removal of the tumor. The development of a chronic inflammatory state and fever secondary to secretion of IL-6 cytokine by the kidney tumor cells may trigger the formation of AA amyloid [1]. An alternate explanation is possible secretion of a precursor of amyloid proteins or enzyme by the tumor, causing subsequent amyloid formation [2]. Fibrillary GN has also been diagnosed with a nephrotic or nephritic syndrome, in the setting of epithelial cancers including stomach, liver, lung and kidney [82] (personal unpublished data). Mucin-producing cancers from several organs (stomach, lung, breast and pancreas) have been implicated to cause endothelial injury and systemic or renal thrombotic microangiopathy [2].

THE HEMATOLOGIC MALIGNANCIES

Paraneoplastic syndromes of hematologic malignancies affect many organ systems including the nervous system, skin, bone marrow and the kidney, and is often associated with autoimmune phenomena [83]. It is also well known that several common autoimmune diseases may be predisposing factors for the development of subsequent lymphoid malignancies. Hematologic malignances are categorized based on their myeloid or lymphoid lineage (Figure 14.7). The frequency of specific types may vary with age, gender, geographical location and any other underlying contributing factors. While the renal involvement is relatively uncommon with some types, virtually all

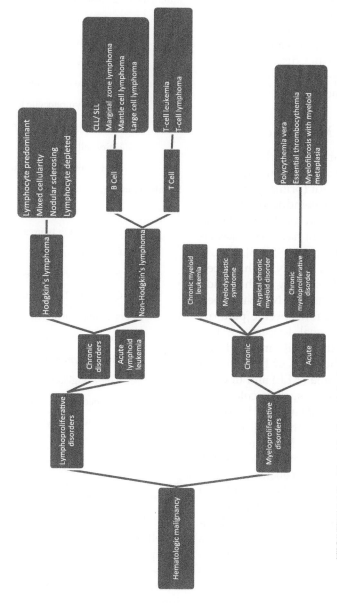

FIGURE 14.7 Classification of the hematologic malignancies according to the 2008 WHO classification.

subtypes of hematologic malignancies affecting the kidney, directly or indirectly, have been reported, in anecdotal case reports or in larger case series. The classifications and subdivisions are useful when discussing PNGNs since the prevalence and type of glomerular pathologies described within the different categories vary significantly. Paraneoplastic disease may be caused by monoclonal proteins, cryoglobulins, autoimmunity or amyloidosis.

PNGN in Lymphoid Malignancies

Lymphoid malignancies including all forms of HL and NHL, both in the immunocompetent and immunodeficient (primary immunodeficiency, age-related, virus-induced HIV, EBV and immunosuppression in post-transplantation and autoimmune states) have been associated with renal disease (Table 14.9) [2,8]. PNGN in patients with CLL, HL and NHL has been documented relatively frequently, with a wide range of glomerular lesions and NS [84], albeit with a predilection for a few specific patterns [1,8,77,85]. In contrast, renal lesions are less commonly observed in cases with myeloid malignancies. Only sporadic cases of PNGN with acute lymphocytic leukemia (ALL) and uncommon lymphoid malignancies such as cutaneous T-cell lymphoma (CTCL) and hairy cell leukemia (HCL) are found in the literature [8]. IgA has been reported with CTCL. PN MN is especially rare among the hematologic malignancies. HL is predominantly a disease of T-cell lineage while CLL, HCL and the majority of NHL are of B-cell lineage. MCD is the most common PNGN associated with HL, followed by FSGS. Hodgkin lymphoma and specific forms of NHL secrete a variety of cytokines that act in an autocrine or a paracrine fashion, to provide growth advantages for the tumor cells [86]. Functional and structural changes of intraglomerular cells have been shown to be influenced by cytokines causing renal disease. MPGN and MN are more commonly associated with the predominantly

TABLE 14.9 PNGN and Lymphoid Malignancies

GN	Tumor type	# cases
Minimal change disease		
	Hodgkin lymphoma	61
	Non-Hodgkin lymphoma	6
	Chronic lymphocytic leukemia	2
Membranoproliferative glomerulonephritis		
	Chronic lymphocytic leukemia	20
	Non-Hodgkin lymphoma	13
	Hairy cell leukemia	5
	Acute lymphocytic leukemia	2
Membranous nephropathy		
	Chronic lymphocytic leukemia	10
	Non-Hodgkin lymphoma	5
	Hodgkin lymphoma	5
	Acute lymphocytic leukemia	1
	Cutaneous T-cell lymphoma	1
Focal segmental glomerular sclerosis		
	Hodgkin lymphoma	7
	Chronic lymphocytic leukemia	6
	Non-Hodgkin lymphoma	3
	Cutaneous T-cell lymphoma	2
	Acute lymphocytic leukemia	1
IgA nephropathy		
	Cutaneous T-cell lymphoma	6
Total		156

B-cell lineage tumors, CLL, HCL and NHL. The composition of the glomerular deposits in the presence of B-lymphocyte lineage tumors is mainly monoclonal proteins, often directly linking to the underlying type of lymphoma [1]. Additionally, a high proportion of cases with some form of glomerular injury secondary to a lymphoma also demonstrate varying amounts

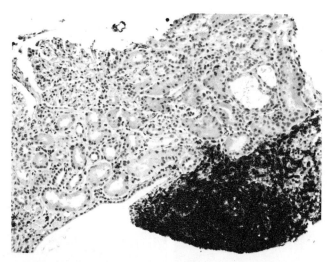

FIGURE 14.8 Paraneoplastic minimal change disease and infiltrating small B-cell lymphoma in the kidney. The figure shows a large lymphoid aggregate in the renal cortex, with positive CD20 and lambda light chain. Adjacent glomeruli appear normal. Immunoperoxidase CD20 × 200. This figure is reproduced in color in the color plate section.

of infiltrating malignant lymphoid cells in the glomeruli and/or in the tubulo-interstitial areas (Figure 14.8). These findings could be responsible for concomitant renal dysfunction [87]. Direct renal parenchymal infiltration of lymphoma may result from a primary lymphoma arising in the kidney or as a part of a disseminated lymphoma from an extrarenal source [88].

PN MCD and PN FSGS

Of the hematologic malignancies, HL represents the majority of cases with PN MCD (see Table 14.4). PN MCD occurs in 0.4–1% of patients with HL [41,83]. Usually, the lymphoma may be apparent at the time of onset of NS. However, the NS can precede the discovery of the malignancy by months to years and not infrequently heralds recurrence of HL [89]. The occurrence of PN FSGS is 1/10 of that of PN MCD. Since the pathogenesis of both entities is based on T-cell-mediated cytokines and other cells, the lower frequency of FSGS may reflect absence of the renal lesions in the early stages of NS or biopsy sampling [90]. In about 50% of cases, MCD has been reported to occur in close proximity with

HL or with disease relapse. In one cohort, HL was diagnosed several months after MCD in five of 21 patients. These patients were initially resistant to cyclosporine (CSA) and CCS but later responded to chemotherapy [41]. While an earlier study demonstrated "mixed cellularity type" as a common form of Hodgkin disease associated with MCD [91], Audard and colleagues reported "nodular sclerosis" as the predominant morphologic subtype with MCD [92]. About 10% of CLL patients with NS are complicated by MCD and rarely by FSGS, and are thought to be connected with functional abnormalities of T-lymphocytes [53,93–96]. Most of these patients have shown clinical resolution of nephrotic syndrome as well as CLL following treatment for the neoplastic condition.

As is the case with solid tumors, a permeability factor (PF), such as cytokines released by the malignant cells or T-lymphocyte activation, acting on the glomerular podocytes, is suspected in the etiopathogenesis of PN MCD and PN FSGS with the hematologic malignancies. HL is associated with T-cell expansion that is directed towards the Th2 phenotype. Importantly, IL-13 expression is increased many fold in

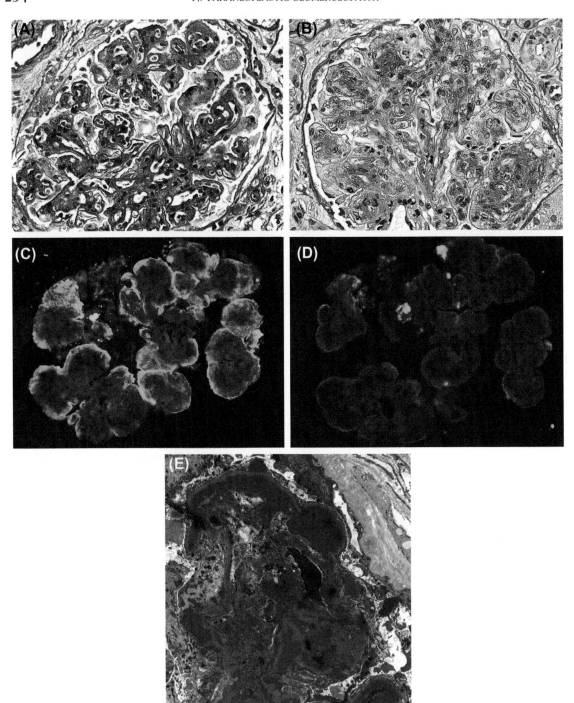

HL-derived cell lines, specifically from Reed—Sternberg (RS) cells. IL-13 is assumed to be the autocrine growth factor for RS cells in HL [97–99]. IL-13 is a Th2 cytokine, whose receptor is expressed in Reed—Sternberg cells in patients with HL. IL-13 in rats induces a MCD-like nephropathy [97]. The possible role of Th2 cytokines in PN MCD has already been discussed in detail above (p. 222) <Subsection IIB.3>.

In addition to IL-13, FSGS serum permeability factor (FSPF) and c-maf-inducing protein (c-mip) have also been examined as possible PFs. Elevated levels of FSPF were measured in a patient who presented with NS. The patient was treated with CSA with no significant drop in FSPF. Subsequently, the patient was diagnosed with HL and FSPF levels decreased following chemotherapy for the HL [100]. These investigators studied eight patients with classic HL and MCD. In previous studies, they had isolated a gene named c-maf-inducing protein (c-mip), which is induced in podocytes of patients with MCD. The protein is thought to be involved in cytoskeleton organization and proximal podocyte signaling. In this study, intense c-mip labeling was observed in the lymphoid follicles of patients with HL with MCD, while it was undetectable in HL patients without MCD [92]. Expression of VEGF and TGF-beta1 by Reed—Sternberg cells has been linked to FSGS in HL [101,102].

PN MN and Lymphoid Malignancies

Unlike PN MN with non-hematologic malignancies or solid tumors (e.g. carcinomas), PN MN in lymphoid malignancies is relatively rare. Occasionally, it has been reported with both Hodgkin and NHL [77,85,91,103,104] as well as CLL [105]. The latter case responded to therapy with fludarabine for CLL with remission of proteinuria.

PN MPGN and Lymphoid Malignancies

A majority of reported cases of PN MPGN (nearly 60%) represent hematologic malignancies involving CLL and NHL (Table 14.8) [2,8]. Even though the incidence of NS in patients with CLL is <1%, MPGN is the most common glomerular pathology in CLL patients with NS, followed by MCD [8]. MPGN in patients with CLL may be caused by cryoglobulins, or by monoclonal immunoglobulins secreted by a B-cell clone, without cryoglobulinemia or complement activation [106]. A few cases of HL have been described with PN MPGN [91,107].

The incidence of renal involvement is less than a third of the cases with type I or type II cryoglobulinemia [85]. In addition to the characteristic glomerular findings of MPGN in these cases, the presence of cryoglobulins or other forms of monoclonal immunoglobulin deposits impart additional distinctive features such as focal or massive intracapillary PAS+, fuscinophilic aggregates along with varying numbers of infiltrating monocytes, which attempt to phagocytose these deposits (Figure 14.9A). Since CLL is a protracted disease, the membranoproliferative pattern of glomerular injury may display varying stages of nodular sclerosing glomerular lesions

FIGURE 14.9 Paraneoplastic membranoproliferative glomerulonephritis and chronic B-cell lymphocytic leukemia (CLL). (A) Glomerulus showing enlargement, increased mesangial cellularity and global thickening of the peripheral capillary walls with frequent double contours and focal cellular interposition. This figure is reproduced in color in the color plate section. (B) Glomerulus from another case of CLL demonstrates hypercellularity and nodular mesangial sclerosing changes leading to narrowing of the capillary lumina with thickening of the capillary walls. PAS × 400. This figure is reproduced in color in the color plate section. (C) Immunofluorescence microscopy shows mainly monoclonal IgG and kappa light chain deposits along the capillary walls and focally in the mesangial areas. FITC kappa LC × 400. This figure is reproduced in color in the color plate section. (D) Immunofluorescence microscopy using FITC lambda light chain is mostly negative in a similar distribution. × 400. This figure is reproduced in color in the color plate section. (E) Electron microscopy discloses abundant subendothelial and mesangial monoclonal deposits. × 15,000.

(Figure 14.9B). While IgM may be the predominant immunoglobulin deposits in CLL, most cases do not have properties of cryoglobulins.

Immunofluorescence microscopy serves to define the composition of the cryoglobulins (often type I or II) and/or monoclonal proteins in the glomeruli. Subtyping of IgG deposits may identify specific isotypes of IgG1, IgG2, IgG3, or IgG4, with or without complement fixation [108]. Cases of mixed or type II cryoglobulinemia demonstrate a monoclonal component IgM kappa (Figure 14.9C and D) or lambda along with polyclonal IgG within the deposits with C3 fixation.

Although the deposits can be localized in the glomerular capillary basement membranes, mesangium, or in the capillary lumina by electron microscopy (Figure 14.9E), the texture or organization of the deposits with a specific substructure can also be recognized [1,85,108,109]. They can have a heterogeneous substructure, depending on the physico-chemical characteristics of the paraprotein deposits such as fibrillar, annular—tubular (Figure 14.10), "finger print" pattern, stacks or randomly arranged microfibrillar/tubular deposits and, more commonly, just finely or coarsely granular appearance. Focal or diffuse tubular basement membrane deposits may be demonstrated in some cases.

Chronic hepatitis C viral infection (HCV), with or without circulating cryoglobulins, is a significant infectious etiology of MPGN. HCV infection is a common cause of MPGN in adults, often associated with type II mixed cryoglobulinemia. It has been postulated that the HCV, which directly infects circulating peripheral blood mononuclear cells and bone marrow cells, stimulates the B-lymphocytes to synthesize the type II mixed cryoglobulin. Using reverse transcriptase/PCR technique, investigators were able to detect IgM-producing clonal B-cells in 38 patients with HCV infection, with and without type II mixed cryoglobulinemia [110]. They hypothesize that

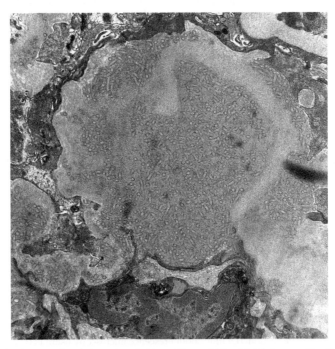

FIGURE 14.10 Organized monoclonal deposits. Same as Figure 14.9 with high magnification of glomerular electron dense deposits showing a tubular configuration, measuring 40—50 nm in diameter. × 40,000.

monoclonal B-cell clones may arise in a minority of patients with more severe lymphocyte dysfunction and a greater impairment of the immunoregulatory mechanisms. These clones then drive the development of both PN MPGN and lymphoproliferative disorders. In one series of 119 consecutive HCV-positive patients diagnosed with mixed cryoglobulinemia, 16 patients had mixed cryoglobulins and MPGN [111]. Bone marrow biopsies performed on patients with MPGN and those without MPGN, showed a higher prevalence of lymphoma in the group with MPGN. This led to the speculation that MPGN in this setting may represent a PNGN due to an occult B-cell lymphoma. These investigators also observed that all of the patients with MPGN died of infection and/or cardiovascular disease, suggesting severe lymphocyte dysfunction in this group [111]. Monoclonal gammopathy, lymphoproliferative disorders and myeloma are recognized etiologies for secondary MPGN and cryoglobulinemia.

While HCV is the major cause of mixed cryoglobulinemia (MC), viral infection may not be required in the pathogenesis of PN MPGN. Matignon et al. looked at a cohort of 20 patients with MC without HCV. All the renal biopsy specimens showed MPGN. Nine patients had primary Sjogren's syndrome [112]. While only one of 20 patients had NHL at the time of the retrospective data collection, four of 20 patients developed B-cell lymphoma during follow-up [112]. Another report on patients with MC without HCV revealed a four-fold increased risk of developing B-cell and NHL [113]. Conversely, a lower incidence of B-cell lymphoma has been reported in patients with HCV-related MC [114]. Furthermore, bone marrow B-cell clonal expansion has been shown to correlate with nephritis in MC syndromes in patients with no clinical or histopathological features of lymphoproliferative disorders, suggesting that MC may be a pre-B-cell lymphoma state, and that routine monitoring for potential transformation to lymphoma in the future may be necessary [115].

Waldenstrom's Macroglobulinemia (WM) and Renal Disease

This entity is characterized by the detection of monoclonal IgM paraproteinemia and may be associated with certain types of B-cell lymphomas and plasma cell myeloma. Occasional monoclonal IgM may be produced in the setting of CLL and benign monoclonal gammopathy. Renal lesions in WM are varied and may present with NS, acute renal failure or hyperviscosity syndrome. Massive intracapillary precipitation of IgM deposits, proliferative glomerulonephritis and/or amyloidosis are the main glomerular findings in WM. The deposits may appear granular or organized by electron microscopy [1,116].

Amyloidosis and Lymphoid Malignancies

Amyloidosis and nephrotic syndrome is a well-known complication of HL, and constitutes about 37% of the cases of paraneoplastic disease involving the kidney [1]. These were predominantly of AA or secondary amyloid type, dating back 2–3 decades ago, and were most probably related to the late inflammatory stage of the disease and not associated with a monoclonal paraprotein (Figure 14.11A–D) [1,8,107]. It is believed that the advances in the treatment protocols for HL later have contributed to the lower incidence of AA amyloidosis. In contrast, though not common, AL type of renal amyloidosis is encountered in patients with monoclonal gammopathy in B-cell lymphomas and Waldenstrom macroglobulinemia, where a single light chain type may be localized within the fibrillar amyloid deposits [117].

Other Forms of PNGN in Lymphoid Malignancies

A variety of other glomerular patterns of injury can occur in several forms of non-Hodgkin lymphoma patients such as proliferative GN (mantle zone lymphoma) [118], focal necrotizing GN (diffuse small cleaved cell lymphocytic

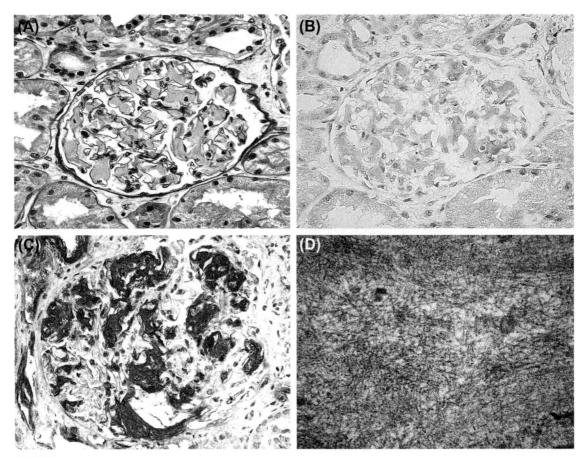

FIGURE 14.11 Paraneoplastic amyloidosis. An 18-year-old girl presented with lymphadenopathy in the neck and axilla of 2 years' duration diagnosed as Hodgkin disease and now has nephrotic syndrome. (A) Glomerular infiltration of pale staining amorphous material, replacing mainly the mesangial areas, without significant proliferative change. PAS × 400. This figure is reproduced in color in the color plate section. (B) Special staining for amyloid (Congo red) is strongly positive in the mesangial areas with amorphous deposits. × 400. This figure is reproduced in color in the color plate section. (C) Amyloid A protein is localized in the glomerulus and small arterial vessels with amyloid deposits. Immunoperoxidase stain × 400. This figure is reproduced in color in the color plate section. (D) Electron microscopy of amyloid with randomly arranged, rigid fibrils measuring 9–11 nm in thickness. × 40,000.

lymphoma) [119], ANCA-mediated crescentic GN (CLL/small lymphocytic lymphoma) [120] and PN MPGN (hairy cell leukemia) [121]. Other un-usual findings include glomerular and peritubu-lar capillary infiltration by lymphoma/leukemia cells (angiotropic lymphomas) [122,123], which have a tendency to grow in small vessels [124] and extensive intraglomerular thrombi of mono-clonal IgM kappa in a case of large cell lymphoma [125]. These cases presented with nephrotic syn-drome and/or renal failure, and showed remis-sion of lymphoma and renal disease following treatment (Figure 14.12A and B). The angiotropic leukemic cells may produce nephrotic syndrome or renal failure due to altered permeability, endothelial damage, small vessel vasculitic lesion, or engorgement of capillaries [126]. "Crystal stor-ing histiocytosis" with a low grade B-cell

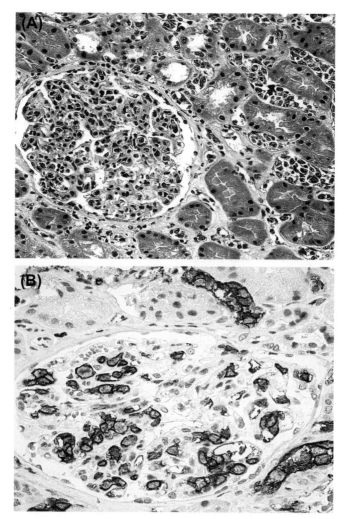

FIGURE 14.12 **Angiotropic B-cell lymphoma/leukemia in the kidney with acute renal failure.** (A) Glomerular and peritubular capillaries occluded and distended by malignant lymphoid cells. PAS × 400. This figure is reproduced in color in the color plate section. (B) Malignant lymphoid cells are positive for monoclonal B-cell markers including CD20 (seen here). × Immunoperoxidase stain × 400. This figure is reproduced in color in the color plate section.

lymphoproliferative disorder infiltrating the glomeruli has been documented, where histiocytes containing crystalline monoclonal proteins lodge within the glomerular capillaries and produce symptoms [127].

Although the preceding sections have been mainly with HL and B-cell origin NHL, T-cells and other lymphocyte cell types have also shown to occasionally produce renal disease. Acute T-lymphocyte leukemia and lymphoma, including those involving the skin (mycosis fungoides/Sezary syndrome) have rarely been reported to cause PNGN [8]. Rare case reports showed glomerular lesions and collapsing glomerulopathy associated with natural killer (NK) cell leukemia/lymphoproliferative disease, and have suggested that soluble factors, elaborated by the malignant cells, may have played a role in the podocyte injury and nephrotic syndrome [128,129].

Myeloproliferative Disorders/ Malignancies

These are a heterogeneous group of diseases which manifest several clonal hematologic entities that arise from clonal expansion of one or more hemopoietic stem cell compartments [8,130]. Based on the molecular pathogenic mechanisms, chronic myeloid neoplasms are classified under three major categories, namely myeloproliferative neoplasms, myelodysplastic syndromes and myelodysplastic—myeloproliferative disorders [8]. The reported prevalence of PNGN with the myeloproliferative neoplasias is 3.6% [131]. Overall, PNGNs are uncommon with both acute and chronic myeloid neoplasia. Chronic myelogenous leukemia (CML), the most common myeloproliferative neoplasm which is associated with the BCR-ABL fusion gene resulting from Philadelphia chromosome translocation (Ph), is seldom linked with PNGN [8]. Given the indolent nature of this disease, glomerulonephritis may well occur coincidentally. In isolated case studies where MCD and RPGN were diagnosed in the setting of CML, the glomerular lesion was treated effectively with immunosuppression without any effect on the underlying CML [132]. Other myeloproliferative diseases (polycythemia vera, essential thrombocythemia and idiopathic myelofibrosis) are more frequently associated with a variety of PNGN, commonly with FSGS and mesangial proliferative GN (Table 14.10) [8,133—135]. Polycythemia vera (PV) and essential thrombocytosis (ET) arise due to expansion of red cell mass and platelet counts, respectively. A leukoerythroblastic picture with bone marrow fibrosis characterizes myelofibrosis with myeloid metaplasia (MMM).

In the sparse case reports of PN RPGN with myeloid malignancies, it is most often reported in association with the myelodysplastic and

TABLE 14.10 PNGN and Myeloid Malignancies

GN	Tumor type	# cases
Focal segmental glomerular sclerosis		
	Polycythemia vera	6
	Essential thrombocytosis	3
	Primary myelofibrosis	2
	Myelodysplastic syndrome	1
	Acute myelogenous leukemia	1
Mesangioproliferative glomerulonephritis		
	Primary myelofibrosis	10
	Polycythemia vera	4
	Essential thrombocytosis	3
	Myelodysplastic syndrome	2
	Chronic myelogenous leukemia	1
Membranous nephropathy		
	Myelodysplastic syndrome	3
	Primary myelofibrosis	1
	Chronic myelomonocytic leukemia	1
	Acute myelogenous leukemia	1
IgA Nephropathy		
	Polycythemia vera	3
	Myelodysplastic syndrome	2
	Chronic myelogenous leukemia	1
Rapidly progressive glomerulonephritis		
	Polycythemia vera	1
	Chronic myelogenous leukemia	1
	Myelodysplastic syndrome	1
Membranoproliferative glomerulonephritis		
	Chronic myelogenous leukemia	1
	Chronic myelomonocytic leukemia	
Minimal change disease		
	Chronic myelogenous leukemia	2
Total		51

myeloproliferative disorders. Renal involvement in myelodysplastic syndrome and chronic myelomonocytic leukemia (CMML) was observed in 2% and 27%, respectively [136]. Severe monocytosis in chronic myelomonocytic or monocytic leukemia promotes lysozymuria, which can produce nephrotic range proteinuria. This is a pseudonephrotic syndrome which resolves with treatment of the primary malignancy. Chronic overproduction of cytokines in myeloproliferative and myelodysplastic syndromes is thought to be responsible for the development of PNGN, secondary to development of autoimmune phenomena.

PN FSGS and Myeloproliferative Malignancies

Cytokines such as TGFb, platelet-derived growth factor (PDGF), basic fibroblast growth factor (bFGF) and vascular endothelial growth factor (VEGF) are thought to produce the histologic changes in the bone marrow affected by myelofibrosis and myeloproliferation [137]. Experimental and human studies have uncovered some of the links between cytokine expression and glomerulopathy. Elements of the PDGF system are induced or constitutively expressed in most renal cells. In cultured mesangial cells, inducers of PDGF synthesis include epidermal growth factor (EGF), fibroblast growth factor (FGF), TNF alpha, TGF beta, angiotensin II, endothelin, thrombin, lipoproteins, phospholipids and PDGF itself. In glomerular endothelial cells, hypoxia induces PDGF. Elements of the PDGF system are involved in multiple pathophysiologic processes, including cell proliferation, extracellular matrix accumulation, regulation of tissue permeability and hemodynamics, and production of pro- and anti-inflammatory cytokines. Almost all experimental and human renal diseases are characterized by modified expression of constituents of the PDGF system [138].

Experimental and *in vivo* data show that high platelet counts in ET are associated with abnormal activation of megakaryocytes and subsequent activation of the PDGF system, which in turn, produces glomerulosclerosis [131]. In the setting of PV, alterations in renal hemodynamics such as renal vasodilation and increased effective renal blood flow could drive the evolution of FSGS via activation of the PDGF and other cytokine systems [139]. In some case reports of PN FSGS with PV, there was partial remission of proteinuria following serial phlebotomies. This lends support to the contention that hyperviscosity and hyperperfusion of the glomeruli incite cytokine pathways which eventually produce glomerulosclerosis [131,140].

TGFb stimulates glomerulosclerosis by increasing synthesis of fibronectin and collagen by mesangial cells [141]. It is considered to be a major profibrotic stimulus in mesangial injury and expansion. TGFb accumulates in experimental animal models of kidney injury and in chronic kidney disease in humans, and increased protein and mRNA levels of TGFb and TGFb2 type II receptors in the glomeruli of FSGS patients have been reported [142,143].

PN Mesangioproliferative GN and Myeloproliferative Malignancies

Mesangioproliferative glomerulopathy is most commonly associated with primary myelofibrosis (Table 14.10) [8,133–135]. On histology, there is mesangial sclerosis and hypercellularity, segmental sclerosis, intracapillary hematopoietic cells (platelet/megakaryocyte aggregation), with segmental subendothelial electron lucency and double contours of the GBM by electronmicroscopy, somewhat resembling chronic thrombotic microangiopathy lesion, secondary to endothelial injury [144] (Figures 14.13 and 14.14). These lesions are referred to as "myeloproliferative neoplasm-related glomerulopathy" occurring in several forms of myeloproliferative disorders, but primary myelofibrosis was the common entity. The same cytokines thought to promote glomerulosclerosis in the myeloproliferative

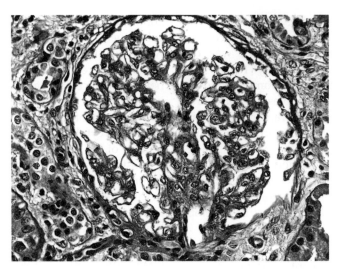

FIGURE 14.13 **Myeloproliferative disorder and mesangial disease presenting as nephrotic range proteinuria.** Glomerulus showing mild mesangial hypercellularity, without immune deposits, but significant epithelial injury by electron microscopy. PAS × 400. This figure is reproduced in color in the color plate section.

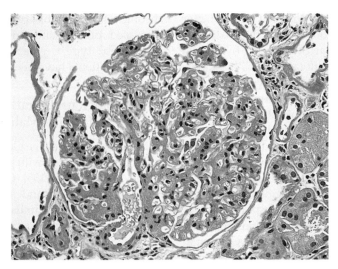

FIGURE 14.14 **Myeloproliferative disorder and glomerular disease with proteinuria and microhematuria.** Glomerulus showing diffuse mesangial sclerosis, focal compromise in capillary lumina and peripheral capillary wall thickening with focal double contours (without immune deposits), suggestive of chronic endothelial injury or thrombotic microangiopathy. PAS × 400. This figure is reproduced in color in the color plate section.

malignancies also produce intraglomerular proliferative changes. PDGF is a potent stimulus of mesangial cell proliferation and extracellular matrix production by them. In rodent models of renal injury showing mesangioproliferative anti-Thy 1.1 GN, PDGF is upregulated. Moreover, in animal and human models of mesangioproliferative GN, PDGF A is overexpressed within mesangial cells

[138]. Additionally, in animal models of cellular injury, PDGF mRNA upregulation is observed in mesangial cells and podocytes and within the interstitium at sites of renal fibrosis [145]. Nephrotic range proteinuria with varying degrees of chronic renal insufficiency are the clinical features of these lesions, often occurring in the later stages of the primary disease and generally refractory to the usual treatment for proteinuria [133].

PN MN and PN MPGN and Myeloproliferative Malignancies

Although PN MGN and MPGN are typically associated with B-lineage lymphoproliferative disorders [77], they can occur with myeloproliferative disorders (Table 14.10) [2,8,134,135].

SCREENING RECOMMENDATIONS FOR PARANEOPLASTIC GLOMERULONEPHRITIS

Overall, PNGN is a rare clinical entity, and when the glomerular disease precedes discovery of the neoplasia, the diagnosis is usually made retrospectively based on age and other risk factors. Arguably, data supporting the relationship between neoplasia and PNGN are most convincing for PN MN with solid tumors and PN MCD with HL. Even so, opinions vary widely regarding an actual link between malignancy and GN. Some investigators believe that the literature has exaggerated the relationship, while others strongly contend that the current data support aggressive screening for malignancy in patients diagnosed with MN in the absence of other clear secondary causes. In the absence of any clear guidelines, it is reasonable to perform age and gender appropriate screening in adult patients with MN after excluding other secondary causes of GN. Colonoscopy, mammography and prostate-specific antigen testing may be adequate. In those with a history of tobacco use, a chest X-ray is appropriate. The positive immunoassay for PLA2R has been generally useful in idiopathic MN to distinguish idiopathic MN from PN MN, although a few cases in their cohort had positive titers [14]. However, it is not presently available outside of the research lab. Screening for malignancy may also be considered in those individuals who fail to respond appropriately to the standard therapy for their primary GN. In a study where eight out of 21 patients had MCD diagnosed months prior to the diagnosis of HL, 2/8 were resistant to steroid therapy or cyclosporine (CSA). The MCD responded to treatment for their HL [41]. Understandably, the numbers here were very small.

Since the risk of a PNGN is not restricted to the onset of the renal disease or the time period immediately surrounding this presentation, ongoing surveillance employing urinalysis and/or renal function tests may be useful to uncover new onset of renal disease, despite quiescence or remission of the malignancy [44]. This may also enable early intervention of both the renal disease as well as the neoplastic condition, when a relationship is established. The duration of surveillance remains ill defined.

Another population that may warrant closer follow-up are those patients with mixed cryoglobulinemia without HCV, since studies have revealed a four-fold increased risk of developing B-cell and NHL, and may represent a pre-B-cell lymphoma state [113]. If a specific tumor is suspected, known circulating tumor markers may be helpful. Serum and urine studies for monoclonal gammopathy, bone marrow, lymph node and peripheral blood testing are essential for confirmation of a hematologic malignancy.

MANAGEMENT OF PARANEOPLASTIC GLOMERULONEPHRITIS

Although the management of symptomatic nephrotic syndrome is similar to those without neoplastic disease, it is generally agreed that the treatment of PNGN is standard/specific therapy indicated for the primary malignancy [8]. In known cases, any recurrences of the glomerular lesion or the malignancy should prompt work-up for the other, to initiate appropriate and timely treatment. Therefore, recognition of PNGN is paramount in avoiding potentially toxic and/or ineffective regimen for the renal disease. Often, the diagnosis is made retrospectively and only after the neoplasia is finally recognized. While almost all the renal lesions associated with lymphoid malignancies mainly require specific anti-neoplastic therapy to induce partial or complete remission, therapy is somewhat varied in PNGN with myeloid malignancies and thymomas, most probably related to the diverse cell types involved [8]. However, some severe glomerular lesions in the setting of solid tumors, such as crescentic GN secondary to ANCA may need aggressive therapy to block the glomerular inflammatory process. Awareness of the renal effects and glomerular lesions of certain chemotherapeutic and biological agents is required to exclude them as potential causes of renal disease [8,144]. A prior history of malignancy could also signal that PNGN needs to be included in the differential diagnosis for GN. In conclusion, a multidisciplinary approach, with participation of nephrologists, oncologists, pathologists and other related members of the medical team may be needed to manage both the paraneoplastic GN and the underlying malignancy [8].

References

[1] Ronco PM. Paraneoplastic glomerulopathies: new insights into an old entity. Kidney Int 1999;56(1): 355—77.

[2] Bacchetta J, Juillard L, Cochat P, Droz JP. Paraneoplastic glomerular diseases and malignancies. Crit Rev Oncol Hematol 2009;70(1):39—58.

[3] Pascal RR, Slovin SF. Tumor directed antibody and carcinoembryonic antigen in the glomeruli of a patient with gastric carcinoma. Hum Pathol 1980;11(6):679—82.

[4] Maesaka JK, Mittal SK, Fishbane S. Paraneoplastic syndromes of the kidney. Semin Oncol 1997;24(3): 373—81.

[5] Kapoor M, Chan GZ. Malignancy and renal disease. Crit Care Clin 2001;17(3):571—98, viii.

[6] Lee JC, Yamauchi H, Hopper Jr J. The association of cancer and the nephrotic syndrome. Ann Intern Med 1966;64(1):41—51.

[7] American Cancer Society. Facts and Figures 2012. http://www.cancer.org/Research/CancerFactsFigures/CancerFactsFigures/cancer-facts-figures-2012.

[8] Lien YH, Lai LW. Pathogenesis, diagnosis and management of paraneoplastic glomerulonephritis. Nat Rev Nephrol 2011;7(2):85—95.

[9] Norris SH. Paraneoplastic glomerulopathies. Semin Nephrol 1993;13(3):258—72.

[10] Kaplan BS, Klassen J, Gault MH. Glomerular injury in patients with neoplasia. Annu Rev Med 1976;27: 117—25.

[11] Lefaucheur C, Stengel B, Nochy D, Martel P, Hill GS, Jacquot C, et al. Membranous nephropathy and cancer: epidemiologic evidence and determinants of high-risk cancer association. Kidney Int 2006;70(8): 1510—7.

[12] Pankhurst T, Savage CO, Gordon C, Harper L. Malignancy is increased in ANCA-associated vasculitis. Rheumatology (Oxford) 2004;43(12):1532—5.

[13] Birkeland SA, Storm HH. Glomerulonephritis and malignancy: a population-based analysis. Kidney Int 2003;63(2):716—21.

[14] Beck Jr LH. Membranous nephropathy and malignancy. Semin Nephrol 2010;30(6):635—44.

[15] Eagen JW. Glomerulopathies of neoplasia. Kidney Int 1977;11(5):297—303.

[16] Alpers CE, Cotran RS. Neoplasia and glomerular injury. Kidney Int 1986;30(4):465—73.

[17] Pascal RR, Iannaccone PM, Rollwagen FM, Harding TA, Bennett SJ. Electron microscopy and immunofluorescence of glomerular immune complex deposits in cancer patients. Cancer Res 1976;36(1):43—7.

[18] Beaufils H, Jouanneau C, Chomette G. Kidney and cancer: results of immunofluorescence microscopy. Nephron 1985;40(3):303—8.

[19] Faria TV, Baptista MA, Burdmann EA, Cury PM. Renal glomerular alterations in patients with cancer: a clinical and immunohistochemical autopsy study. Ren Fail 2010;32(8):918—22.

[20] Rossen RD, Reisberg MA, Singer D, Suki WN, Duffy J, Hersh EM, et al. The effect of age on the character of immune complex disease: a comparison of the incidence and relative size of materials

reactive with Clq in sera of patients with glomerulonephritis and cancer. Medicine 1979;58(1):65—79.

[21] Ozawa T, Pluss R, Lacher J, Boedecker E, Guggenheim S, Hammond W, et al. Endogenous immune complex nephropathy associated with malignancy. I. Studies on the nature and immunopathogenic significance of glomerular bound antigen and antibody, isolation and characterization of tumor specific antigen and antibody and circulating immune complexes. Q J Med 1975;44(176):523—41.

[22] Ohtani H, Wakui H, Komatsuda A, Okuyama S, Masai R, Maki N, et al. Distribution of glomerular IgG subclass deposits in malignancy-associated membranous nephropathy. Nephrol Dial Transplant 2004;19(3):574—9.

[23] Keaney CM, Springate JE. Cancer and the kidney. Adolesc Med Clin 2005;16(1):121—48.

[24] Brueggemeyer CD, Ramirez G. Membranous nephropathy: a concern for malignancy. Am J Kidney Dis 1987;9(1):23—6.

[25] Burstein DM, Korbet SM, Schwartz MM. Membranous glomerulonephritis and malignancy. Am J Kidney Dis 1993;22(1):5—10.

[26] Sultan-Bichat N, Vuiblet V, Winckel A, Journet J, Goedel AL, Khoury A, et al. Membranous glomerulonephritis as a paraneoplastic manifestation of melanoma. Ann Dermatol Venereol 2011;138(1):46—9.

[27] Ito C, Akimoto T, Nakazawa E, Komori S, Sugase T, Chinda J, et al. A case of cervical cancer-related membranous nephropathy treated with radiation therapy. Intern Med 2011;50(1):47—51.

[28] Matsui S, Tsuji H, Takimoto Y, Ono S. Clinical improvement of membranous nephropathy after endoscopic resection of double early gastrointestinal cancers. Clin Exp Nephrol 2011;15(2):285—8.

[29] Arenas MD, Gil MT, Malek T, Farre J, Fernandez Morejon FJ, Arriero JM, et al. Nephrotic syndrome as paraneoplastic manifestation of a primary pulmonary lymphoepithelioma-like carcinoma. Clin Nephrol 2009;72(3):206—10.

[30] Heymann W, Hackel DB, Harwood S, Wilson SG, Hunter JL. Production of nephrotic syndrome in rats by Freund's adjuvants and rat kidney suspensions. Proc Soc Exp Biol Med 1959;100(4):660—4.

[31] Beck Jr LH, Bonegio RG, Lambeau G, Beck DM, Powell DW, Cummins TD, et al. M-type phospholipase A2 receptor as target antigen in idiopathic membranous nephropathy. N Engl J Med 2009;361(1):11—21.

[32] Wakashin M, Wakashin Y, Iesato K, Ueda S, Mori Y, Tsuchida H, et al. Association of gastric cancer and nephrotic syndrome. An immunologic study in three patients. Gastroenterology 1980;78(4):749—56.

[33] Costanza ME, Pinn V, Schwartz RS, Nathanson L. Carcinoembryonic antigen—antibody complexes in a patient with colonic carcinoma and nephrotic syndrome. N Engl J Med 1973;289(10):520—2.

[34] Borochovitz D, Kam WK, Nolte M, Graner S, Kiss J. Adenocarcinoma of the palate associated with nephrotic syndrome and epimembranous carcinoembryonic antigen deposition. Cancer 1982;49(10): 2097—102.

[35] Lewis MG, Loughridge LW, Phillips TM. Immunological studies in nephrotic syndrome associated with extrarenal malignant disease. Lancet 1971; 2(7716):134—5.

[36] Mellors RC, Shirai T, Aoki T, Huebner RJ, Krawczynski K. Wild-type gross leukemia virus and the pathogenesis of the glomerulonephritis of New Zealand mice. J Exp Med 1971;133(1):113—32.

[37] Oldstone MB, Aoki T, Dixon FJ. The antibody response of mice to murine leukemia virus in spontaneous infection: absence of classical immunologic tolerance (AKR mice—complement-fixing antibodies—lymphocytic choriomeningitis virus—immunofluorescence—glomerular deposits of antigen—antibody complexes). Proc Natl Acad Sci U S A 1972;69(1):134—8.

[38] Pascal RR, Rollwagen FM, Harding TA, Schiavone WA. Glomerular immune complex deposits associated with mouse mammary tumor. Cancer Res 1975;35(2):302—4.

[39] Takeda S, Chinda J, Murakami T, Numata A, Iwazu Y, Akimoto T, et al. Development of features of glomerulopathy in tumor-bearing rats: a potential model for paraneoplastic glomerulopathy. Nephrol Dial Transplant 2012;27(5):1786—92.

[40] Cameron JS. The nephrotic syndrome and its complications. Am J Kidney Dis 1987;10(3):157—71.

[41] Audard V, Larousserie F, Grimbert P, Abtahi M, Sotto JJ, Delmer A, et al. Minimal change nephrotic syndrome and classical Hodgkin's lymphoma: report of 21 cases and review of the literature. Kidney Int 2006;69(12):2251—60.

[42] Ishimoto T, Shimada M, Araya CE, Huskey J, Garin EH, Johnson RJ. Minimal change disease: a CD80 podocytopathy? Semin Nephrol 2011;31(4):320—5.

[43] Shankland SJ. The podocyte's response to injury: role in proteinuria and glomerulosclerosis. Kidney Int 2006;69(12):2131—47.

[44] Karras A, de Montpreville V, Fakhouri F, Grunfeld JP, Lesavre P. Renal and thymic pathology in thymoma-associated nephropathy: report of 21 cases and review of the literature. Nephrol Dial Transplant 2005;20(6):1075—82.

[45] Lai KW, Wei CL, Tan LK, Tan PH, Chiang GS, Lee CG, et al. Overexpression of interleukin-13

induces minimal-change-like nephropathy in rats. J Am Soc Nephrol 2007;18(5):1476–85.

[46] Garin EH, Blanchard DK, Matsushima K, Djeu JY. IL-8 production by peripheral blood mononuclear cells in nephrotic patients. Kidney Int 1994;45(5):1311–7.

[47] Laflam PF, Haraguchi S, Garin EH. Cytokine mRNA profile in lipoid nephrosis: evidence for increased IL-8 mRNA stability. Nephron 2002;91(4):620–6.

[48] Cheong HI, Lee JH, Hahn H, Park HW, Ha IS, Choi Y. Circulating VEGF and TGF-beta1 in children with idiopathic nephrotic syndrome. J Nephrol 2001;14(4):263–9.

[49] Kuriyama M, Taniguchi T, Shirai Y, Sasaki A, Yoshimura A, Saito N. Activation and translocation of PKCdelta is necessary for VEGF-induced ERK activation through KDR in HEK293T cells. Biochem Biophys Res Commun 2004;325(3):843–51.

[50] Yang JC, Haworth L, Sherry RM, Hwu P, Schwartzentruber DJ, Topalian SL, et al. A random-ized trial of bevacizumab, an anti-vascular endo-thelial growth factor antibody, for metastatic renal cancer. N Engl J Med 2003;349(5):427–34.

[51] Wu S, Kim C, Baer L, Zhu X. Bevacizumab increases risk for severe proteinuria in cancer patients. J Am Soc Nephrol 2010;21(8):1381–9.

[52] D'Agati VD, Kaskel FJ, Falk RJ. Focal segmental glomerulosclerosis. N Engl J Med 2011;365(25): 2398–411.

[53] Arampatzis S, Giannakoulas N, Liakopoulos V, Eleftheriadis T, Kourti P, Karasavvidou F, et al. Simultaneous clinical resolution of focal segmental glomerulosclerosis associated with chronic lympho-cytic leukaemia treated with fludarabine, cyclo-phosphamide and rituximab. BMC Nephrology 2011;12:33.

[54] Wei C, El Hindi S, Li J, Fornoni A, Goes N, Sageshima J, et al. Circulating urokinase receptor as a cause of focal segmental glomerulosclerosis. Nat Med 2011;17(8):952–60.

[55] Nakamura T, Matsuyama M, Kojima A, Ogiu T, Kubota A, Suzuki Y, et al. The effect of thymectomy on the development of nephropathy in spontaneous thymoma rats of the BUF/Mna strain. Clin Exp Immunol 1988;71(2):350–2.

[56] Le Berre L, Godfrin Y, Gunther E, Buzelin F, Perretto S, Smit H, et al. Extrarenal effects on the pathogenesis and relapse of idiopathic nephrotic syndrome in Buffalo/Mna rats. J Clin Invest 2002;109(4):491–8.

[57] Le Berre L, Herve C, Buzelin F, Usal C, Soulillou JP, Dantal J. Renal macrophage activation and Th2 polarization precedes the development of nephrotic syndrome in Buffalo/Mna rats. Kidney Int 2005;68(5):2079–90.

[58] Mimura I, Tojo A, Kinugasa S, Uozaki H, Fujita T. Renal cell carcinoma in association with IgA ne-phropathy in the elderly. Am J Med Sci 2009; 338(5):431–2.

[59] Roberts IS, Cook HT, Troyanov S, Alpers CE, Amore A, Barratt J, et al. The Oxford classification of IgA nephropathy: pathology definitions, correlations, and reproducibility. Kidney Int 2009;76(5):546–56.

[60] Floege J. The pathogenesis of IgA nephropathy: what is new and how does it change therapeutic ap-proaches? Am J Kidney Dis 2011;58(6):992–1004.

[61] Suzuki H, Kiryluk K, Novak J, Moldoveanu Z, Herr AB, Renfrow MB, et al. The pathophysiology of IgA nephropathy. J Am Soc Nephrol 2011;22(10): 1795–803.

[62] Magyarlaki T, Kiss B, Buzogany I, Fazekas A, Sukosd F, Nagy J. Renal cell carcinoma and paraneo-plastic IgA nephropathy. Nephron 1999;82(2):127–30.

[63] Mustonen J, Pasternack A, Helin H. IgA mesangial nephropathy in neoplastic diseases. Contrib Nephrol 1984;40:283–91.

[64] Pertuiset E, Liote F, Launay-Russ E, Kemiche F, Cerf-Payrastre I, Chesneau AM. Adult Henoch–Schonlein purpura associated with malignancy. Semin Arthritis Rheum 2000;29(6):360–7.

[65] Kellerman PS. Henoch–Schonlein purpura in adults. Am J Kidney Dis 2006;48(6):1009–16.

[66] Henry Jr CL, Ogletree ML, Brigham KL, Hammon Jr JW. Attenuation of the pulmonary vascular response to endotoxin by a thromboxane synthesis inhibitor (UK-38485) in unanesthetized sheep. J Surg Res 1991;50(1):77–81.

[67] Haas M, Eustace JA. Immune complex deposits in ANCA-associated crescentic glomerulonephritis: a study of 126 cases. Kidney Int 2004;65(6):2145–52.

[68] Rutgers A, Sanders JS, Stegeman CA, Kallenberg CG. Pauci-immune necrotizing glomerulonephritis. Rheum Dis Clin North Am 2010;36(3):559–72.

[69] Tarzi RM, Cook HT, Pusey CD. Crescentic glomer-ulonephritis: new aspects of pathogenesis. Semin Nephrol 2011;31(4):361–8.

[70] Falk RJ, Gross WL, Guillevin L, Hoffman GS, Jayne DR, Jennette JC, et al. Granulomatosis with polyangiitis (Wegener's): an alternative name for Wegener's granulomatosis. Arthritis Rheum 2011; 63(4):863–4.

[71] Tatsis E, Reinhold-Keller E, Steindorf K, Feller AC, Gross WL. Wegener's granulomatosis associated with renal cell carcinoma. Arthritis Rheum 1999;42(4): 751–6.

[72] Knight A, Askling J, Ekbom A. Cancer incidence in a population-based cohort of patients with Wegener's granulomatosis. Int J Cancer 2002;100(1):82–5.

[73] Edgar JD, Rooney DP, McNamee P, McNeill TA. An association between ANCA positive renal disease and malignancy. Clin Nephrol 1993;40(1):22–5.

[74] Chen M, Daha MR, Kallenberg CG. The complement system in systemic autoimmune disease. J Autoimmun 2010;34(3):J276–86.

[75] Ahmed M, Solangi K, Abbi R, Adler S. Nephrotic syndrome, renal failure, and renal malignancy: an unusual tumor-associated glomerulonephritis. J Am Soc Nephrol 1997;8(5):848–52.

[76] Reshi AR, Mir SA, Gangoo AA, Shah S, Banday K. Nephrotic syndrome associated with transitional cell carcinoma of urinary bladder. Scand J Urol Nephrol 1997;31(3):295–6.

[77] Da'as N, Polliack A, Cohen Y, Amir G, Darmon D, Kleinman Y, et al. Kidney involvement and renal manifestations in non-Hodgkin's lymphoma and lymphocytic leukemia: a retrospective study in 700 patients. Eur J Haematol 2001;67(3):158–64.

[78] Ahmed MS, Wong CF, Abraham KA. Membranoproliferative glomerulonephritis associated with metastatic prostate carcinoma – should immunosuppressive therapy be considered? Nephrol Dial Transplant 2008;23(2):777.

[79] Sartelet H, Melin JP, Wynckel A, Lallemand A, Brambilla E, Chanard J. Membranoproliferative glomerulonephritis (MPGN) and pulmonary carcinoid tumour. Nephrol Dial Transplant 1997;12(11): 2405–6.

[80] Vanatta PR, Silva FG, Taylor WE, Costa JC. Renal cell carcinoma and systemic amyloidosis: demonstration of AA protein and review of the literature. Hum Pathol 1983;14(3):195–201.

[81] Davison AM. Renal diseases associated with malignancies. Nephrol Dial Transplant 2001;16(Suppl. 6):13–4.

[82] Brady HR. Fibrillary glomerulopathy. Kidney Int 1998;53(5):1421–9.

[83] Hagler KT, Lynch Jr JW. Paraneoplastic manifestations of lymphoma. Clin Lymphoma 2004;5(1):29–36.

[84] Cohen LJ, Rennke HG, Laubach JP, Humphreys BD. The spectrum of kidney involvement in lymphoma: a case report and review of the literature. Am J Kidney Dis 2010;56(6):1191–6.

[85] Moulin B, Ronco PM, Mougenot B, Francois A, Fillastre JP, Mignon F. Glomerulonephritis in chronic lymphocytic leukemia and related B-cell lymphomas. Kidney Int 1992;42(1):127–35.

[86] Hsu SM, Waldron Jr JW, Hsu PL, Hough Jr AJ. Cytokines in malignant lymphomas: review and prospective evaluation. Hum Pathol 1993;24(10):1040–57.

[87] Kowalewska J, Nicosia RF, Smith KD, Kats A, Alpers CE. Patterns of glomerular injury in kidneys infiltrated by lymphoplasmacytic neoplasms. Hum Pathol 2011;42(6):896–903.

[88] Ferry JA, Harris NL, Papanicolaou N, Young RH. Lymphoma of the kidney. A report of 11 cases. Am J Surg Pathol 1995;19(2):134–44.

[89] Korzets Z, Golan E, Manor Y, Schneider M, Bernheim J. Spontaneously remitting minimal change nephropathy preceding a relapse of Hodgkin's disease by 19 months. Clin Nephrol 1992;38(3): 125–7.

[90] Mallouk A, Pham PT, Pham PC. Concurrent FSGS and Hodgkin's lymphoma: case report and literature review on the link between nephrotic glomerulopathies and hematological malignancies. Clin Exp Nephrol 2006;10(4):284–9.

[91] Cale WF, Ullrich IH, Jenkins JJ. Nodular sclerosing Hodgkin's disease presenting as nephrotic syndrome. South Med J 1982;75(5):604–6.

[92] Audard V, Zhang SY, Copie-Bergman C, Rucker-Martin C, Ory V, Candelier M, et al. Occurrence of minimal change nephrotic syndrome in classical Hodgkin lymphoma is closely related to the induction of c-mip in Hodgkin–Reed Sternberg cells and podocytes. Blood 2010;115(18):3756–62.

[93] Platsoucas CD, Galinski M, Kempin S, Reich L, Clarkson B, Good RA. Abnormal T lymphocyte subpopulations in patients with B cell chronic lymphocytic leukemia: an analysis by monoclonal antibodies. J Immunol 1982;129(5):2305–12.

[94] Mc'Ligeyo SO, Notghi A, Thomson D, Anderton JL. Nephrotic syndrome associated with chronic lymphocytic leukaemia. Nephrol Dial Transplant 1993; 8(5):461–3.

[95] Aslam N, Nseir NI, Viverett JF, Bastacky SI, Johnson JP. Nephrotic syndrome in chronic lymphocytic leukemia: a paraneoplastic syndrome? Clin Nephrol 2000;54(6):492–7.

[96] Alzamora MG, Schmidli M, Hess U, Cathomas R, von Moos R. Minimal change glomerulonephritis in chronic lymphocytic leukemia: pathophysiological and therapeutic aspects. Onkologie 2006;29(4):153–6.

[97] Ohshima K, Akaiwa M, Umeshita R, Suzumiya J, Izuhara K, Kikuchi M. Interleukin-13 and interleukin-13 receptor in Hodgkin's disease: possible autocrine mechanism and involvement in fibrosis. Histopathology 2001;38(4):368–75.

[98] Skinnider BF, Mak TW. The role of cytokines in classical Hodgkin lymphoma. Blood 2002;99(12):4283–97.

[99] Skinnider BF, Kapp U, Mak TW. The role of interleukin 13 in classical Hodgkin lymphoma. Leuk Lymphoma 2002;43(6):1203–10.

[100] Aggarwal N, Batwara R, McCarthy ET, Sharma R, Sharma M, Savin VJ. Serum permeability activity in

steroid-resistant minimal change nephrotic syndrome is abolished by treatment of Hodgkin disease. Am J Kidney Dis 2007;50(5):826–9.

[101] Doussis-Anagnostopoulou IA, Talks KL, Turley H, Debnam P, Tan DC, Mariatos G, et al. Vascular endothelial growth factor (VEGF) is expressed by neoplastic Hodgkin–Reed–Sternberg cells in Hodgkin's disease. J Pathol 2002;197(5):677–83.

[102] Newcom SR, Gu L. Transforming growth factor beta 1 messenger RNA in Reed–Sternberg cells in nodular sclerosing Hodgkin's disease. J Clin Pathol 1995;48(2):160–3.

[103] Dabbs DJ, Striker LM, Mignon F, Striker G. Glomerular lesions in lymphomas and leukemias. Am J Med 1986;80(1):63–70.

[104] Rault R, Holley JL, Banner BF, el-Shahawy M. Glomerulonephritis and non-Hodgkin's lymphoma: a report of two cases and review of the literature. Am J Kidney Dis 1992;20(1):84–9.

[105] Butty H, Asfoura J, Cortese F, Doyle M, Rutecki G. Chronic lymphocytic leukemia-associated membranous glomerulopathy: remission with fludarabine. Am J Kidney Dis 1999;33(2):E8.

[106] Favre G, Courtellemont C, Callard P, Colombat M, Cabane J, Boffa JJ, et al. Membranoproliferative glomerulonephritis, chronic lymphocytic leukemia, and cryoglobulinemia. Am J Kidney Dis 2010;55(2): 391–4.

[107] Buyukpamukcu M, Hazar V, Tinaztepe K, Bakkaloglu A, Akyuz C, Kutluk T. Hodgkin's disease and renal paraneoplastic syndromes in childhood. Turk J Pediatr 2000;42(2):109–14.

[108] Guiard E, Karras A, Plaisier E, Duong Van Huyen JP, Fakhouri F, Rougier JP, et al. Patterns of noncryoglobulinemic glomerulonephritis with monoclonal Ig deposits: correlation with IgG subclass and response to rituximab. Clin J Am Soc Nephrol 2011; 6(7):1609–16.

[109] Touchard G, Bauwens M, Goujon JM, Aucouturier P, Patte D, Preud'homme JL. Glomerulonephritis with organized microtubular monoclonal immunoglobulin deposits. Adv Nephrol Necker Hosp 1994;23: 149–75.

[110] Franzin F, Efremov DG, Pozzato G, Tulissi P, Batista F, Burrone OR. Clonal B-cell expansions in peripheral blood of HCV-infected patients. Br J Haematol 1995;90(3):548–52.

[111] Mazzaro C, Panarello G, Tesio F, Santini G, Crovatto M, Mazzi G, et al. Hepatitis C virus risk: a hepatitis C virus related syndrome. J Intern Med 2000;247(5):535–45.

[112] Matignon M, Cacoub P, Colombat M, Saadoun D, Brocheriou I, Mougenot B, et al. Clinical and morphologic spectrum of renal involvement in patients with mixed cryoglobulinemia without evidence of hepatitis C virus infection. Medicine 2009;88(6):341–8.

[113] Saadoun D, Sellam J, Ghillani-Dalbin P, Crecel R, Piette JC, Cacoub P. Increased risks of lymphoma and death among patients with non-hepatitis C virus-related mixed cryoglobulinemia. Arch Intern Med 2006;166(19):2101–8.

[114] Ferri C, Sebastiani M, Giuggioli D, Cazzato M, Longombardo G, Antonelli A, et al. Mixed cryoglobulinemia: demographic, clinical, and serologic features and survival in 231 patients. Semin Arthritis Rheum 2004;33(6):355–74.

[115] Quartuccio L, Fabris M, Salvin S, Isola M, Soldano F, Falleti E, et al. Bone marrow B-cell clonal expansion in type II mixed cryoglobulinaemia: association with nephritis. Rheumatology (Oxford) 2007;46(11):1657–61.

[116] Morel-Maroger L, Basch A, Danon F, Verroust P, Richet G. Pathology of the kidney in Waldenstrom's macroglobulinemia. Study of sixteen cases. N Engl J Med 1970;283(3):123–9.

[117] Pamuk GE, Demir M, Orum H, Turgut B, Ozyilmaz F, Tekgunduz E. Secondary amyloidosis causing nephrotic syndrome in a patient with non-Hodgkin's lymphoma: quite a rare diagnosis. Clin Lab Haematol 2006;28(4):259–61.

[118] Karim M, Hill P, Pillai G, Gatter K, Davies DR, Winearls CG. Proliferative glomerulonephritis associated with mantle cell lymphoma — natural history and effect of treatment in 2 cases. Clin Nephrol 2004;61(6):422–8.

[119] Pollock CA, Ibels LS, Levi JA, Eckstein RP, Wakeford P. Acute renal failure due to focal necrotizing glomerulonephritis in a patient with non-Hodgkin's lymphoma. Resolution with treatment of lymphoma. Nephron 1988;48(3):197–200.

[120] Henriksen KJ, Hong RB, Sobrero MI, Chang A. Rare association of chronic lymphocytic leukemia/small lymphocytic lymphoma, ANCAs, and pauciimmune crescentic glomerulonephritis. Am J Kidney Dis 2011;57(1):170–4.

[121] Abboud I, Galicier L, De Labarthe A, Dossier A, Glotz D, Verine J. A paraneoplastic membranoproliferative glomerulonephritis with isolated C3 deposits associated with hairy cell leukaemia. Nephrol Dial Transplant 2010;25(6):2026–8.

[122] Cossu A, Deiana A, Lissia A, Satta A, Cossu M, Dedola MF, et al. Nephrotic syndrome and angiotropic lymphoma report of a case. Tumori 2004;90(5): 510–3.

[123] Kusaba T, Hatta T, Tanda S, Kameyama H, Tamagaki K, Okigaki M, et al. Histological analysis

on adhesive molecules of renal intravascular large B cell lymphoma treated with CHOP chemotherapy and rituximab. Clin Nephrol 2006;65(3):222−6.

[124] Tornroth T, Heiro M, Marcussen N, Franssila K. Lymphomas diagnosed by percutaneous kidney biopsy. Am J Kidney Dis 2003;42(5):960−71.

[125] Oyama Y, Komatsuda A, Ohtani H, Imai H, Kitabayashi A, Yamaguchi A, et al. Extensive intraglomerular thrombi of monoclonal IgM-kappa in a patient with malignant lymphoma. Am J Kidney Dis 2000;35(3):E11.

[126] Nishikawa K, Sekiyama S, Suzuki T, Ito Y, Matsukawa W, Tamai H, et al. A case of angiotropic large cell lymphoma manifesting nephrotic syndrome and treated successfully with combination chemotherapy. Nephron 1991;58(4):479−82.

[127] Sethi S, Cuiffo BP, Pinkus GS, Rennke HG. Crystal-storing histiocytosis involving the kidney in a low-grade B-cell lymphoproliferative disorder. Am J Kidney Dis 2002;39(1):183−8.

[128] Bassan R, Rambaldi A, Abbate M, Biondi A, Allavena P, Barbui T, et al. Association of NK-cell lymphoproliferative disease and nephrotic syndrome. Am J Clin Pathol 1990;94(3):334−8.

[129] Palma Diaz MF, Pichler RH, Nicosia RF, Alpers CE, Smith KD. Collapsing glomerulopathy associated with natural killer cell leukemia: a case report and review of the literature. Am J Kidney Dis 2011;58(5):855−9.

[130] Campbell PJ, Green AR. The myeloproliferative disorders. N Engl J Med 2006;355(23):2452−66.

[131] Au WY, Chan KW, Lui SL, Lam CC, Kwong YL. Focal segmental glomerulosclerosis and mesangial sclerosis associated with myeloproliferative disorders. Am J Kidney Dis 1999;34(5):889−93.

[132] Sudholt BA, Heironimus JD. Chronic myelogenous leukemia with nephrotic syndrome. Arch Intern Med 1983;143(1):168−9.

[133] Said SM, Leung N, Sethi S, Cornell LD, Fidler ME, Grande JP, et al. Myeloproliferative neoplasms cause glomerulopathy. Kidney Int 2011;80(7):753−9.

[134] Subramanian M, Kilara N, Manjunath R, Mysorekar V. Membranoproliferative glomerulonephritis secondary to chronic myeloid leukemia. Saudi Journal of Kidney Diseases and Transplantation: an official publication of the Saudi Center for Organ Transplantation. Saudi Arabia 2010;21(4):738−41.

[135] Fernando BK, Ruwanpathirana HS, Veerasuthen T. A patient with polycythaemia vera associated with membranoproliferative glomerulonephritis. Ceylon Med J 2011;56(3):119−20.

[136] Saitoh T, Murakami H, Uchiumi H, Moridaira K, Maehara T, Matsushima T, et al. Myelodysplastic syndromes with nephrotic syndrome. Am J Hematol 1999;60(3):200−4.

[137] Kaygusuz I, Koc M, Arikan H, Adiguzel C, Cakalagaoglu F, Tuglular TF, et al. Focal segmental glomerulosclerosis associated with idiopathic myelofibrosis. Ren Fail 2010;32(2):273−6.

[138] Floege J, Eitner F, Alpers CE. A new look at platelet-derived growth factor in renal disease. Journal of the American Society of Nephrology: JASN 2008;19(1): 12−23.

[139] Okuyama S, Hamai K, Fujishima M, Ohtani H, Komatsuda A, Sawada K, et al. Focal segmental glomerulosclerosis associated with polycythemia vera: report of a case and review of the literature. Clin Nephrol 2007;68(6):412−5.

[140] Kosch M, August C, Hausberg M, Kisters K, Gabriels G, Matzkies F, et al. Focal sclerosis with tip lesions secondary to polycythaemia vera. Nephrol Dial Transplant 2000;15(10):1710−1.

[141] Floege J, Burns MW, Alpers CE, Yoshimura A, Pritzl P, Gordon K, et al. Glomerular cell proliferation and PDGF expression precede glomerulosclerosis in the remnant kidney model. Kidney Int 1992;41(2):297−309.

[142] Haraguchi K, Shimura H, Ogata R, Inoue H, Saito T, Kondo T, et al. Focal segmental glomerulosclerosis associated with essential thrombocythemia. Clin Exp Nephrol 2006;10(1):74−7.

[143] Kim JH, Kim BK, Moon KC, Hong HK, Lee HS. Activation of the TGF-beta/Smad signaling pathway in focal segmental glomerulosclerosis. Kidney Int 2003;64(5):1715−21.

[144] Haas M, VanBeek C. Glomerular diseases associated with hematopoietic neoplasms: an expanding spectrum. Kidney Int 2011;80(7):701−3.

[145] Iida H, Seifert R, Alpers CE, Gronwald RG, Phillips PE, Pritzl P, et al. Platelet-derived growth factor (PDGF) and PDGF receptor are induced in mesangial proliferative nephritis in the rat. Proc Natl Acad Sci U S A 1991;88(15):6560−4.

15

Pharmacokinetics of Anti-cancer Chemotherapy in Renal Insufficiency and Dialysis

William H. Fissell, IV, Marc Earl

Cleveland Clinic, Cleveland, OH, USA

INTRODUCTION

As the United States population ages and as treatment for cardiovascular disease improves, the prevalence of chronic kidney disease (CKD) and end stage renal disease (ESRD) has increased dramatically. As of December 2009, the United States Renal Data System reported that approximately 15% of subjects in the National Health and Nutrition Examination Survey had CKD, as defined by a glomerular filtration rate less than 60 ml/min, and there are 613,432 patients in the United States with ESRD [1]. The American Cancer Society estimated 1.6 million new cancer diagnoses and 577,000 deaths from cancer in 2012 [2]. The risk of developing renal disease or invasive cancer increases with age, suggesting that the number of patients with simultaneous renal insufficiency and cancer may be significant and growing [1,2]. The opportunities for nephrologists to encounter cancer patients in acute consults or during longitudinal care are considerable, as evidenced by a recent special issue of *Seminars in Nephrology* dedicated to "Onco-Nephrology" [3]. The vast majority of drugs are dosed by any combination of three methods: a one-size fits all approach made possible by a drug's low toxicity and high therapeutic index (consider standardized dosage packs of azithromycin or solumedrol), gradual titration to effect (consider JNC VII guidelines on titration of anti-hypertensives [4]), or through intensive therapeutic drug monitoring (TDM) when the therapeutic index is low, as in calcineurin inhibitors for transplant immunosuppression. For cancer chemotherapy, therapeutic indices are low, overdoses life-threatening or fatal, drug effect delayed and therapeutic drug monitoring frequently problematic as many drugs are rapidly taken up into tissues, complicating interpretation of plasma estimates. Accurate, individualized dosing of antineoplastics is essential to optimize risk/benefit ratios in the use of these agents.

Renal Disease in Cancer Patients
http://dx.doi.org/10.1016/B978-0-12-415948-8.00015-5

DRUG PROPERTIES THAT INFLUENCE RENAL AND EXTRACORPOREAL ELIMINATION

The physicochemical properties of a drug that dictate whether dosage adjustment is required in renal insufficiency or dialysis can be grouped into a few characteristics that can be easily determined from a drug reference or the package insert. Idiosyncratic exceptions to these general rules are uncommon, but recommendations will differ between renal insufficiency and dialysis. To orient the reader to the concepts, examples familiar to most nephrologists will be used to highlight each factor influencing drug disposition.

The molecular weight of the drug will strongly influence renal clearance and dialyzability. For example, ceftazidime (molecular weight 547), a third generation cephalosporin antibiotic, is almost exclusively excreted by the kidney and is highly dialyzable; vancomycin, a glycopeptide antibiotic (molecular weight 1449), is also nearly freely filtered by the glomerulus, but is much less dialyzable. Increasing the molecular weight of a drug through conjugation with a comparatively inert macromolecule, such as poly(ethylene glycol) or dextran, is a common strategy to reduce renal clearance of an expensive or difficult to administer drug. Protein binding of a drug (covered below) also influences the renal and extracorporeal clearance of the drug, as the protein-bound fraction is too large to be filtered.

When a dose drug is administered, either orally or parenterally, some concentration is achieved in plasma after the distribution of the drug is complete. The "volume of distribution" is conceptualized as the equivalent volume of water into which one would have to dissolve the same dose to achieve the same concentration. In theory and in practice, most drugs distribute into several anatomic or physiologic compartments with distinct equilibration times and volumes, which motivates the discipline of multicompartment kinetic modeling. This is familiar material, although in a different context, to nephrologists comparing single-pool and equilibrated Kt/V. To be clear, the volume of distribution of a drug is generally not in any way correlated to a specific anatomical space. Volume of distribution of a drug is a complex function of the availability of potential binding sites and the lipophilicity of the drug. Drugs that are lipophilic can freely cross cell membranes and enter not only vascular and interstitial water, but also intracellular water. Drugs that are highly protein bound, either to albumin or to other structures, may not achieve significant plasma-free drug levels or renal clearance. Thus, the volume of distribution has a significant influence on whether dialysis can effectively change the plasma concentrations of the drug for two reasons: first, large volumes of distribution are usually associated with high degrees of protein binding and thus low glomerular filtration or dialyzability; second, for the same clearance rate, a drug with a larger volume of distribution will have a longer half-life.

Lastly, and often most importantly for cancer chemotherapy agents, renal or dialytic clearance of a drug can have a clinically significant impact on levels in the body only if the renal or dialytic clearance of the drug is comparable or greater than other clearance routes. Classic examples of drugs that are highly similar in structure and indication, but differ in dosing recommendations, are well known to nephrologists. For example, atenolol (molecular weight 266.3) requires dosage adjustment in renal failure, yet metoprolol (molecular weight 267.3) does not. Metoprolol undergoes extensive hepatic metabolism to biologically inactive metabolites, which are then excreted in urine. Atenolol, despite a highly similar structure and molecular weight, has negligible hepatic clearance and is excreted unchanged in urine. Neither drug is extensively protein bound, both have similar volumes of distribution, and both drugs are dialyzable, but only atenolol requires dose adjustment in renal failure, as the hepatic route of clearance is dominant for metoprolol.

In considering dose adjustments for chronic kidney disease and dialysis, the molecular weight of the drug, its protein binding, its volume of distribution and primary clearance mechanisms can provide immediate guidance to the clinician. Peer-reviewed literature on renal dose adjustment is available for a wide array of chemotherapeutic agents, and a useful resource is Aronoff's *Drug Prescribing in Renal Failure*, now in its fifth edition, colloquially known as "the green book" [5]. The "green book" provides dose-adjustment information and references for 25 commonly used antineoplastic agents. We have documented the original source materials for pharmacokinetic data we present, often the package insert or the relevant journal articles. The general paucity of primary data speaks to the need for practitioners to measure pharmacokinetics wherever possible in patients with renal disease receiving chemotherapy agents.

HEMODIALYSIS AND ANTINEOPLASTIC AGENTS

The literature on cancer chemotherapy in maintenance hemodialysis is sparse and largely consists of case reports and small case series, and one suspects that, in contrast to CKD, concomitant treatment for cancer and for ESRD is uncommon. There is an emerging literature on conservative medical management of elderly patients approaching ESRD indicating that dialytic treatment of renal failure does not prolong life in high-risk patients, and is associated with increased hospitalizations [6]. Unsurprisingly, poorer performance status predicts higher mortality in dialysis [7]. In the acute setting, mortality is very high for patients with acute renal failure in the setting of cancer, with estimates ranging between 50 and 83% in recent studies [8–10]. The very real concern that initiating or continuing concomitant aggressive therapies for renal failure and cancer may be futile limits the clinical experience with dosing antineoplastic agents in patients with acute or chronic renal failure. A search of the Ovid medical literature database between 1996 and 2012 for "Renal Dialysis" and "Antineoplastic Agents" revealed 100 citations, of which 40 were case reports regarding single patients, 10 citations were specifically regarding sunitinib, and seven were discussions of tumor lysis syndrome. The literature on chemotherapy dose adjustments for renal failure and dialysis remains sparse, except in special cases where cancer and renal failure coincide, such as myeloma and renal cell cancers.

This chapter provides an overview of the various classes of agents and tabulates the pharmacokinetic data, where known, that allows a clinician insight into whether dose adjustment is needed, and whether rescue dialysis is a plausible strategy for managing overdoses. Paradoxically, the oldest agents are also sometimes the ones about which least is known, while new molecular entities are accepted only after extensive scrutiny. We have avoided specific dose-adjustment recommendations, as the literature evolves quickly. References are provided to facilitate the clinician's initial search in the medical literature.

CELL KINETIC THEORY OF CHEMOTHERAPY

Chemotherapy of malignancy is based on the premise that exposure to an anti-cancer agent will kill a particular fraction of cells in the tumor, based on the mechanism of action of the drug and the fraction of malignant cells in each stage of the cell cycle, or the growth fraction. Repeated doses of the agent eventually reduce the number of malignant cells to less than one. For example, a tumor with 10^9 cells might be treated by a combination drug protocol that achieves a 99% or 2 log kill rate. After five cycles, 10^9 cells $\times (10^{-2})^5$ yields 10^{-1} cells, or complete obliteration of the tumor. In practice, incomplete drug penetration, growth fraction, dose-limiting toxicities and acquired resistance to individual agents undermine treatment success. The sensitive balance between achieving the kill fraction necessary to effect a cure and the toxicities associated with selectivities based on cell division speak to the need for precise dosing.

CLASSES OF ANTINEOPLASTIC AGENTS

The array of antineoplastic agents in use today may be bewildering to consultants from other disciplines who may be assisting in the care of the cancer patient. Fortunately, almost all agents belong to a class of agents with similar

mechanisms of action, kinetics and toxicities. A nosology based on mechanism of action provides a system for the nonspecialist to begin consideration of kinetics, dose adjustments and toxicities.

Nucleotide and Nucleoside Analogs (Table 15.1)

Several antineoplastic agents interfere with cell division by acting as noncanonical substrates for DNA or RNA polymerase. Incorporation of these agents into the polynucleotide chain interferes with chain elongation and thus activates damage pathways leading to apoptosis, or results in early termination of messenger RNA and failure to produce the corresponding peptide chain. Among these are

TABLE 15.1   Nucleoside and Nucleotide Analogs

Name	Molecular weight (Da)	Protein binding	Volume of distribution	Primary elimination	Renal and dialytic clearance
5-FU [12]	130.8	Negligible	4–9 L/m²	Hepatic dihydropyrimidine dehydrogenase	170–180 ml/min; 5-FU and metabolites cleared by hemodialysis but precise PK not reported. Hepatic DPD possibly inhibited by metabolites that accumulate in renal failure [13–18]
Cytarabine (Ara-C) [19]	244	NR	0.6–1 L/kg	Hepatic cytidine deaminase	Ara-C and metabolite Ara-U removed by hemodialysis [20–22]
Gemcitabine [23]	300	Negligible	50–370L/m²	Intracellular nucleoside kinases	<10% unchanged. No change in PK in patients with ESRD, but metabolite dFdU effectively dialyzed [24–26]
Azathioprine, 6-MP [27]	277 171	30% 19%	0.8 L/kg 0.9 L/kg	Hepatic xanthine oxidase	50 ml/min; drug and its metabolite dialyzable [28]. Majority of data in CKD from extensive transplant literature
6-TG [29]	167	NR	NR	Hepatic HGPRT	No data. 6-TG rapidly taken up intracellularly with little residence in circulation. Minor metabolite 2-amino-6-methylthiopurine inactive and renally excreted
Fludarabine [30]	365	19–29%	98 L/m²	Hepatic	40% of metabolite renally cleared and metabolite is cleared by dialysis. Dose reduction recommended in renal insufficiency [31,32]

some of the earliest anti-cancer agents, and background pharmacokinetic data that would be standard for a new drug today is not available. These agents are all small molecules which are very rapidly converted to their active forms by hepatic or erythrocytic enzymes and incorporated into intracellular nucleic acid chains. Metabolism broadly occurs by the same pathways that cycle purine and pyrimidine nucleotides, so purine analogs are affected by allopurinol. The end products of the nucleotide pathway metabolism of these drugs are often renally excreted, although accumulation in renal failure is not generally clinically problematic. Dosage adjustment for renal failure or dialysis is not warranted, and extracorporeal removal in overdose situations would not be expected to be helpful. One exception is the use of cytarabine. While low doses ($\leq$400 mg/m^2/ day) generally do not need dose reduction, high doses >1 g/m^2/day may require dose reduction or change of therapy. It has been shown that renal dysfunction is a risk factor for neurotoxicity and that reducing the dose (3 g/m^2/dose to 1 or 2 g/m^2/dose) or lengthening the dosing interval (q12 hours to q24 hours) may reduce this risk [11]. Little safety data exist for the use of high-dose cytarabine with dialysis.

Microtubule Inhibitors (Table 15.2)

This class of agents derive their anti-tumor specificity by arresting dividing cells in metaphase, but also arrest other rapidly dividing cells, such as those found in intestinal mucosa and hair follicles. Both classes — the vinca alkaloids and the taxanes — are about 1 kilodalton in molecular weight with multiple ring structures, and, interestingly, both are derived from unrelated evergreen shrubs. The vinca alkaloids were discovered in the periwinkle *Catharanthus roseus*, a flowering plant (and not the littoral mollusk by the same common name), and the

TABLE 15.2 Microtubule Inhibitors

Name	Molecular weight (Da)	Protein binding	Volume of distribution	Primary elimination	Renal and dialytic clearance
Vincristine [33]	923	NR	137–1241 L/m^2 [34]	CYP3A followed by biliary excretion	Negligible data. Very large volumes of distribution and non-renal mechanisms suggest dose adjustment not necessary
Vinblastine [35]	909	NR	NR	CYP3A4 and biliary excretion	Package insert suggests no need for renal dose adjustment
Vinorelbine [36]	1079	80–90%	25–40 L/kg	CYP3A4 and biliary excretion	Package insert suggests no need for renal dose adjustment
Paclitaxel [37]	854	89–98%	227–688 L/m^2	CYP2C8 CYP3A4	Minimal recovery from urine. Extensive protein binding suggests negligible dialytic clearance. Case reports suggest no dose adjustment for renal failure or dialysis [38,39]
Docetaxel [40]	862	97%	113 L	CYP3A4	Minimal recovery from urine. Extensive protein binding suggests negligible dialytic clearance. Case reports suggest no dose adjustment for renal failure or dialysis [41,42]

taxanes are derived from the Pacific yew *Taxus brevifolia*, a conifer. The molecules bind to tubulin dimers, preventing further polymerization of tubulin into microtubules necessary to form the mitotic spindle. Although pharmacokinetic data in relation to renal function is somewhat sparse for the earliest agents, in general they are highly protein bound with very large volumes of distribution, and thus have insignificant renal or dialytic clearance. Rescue dialysis for overdose is unlikely to affect plasma concentrations.

Alkylating Agents (Table 15.3)

Alkylating agents were first developed immediately after the Second World War by Brock and colleagues, who developed the idea of a transport form and an active form for nitrogen mustards [43]. These drugs achieve their therapeutic action through the irreversible covalent modification of intracellular molecules, particularly nucleic acids. These agents are among the oldest anti-cancer agents in clinical use, and, paradoxically, for some agents basic pharmacokinetics, such as protein binding and identification of enzymes involved in elimination, remain underreported. Most agents are relatively stable prodrugs which are converted to highly reactive species which crosslink DNA, interrupting transcription and cell division. As a group they are active in both stable and dividing cells. The parent drugs are rapidly metabolized to the active agents by hepatic enzymes or enzyme-free hydrolysis. Volumes of distribution are similar to total body water. Protein binding, if known, is highly variable from drug to drug. Typical dose-limiting toxicities are hematologic suppression and, in the case of cyclophosphamide and ifosfamide, hemorrhagic cystitis, and the nitrosoureas are associated with pulmonary fibrosis.

Platinum Agents (Table 15.4)

Platinum salts were discovered to prevent cell division in *E. coli*, which stimulated further inquiry into their therapeutic uses [64,65]. Cisplatin was discovered to have activity against eukaryotic cell division, initiating a new class of anti-cancer drugs [66]. The agents as a class exert their action by crosslinking DNA via covalent bonds to guanine nucleotide bases, preventing mitosis, much as the alkylating agents do. In each case, the drug is a parent compound releasing the active platinum, which is rapidly bound to proteins and tissues. Renal and dialytic clearances are significant and multiple formulas for dose adjustment exist for each drug. The high degree of protein/tissue binding probably makes rescue hemodialysis for overdose impractical [67]. There are case reports of plasma exchange for overdose [68].

Anti-tumor Antibiotics: Glycopeptides and Anthracyclines (Table 15.5)

Although other antineoplastics are also structurally similar to antibiotics, these drugs are grouped together here as they are thought to share common mechanisms of action [84]. These drugs are among the earliest antineoplastic agents, and mechanisms of action continue to be debated [84,85]. They are thought to act via intercalation between base pairs in the DNA double-helix and thus inhibit DNA and RNA polymerases, resulting in failure of chain elongation and either mitotic arrest or decreased message. However, free radical formation is thought to play a role in cardiotoxicity and possibly also DNA damage [85]. Bleomycin is thought to act via induction of single-strand DNA breaks. Doxorubicin, and possibly others, is also thought to act via inhibition of topoisomerase II, resulting in unrepaired breaks to DNA. The glycopeptides have moderately large volumes of distribution and low or uncertain protein binding. Attempts at dialytic removal of these agents should probably be accompanied by pharmacokinetic measurements with which to guide treatment. The anthracyclines have very short half-lives and extraordinarily large

TABLE 15.3 Alkylating Agents

Name	Molecular weight (Da)	Protein binding	Volume of distribution	Primary elimination	Renal and dialytic clearance
Cyclophosphamide [44,45]	279	NR	0.36—0.49 L/kg [46]	Hepatic CYP2B6 (predominant) and CYP2C9 convert to active metabolite; 20—30% of drug and metabolite cleared renally [45,46]	Extensive experience from treatment of ANCA vasculitides. Specific case reports and case series on PK in dialysis and CKD. Exposure to drug and alkylating metabolite increased in CKD and ESRD. Both drug and alkylating metabolite removed by dialysis, but significant rebound occurs. Exposure in normal subjects and well-dialyzed ESRD may be similar [45—49]. Acrolein metabolite causes hemorrhagic cystitis which can be ameliorated with MESNA
Ifosfamide [45,50]	261	NR	40—50 L [51]; 0.23—0.8 L/kg in children [52]	Hepatic CYP3A4 (predominant) and CYP2C9 convert to active metabolite; 61% of drug and metabolite cleared renally [45,50]	Significant nephrotoxicity attributed to chloroacetaldehyde (CAA), which causes a Fanconi syndrome. Acrolein metabolite causes hemorrhagic cystitis which can be ameliorated with MESNA [45]. Package insert states safety in children not established, but extensive literature available. Single case report in an anephric 20-m-old treated with dialysis suggested parent drug dialyzable, as is nephrotoxic metabolite; active 4-OH metabolite removed less well
Melphalan [32,53—55]	305	60—90%	0.5 L/kg	Nonenzymatic hydrolysis and renal excretion	Short half-life suggests dialysis unlikely to remove significant drug; case reports of use in dialysis patients with and without dose adjustment [32,56]
Busulphan [57]	246	32%	0.64 L/kg	Glutathione-S-transferase and partial renal excretion	Partially removed with dialysis [58]
(Carmustine) BiCNU [59—61]	214	77% [62]	3—5 L/kg [62]	Hepatic microsomes; P450 [63]	Rapidly metabolized; no data regarding dialysis or renal insufficiency [59—62]

TABLE 15.4 Platinum Agents

Name	Molecular weight (Da)	Protein binding	Volume of distribution	Primary elimination	Renal and dialytic clearance
Cisplatin [69]	300	Negligible (cisplatin) 90% (platinum)	11–12 L/m^2	Renal. Both cisplatin and free platinum appear to be filtered and undergo tubular secretion [69]	Platinum, not cisplatin, is protein bound [69]. Drug appears to accumulate in renal failure and unbound platinum is cleared by dialysis [70–74]. High protein binding of platinum suggests emergency or salvage dialysis after overdose will be ineffective
Carboplatin [75]	371	Negligible (carboplatin) 90% (platinum)	16 L	Renal. Package insert reports that the only platinum in urine was as carboplatin	Package insert recommends dosage reduction in CKD. Doses adjusted for renal failure according to Calvert formula appear to work well in hemodialysis as long as dialysis delayed until initial distribution phase is complete [76–80]
Oxaliplatin [81]	397	Rapid distribution of oxaliplatin into tissues (85%). Free platinum bound to plasma proteins		Rapid nonenzymatic modification, followed by renal excretion of modified oxaliplatin and free platinum. Free platinum almost completely bound to plasma proteins	Multiple reports of oxaliplatin use in ESRD. Oxaliplatin removed by hemodialysis, as was free platinum, but free platinum showed large rebound not seen with other agents [13,82,83]. Package insert states no dose reduction in subjects with GFR >30 ml/min, advises dose reduction in severe renal impairment but does not provide suggested dose modifications

TABLE 15.5   Anti-tumor Antibiotics

Name	Molecular weight (Da)	Protein binding	Volume of distribution	Primary elimination	Renal and dialytic clearance
GLYCOPEPTIDES					
Dactinomycin [86]	1255	NR	NR	Biliary and renal	NR. Very little published data. What is published is inconsistent [86,87]. 30–50% excreted unchanged in feces and urine [88]
Mitomycin [88,89]	334	22%	7 L/m^2, 11–48 L/m^2	Biliary	Pharmacokinetics reported have high interindividual variability and to be independent of renal function [88,89]
Bleomycin [90]	1425	NR	17.5 L/m^2	60–70% of drug is excreted in urine as unchanged drug	Clearance decreases with increased creatinine [91]. Reported as not dialyzable, but presumably with low-flux membranes
ANTHRACYCLINES					
Doxorubicin [92]	580	75%	$809–1214 \text{ L/m}^2$; 24.6 L/kg	Renal aldo-keto reductase, biliary excretion	Half-life and AUC increased in hemodialysis. Dialytic clearance negligible [93,94]
Daunorubicin [95]	564	NR	39.2 L/kg	Renal and hepatic aldo-keto reductase, biliary excretion	Package insert states to reduce dose by 50% if patients with creatinine >3 mg/dL
Idarubicin [96,97]	534	97%	$362–2550 \text{ L/m}^2$ [97]	Hepatic aldo-keto reductase followed by biliary excretion	No data in dialysis or renal failure

NR = Not reported.

volumes of distribution, suggesting extracorporeal therapy would neither assist in management of overdoses nor require dose adjustment in clinical use.

Topoisomerase Inhibitors (Table 15.6)

Topoisomerases are enzymes essential to DNA replication and transcription by temporarily cleaving one or both strands of the double-helix and re-ligating them, allowing relief of torsional stresses induced by DNA and RNA polymerases. Bacterial topoisomerases are targets for fluoroquinolone antibiotics, and drug-induced failure to re-ligate the cleaved DNA strands in eukaryotic cells triggers DNA repair mechanisms or apoptosis. As a group, these drugs are initially metabolized or glucuronidated by hepatic enzymes and secreted into bile. These small molecules are only partially protein bound and both they and their metabolites are renally cleared. All of these agents except doxorubicin (discussed above) require dose adjustment in renal insufficiency. Volumes of distribution are fairly high, but moderate protein binding and low molecular weights suggest that dialysis rescue after overdose might be reasonable to

TABLE 15.6 Topoisomerase Inhibitors

Name	Molecular weight (Da)	Protein binding	Volume of distribution	Primary elimination	Renal and dialytic clearance
TOPOISOMERASE I					
Irinotecan [98]	677	30–68%; active metabolite SN-38 95% bound	110–234 L/m²	Hepatic carboxylesterase; metabolite SN-38 glucuronidated by UGT1A1	Package insert states: "is not recommended for use in patients on dialysis." Delayed clearance of metabolites seen in renal failure; possible competitive inhibition by uremic organic anions [99–101]
Topotecan [102]	458	35%	45 L/m²	About half of drug excreted unchanged in urine; balance hepatic CYP3A4/5	Prolonged half-life in dialysis and rebound after dialysis [103,104]. Package insert recommends 50% dose reduction for subjects with creatinine clearance <40 ml/min. Creatinine predicts topotecan clearance and dose-limiting toxicity [105]
TOPOISOMERASE II					
Teniposide [106]	656	>99%	8–44 L/m² (adults); 3–11 L/m² (children)	NR	Renal clearance 2–3 ml/min; 86% metabolized but site not specified in package insert or in manuscripts [107]
Etoposide [108]	588.6	97%	7–17 L/m²	Hepatic and renal clearance	PK similar in ESRD as in normal subjects [74,109,110]. Dose adjustments in CKD largely empiric [111]
Doxorubicin* [92]	580	75%	809–1214 L/m²; 24.6 L/kg	Renal aldo-keto reductase, biliary excretion	Half-life and AUC increased in hemodialysis. Dialytic clearance negligible [93,94]

Doxorubicin is listed under anti-tumor antibiotics and under topoisomerase inhibitors as it is thought to have two mechanisms of action.

attempt, although literature supporting this approach could not be located.

Tyrosine Kinase Inhibitors (Table 15.7)

Mammalian cells express a variety of transmembrane growth factor receptors, among them tyrosine kinases that appear critical for cell-cycle signaling, such as the vascular endothelial growth factor receptor (VEGFR) and the epidermal growth factor receptor (EGFR). The discovery that chronic myelogenous leukemias frequently were associated with a specific chromosomal translocation, t(9;22), and a constitutively activated fusion protein BCR-ABL, which was a tyrosine kinase, drove a rational drug design program seeking small-molecule inhibitors, the first of which was imatinib, marketed as Gleevec (USA) or Glivec (outside the USA). A second well-known example of a cancer-related growth factor receptor tyrosine kinase is the HER2/Neu protein overexpressed in some breast cancers, against which a monoclonal antibody, trastuzimab, is directed. The family of small-molecule inhibitors of membrane receptor tyrosine kinases continues to grow. These agents are small, highly protein bound, and all metabolized by hepatic cytochrome P-450 enzymes. Available literature does not support roles for dose adjustment in renal failure or dialysis.

Unique Agents (Table 15.8)

There are a number of anti-tumor agents which uniquely exploit some feature of a specific malignancy, or remain the only entity with a particular mechanism of action or the only approved agent in its class. Methotrexate is a small-molecule inhibitor of dihydrofolate reductase, blocking a key step in purine synthesis, thus preventing DNA and RNA synthesis. It is cytotoxic to cells in S-phase, and exerts its anti-tumor selectivity solely by targeting cells that divide rapidly. It is moderately protein bound with a volume of distribution approximating body water, so it would be expected to be incompletely removed by dialysis, and to require multiple sessions of dialysis to significantly alter the time-average concentration. Hydroxyurea is a small-molecule agent first synthesized in the 19th century and noted to have activity against certain leukemias, and later essential thrombocytosis and sickle cell anemia, although the precise mechanism of action continues to be debated [127,128]. Hydroxyurea is thought to act by inhibition of ribonucleotide reductase, interfering with nucleic acid synthesis and thus acting with selectivity against rapidly dividing cells [128]. One would anticipate removal with dialysis and the need for an additional dose post dialysis. Asparaginase is an enzyme produced by *E. coli* that hydrolyzes asparagine to aspartic acid. Certain leukemic cells may be unable to synthesize asparagine and thus are sensitive to depletion of the extracellular asparagine pool, while healthy cells are able to synthesize asparagine. It is a large (31 kD) protein that distributes into plasma volume and is not dialyzable. Thalidomide and lenalidomide are small-molecule antiangiogenic and anti-tumor agents with pleiotrophic mechanisms of action, among them interference with signaling downstream from the vascular endothelial growth factor receptor and upregulation of apoptotic pathways [129]. Both are small molecules with moderate protein binding, and quite different routes of elimination; thalidomide is hydrolyzed, whereas lenalidomide is excreted largely unchanged in urine, and requires dose adjustments in renal insufficiency and dialysis. Bortezomib is a small-molecule inhibitor of the 26S proteosome, an element of the intracellular machinery responsible for degrading damaged and ubiquinated proteins. In rapidly dividing cells this manifests as cell-cycle arrest and death; additional pro-apoptotic and antiangiogenic effects are thought to be specific to myeloma [130,131]. It has a high degree of protein binding and an

TABLE 15.7 Tyrosine Kinase Inhibitors

Name	Molecular weight (Da)	Protein binding	Volume of distribution	Primary elimination	Renal and dialytic clearance
Imatinib [112]	493	95%	NR	CYP3A4, biliary excretion	Minimal change in PK in one hemodialysis patient compared to published values for normal renal function. Primary metabolite also active [112,113]
Gefitinib [114]	447	90%	NR	CYP3A4, CYP2D6, biliary excretion	Minimal change in PK in one hemodialysis patient compared to published values for normal renal function [115]
Sunitinib [116]	398	95%	NR	CYP3A4 biliary excretion	Minimal change in PK in hemodialysis patients compared to published values for normal renal function [117–119]
Sorafenib [120]	465	99.5	NR	CYP3A4, UGT1A9 biliary excretion	Used for renal cell cancer in hemodialysis patients with minimal dose adjustments. Sorafenib levels appear to rise slightly during dialysis session [121–124]
Dasatinib [125]	488	96%	2505 L	CYP3A4, biliary excretion	NR
Nilotinib [126]	530	98% based on *in vitro* experiments	NR	CYP3A4, excreted largely unchanged in feces. CYP3A4 inhibitor	NR. Package insert suggests untested in subjects with creatinine >1.5 mg/dL

NR = Not reported.

TABLE 15.8 Unique Agents

Name	Molecular weight (Da)	Protein binding	Volume of distribution	Primary elimination	Renal and dialytic clearance
Methotrexate [132]	454	50%	0.4–0.8 L/kg	80–90% excreted unchanged in urine	High-flux membrane dialysis removes up to 75% of serum methotrexate. Repeat dialysis sessions may be necessary due to intracellular redistribution [133]
Hydroxyurea [134]	76	0% [135]	Total body water; 20 L/m^2 [128]	60% hepatic; 40% renal	Renal failure associated with 60% increase in AUC. Administer after dialysis. Literature reports rare
Asparaginase [136]	31,731	NR	Plasma volume	Very little data, apparently not excreted into urine	Very little data. One would not expect dialytic clearance of a 31 kD protein
Thalidomide [137]	258	55–60%	0.88 L/kg [138]	Package insert states no P450 metabolism. [138] states minimal excretion of metabolites in urine. Possible hepatic CYP2C19 [139]	Considerable variation in reports on metabolism and elimination. Probably no requirement for dose adjustment in CKD. Supplement after dialysis [138]
Lenalidomide [140]	259	30% [140] 40% [141]	50–60 L	Drug excreted unchanged in urine	Increased exposure in renal insufficiency. Package insert suggests 40% dose removed in single dialysis session; another manuscript states 31% [141], contains specific dosing suggestions for CKD and hemodialysis
Bortezomib [142]	384	83%	498–1884 L/m^2	CYP3A4 CYP2C19 CYP1A2	Metabolites inactive. Elimination routes poorly described. Adverse events more common in renal insufficiency [143]. Systemic exposure (AUCs) reported as similar in subjects with normal renal function, CKD, and on dialysis [142]

NR = Not reported.

extraordinarily large volume of distribution, and is not thought to require dose adjustment in renal failure or dialysis; nor is dialysis likely to assist in overdose.

SUMMARY

The number and variety of anti-cancer agents in common use today is quite large and growing quickly, as is the number of patients with dual diagnoses of cancer and renal disease. This chapter has presented pharmacokinetic data on 42 of the most commonly used agents in order to provide broad guidance to nephrologists and oncologists caring for patients with renal insufficiency and cancer. The number of agents for which definitive data exist guiding prospective dose adjustment remains few. Wherever possible, concomitant pharmacokinetic measurements should be attempted to guide therapy, and the data published, particularly for older agents for which organ-specific pharmacokinetic data are sparse.

References

[1] US Renal Data System. USRDS 2011 annual data report. Atlas of Chronic Kidney Disease and End-stage Renal Disease in the United States. Bethesda, Maryland: National Institutes of Health, National Institute of Diabetes and Digestive and Kidney Diseases; 2012.

[2] American Cancer Society. Cancer Facts & Figures 2012. Atlanta, Georgia: American Cancer Society; 2012.

[3] Humphreys BD. Onco-nephrology: kidney disease in the cancer patient: introduction. Semin Nephrol 2010;30:531−3.

[4] Chobanian A. The Seventh Report of the Joint National Committee on Prevention, Detection, Evaluation, and Treatment of High Blood Pressure. Bethesda, MD: National Heart, Lung, and Blood Institute; 2003.

[5] Aronoff G, Bennett W, Berns J, Brier M, Kasbekar N, Mueller BA, et al. Drug prescribing in renal failure. 5th ed. Philadelphia: American College of Physicians; 2007.

[6] Smith C, Da Silva-Gane M, Chandna S, Warwicker P, Greenwood R, Farrington K, et al. Choosing not to dialyse: evaluation of planned non-dialytic management in a cohort of patients with end-stage renal failure. Nephron 2003;95:c40−6.

[7] Ifudu O, Paul HR, Homel P, Friedman EA. Predictive value of functional status for mortality in patients on maintenance hemodialysis. Am J Nephrol 1998;18:109−16.

[8] Soares M, Salluh JI, Carvalho MS, Darmon M, Rocco JR, Spector N, et al. Prognosis of critically ill patients with cancer and acute renal dysfunction. J Clin Oncol 2006;24:4003−10.

[9] Groeger JS. Aurora RN. Intensive care, mechanical ventilation, dialysis, and cardiopulmonary resuscitation. Implications for the patient with cancer. Crit Care Clin 2001;17:791−803.

[10] Groeger JS, Glassman J, Nierman DM, Wallace SK, Price K, Horak D, et al. Probability of mortality of critically ill cancer patients at 72 h of intensive care unit (ICU) management. Support Care Cancer 2003;11:686−95.

[11] Smith GA, Damon LE, Rugo HS, Ries CA, Linker CA. High-dose cytarabine dose modification reduces the incidence of neurotoxicity in patients with renal insufficiency. J Clin Oncol 1997;15:833−9.

[12] Iyer L. Ratain MJ. 5-Fluorouracil pharmacokinetics: causes for variability and strategies for modulation in cancer chemotherapy. Cancer Invest 1999;17:494−506.

[13] Watayo Y, Kuramochi H, Hayashi K, Nakajima G, Kamikozuru H, Yamamoto M, et al. Drug monitoring during folfox6 therapy in a rectal cancer patient on chronic hemodialysis. Jpn J Clin Oncol 2010;40:360−4.

[14] Gusella M, Rebeschini M, Cartei G, Ferrazzi E, Ferrari M, Padrini R, et al. Effect of hemodialysis on the metabolic clearance of 5-fluorouracil in a patient with end-stage renal failure. Ther Drug Monit 2005;27:816−8.

[15] Keller F, Gallkowski U, Roth W, Boese-Landgraf J. Combined haemoperfusion, haemofiltration and haemodialysis for systemic detoxification in locoregional 5-fluorouracil therapy. Cancer Chemother Pharmacol 1991;29:164−6.

[16] Rengelshausen J, Hull WE, Schwenger V, Goggelmann C, Walter-Sack I, Bommer J, et al. Pharmacokinetics of 5-fluorouracil and its catabolites determined by 19f nuclear magnetic resonance spectroscopy for a patient on chronic hemodialysis. Am J Kidney Dis 2002;39:E10.

[17] Tomiyama N, Hidaka M, Hidaka H, Kawano Y, Hanada N, Kawaguchi H, et al. Safety, efficacy and

pharmacokinetics of s-1 in a hemodialysis patient with advanced gastric cancer. Cancer Chemother Pharmacol 2010;65:807−9.

[18] Venat-Bouvet L, Saint-Marcoux F, Lagarde C, Peyronnet P, Lebrun-Ly V, Tubiana-Mathieu N. Irinotecan-based chemotherapy in a metastatic colorectal cancer patient under haemodialysis for chronic renal dysfunction: two cases considered. Anticancer Drugs 2007;18:977−80.

[19] Laliberte J, Momparier RL. Human cytidine deaminase: purification of enzyme, cloning, and expression of its complementary DNA. Cancer Res 1994;54:5401−7.

[20] Poschl JM, Klaus G, Querfeld U, Ludwig R, Mehls O. Chemotherapy with cytosine arabinoside in a child with Burkitt's lymphoma on maintenance hemodialysis and hemofiltration. Ann Hematol 1993;67:37−9.

[21] Radeski D, Cull GM, Cain M, Hackett LP, Ilett KF. Effective clearance of ara-u the major metabolite of cytosine arabinoside (ara-c) by hemodialysis in a patient with lymphoma and end-stage renal failure. Cancer Chemother Pharmacol 2011;67:765−8.

[22] Tsuchiya Y, Ubara Y, Suwabe T, Hoshino J, Sumida K, Hiramatsu R, et al. Successful treatment of acute promyelocytic leukemia in a patient on hemodialysis. Clin Exp Nephrol 2011;15:434−7.

[23] Eli Lilly and Company. Highlights of prescribing information: Gemzar powder, lyophilized, for solution intravenous use. Indianapolis, IN: Eli Lilly and Company; 2011.

[24] Kiani A, Kohne CH, Franz T, Passauer J, Haufe T, Gross P, et al. Pharmacokinetics of gemcitabine in a patient with end-stage renal disease: effective clearance of its main metabolite by standard hemodialysis treatment. Cancer Chemother Pharmacol 2003;51:266−70.

[25] Koolen SL, Huitema AD, Jansen RS, van Voorthuizen T, Beijnen JH, Smit WM, et al. Pharmacokinetics of gemcitabine and metabolites in a patient with double-sided nephrectomy: a case report and review of the literature. Oncologist 2009;14:944−8.

[26] Masumori N, Kunishima Y, Hirobe M, Takeuchi M, Takayanagi A, Tsukamoto T, et al. Measurement of plasma concentration of gemcitabine and its metabolite dFdU in hemodialysis patients with advanced urothelial cancer. Jpn J Clin Oncol 2008;38:182−5.

[27] Triton Pharma Inc. Product monograph imuran azathioprine tablets. Concord, ON: Triton Pharma, Inc; 2010.

[28] Schusziarra V, Ziekursch V, Schlamp R, Siemensen HC. Pharmacokinetics of azathioprine under haemodialysis. Int J Clin Pharmacol Biopharm 1976;14:298−302.

[29] GlaxoSmithKline. Tabloid® prescribing information. Research Triangle Park, NC: GlaxoSmithKline; 2009.

[30] Bayer HealthCare Pharmaceuticals Inc. Fludara package insert. Wayne, NJ: Bayer HealthCare Pharmaceuticals Inc; 2007.

[31] Kielstein JT, Stadler M, Czock D, Keller F, Hertenstein B, Radermacher J. Dialysate concentration and pharmacokinetics of 2f-ara-a in a patient with acute renal failure. Eur J Haematol 2005;74:533−4.

[32] Tendas A, Cupelli L, Dentamaro T, Scaramucci L, Palumbo R, Niscola P, et al. Feasibility of a dose-adjusted fludarabine-melphalan conditioning prior autologous stem cell transplantation in a dialysis-dependent patient with mantle cell lymphoma. Ann Hematol 2009;88:285−6.

[33] Hospira Inc. Vincristine sulfate injection, USP. Lake Forest, IL: Hospira, Inc; 2007.

[34] Lonnerholm G, Frost BM, Soderhall S, de Graaf SS. Vincristine pharmacokinetics in children with down syndrome. Pediatr Blood Cancer 2009;52:123−5.

[35] Bedford Laboratories. Vinblastine sulfate for injection USP. Bedford, Ohio: Bedford Laboratories; 2001.

[36] Bedford Laboratories: Vinorelbine injection USP. Bedford, Ohio: Bedford Laboratories; July, 2005.

[37] Bristol-Myers Squibb Company. Taxol® (paclitaxel) injection. Princeton, NJ: Bristol-Myers Squibb Company; 2011.

[38] Baur M, Fazeny-Doerner B, Olsen SJ, Dittrich C. High dose single-agent paclitaxel in a hemodialysis patient with advanced ovarian cancer: a case report with pharmacokinetic analysis and review of the literature. Int J Gynecol Cancer 2008;18:564−70.

[39] Ide H, Satou A, Hoshino K, Yasumizu Y, Uchida Y, Tasaka Y, et al. Successful management of metastatic urothelial carcinoma with gemcitabine and paclitaxel chemotherapy in a hemodialysis patient. Urol Int 2011;87:245−7.

[40] sanofi-aventis US LLC. Taxotere® prescribing information. Bridgewater, NJ: sanofi-aventis US LLC; 2010.

[41] Hochegger K, Lhotta K, Mayer G, Czejka M, Hilbe W. Pharmacokinetic analysis of docetaxel during haemodialysis in a patient with locally advanced non-small cell lung cancer. Nephrol Dial Transplant 2007;22:289−90.

[42] Mencoboni M, Olivieri R, Vannozzi MO, Schettini G, Viazzi F, Ghio R. Docetaxel pharmacokinetics with pre- and post-dialysis administration in a hemodyalized patient. Chemotherapy 2006;52:147−50.

[43] Brock N. Oxazaphosphorine cytostatics: past-present-future. Cancer Res 1989;49:1−7.

[44] Baxter Healthcare Corporation. Cyclophosphamide for injection, USP. Deerfield, IL: Baxter Healthcare Corporation; 2007.

[45] Giraud B, Hebert G, Deroussent A, Veal GJ, Vassal G, Paci A. Oxazaphosphorines: new therapeutic strategies for an old class of drugs. Expert Opin Drug Metab Toxicol 2010;6:919–38.

[46] Haubitz M, Bohnenstengel F, Brunkhorst R, Schwab M, Hofmann U, Busse D. Cyclophosphamide pharmacokinetics and dose requirements in patients with renal insufficiency. Kidney Int 2002;61:1495–501.

[47] McCune JS, Adams D, Homans AC, Guillot A, Iacono L, Stewart CF. Cyclophosphamide disposition in an anephric child. Pediatr Blood Cancer 2006;46:99–104.

[48] Perry JJ, Fleming RA, Rocco MV, Petros WP, Bleyer AJ, Radford Jr JE, et al. Administration and pharmacokinetics of high-dose cyclophosphamide with hemodialysis support for allogeneic bone marrow transplantation in acute leukemia and end-stage renal disease. Bone Marrow Transplant 1999;23:839–42.

[49] Wang LH, Lee CS, Majeske BL, Marbury TC. Clearance and recovery calculations in hemodialysis: application to plasma, red blood cell, and dialysate measurements for cyclophosphamide. Clin Pharmacol Ther 1981;29:365–72.

[50] Baxter Healthcare Corporation. Ifex (ifosfamide for injection). Deerfield, IL: Baxter Healthcare Corporation; 2007.

[51] van Putten JW, Kerbush T, Smit EF, van Rijswijk R, Beijnen JH, Sleijfer DT, et al. Dose-finding and pharmacological study of ifosfamide in combination with paclitaxel and carboplatin in resistant small-cell lung cancer. Ann Oncol 2001;12:787–92.

[52] Carlson L, Goren MP, Bush DA, Griener JC, Quigley R, Tkaczewski I, et al. Toxicity, pharmacokinetics, and in vitro hemodialysis clearance of ifosfamide and metabolites in an anephric pediatric patient with Wilms' tumor. Cancer Chemother Pharmacol 1998;41:140–6.

[53] Celgene Corporation. Alkeran (melphalan) tablets. Warren, NJ: Celgene Coporation; 2004.

[54] Nath CE, Shaw PJ, Trotman J, Zeng L, Duffull SB, Hegarty G, et al. Population pharmacokinetics of melphalan in patients with multiple myeloma undergoing high dose therapy. Br J Clin Pharmacol 2010;69:484–97.

[55] Pinguet F, Culine S, Bressolle F, Astre C, Serre MP, Chevillard C, et al. A phase I and pharmacokinetic study of melphalan using a 24-hour continuous infusion in patients with advanced malignancies. Clin Cancer Res 2000;6:57–63.

[56] Hamaki T, Katori H, Kami M, Yamato T, Yamakado H, Itoh T, et al. Successful allogeneic blood stem cell transplantation for aplastic anemia in a patient with renal insufficiency requiring dialysis. Bone Marrow Transplant 2002;30:195–8.

[57] Otsuka America Pharmaceutical Inc. IV busulfex (busulfan injection) prescribing information. Tokyo: Otsuka America Pharmaceutical Inc; 2011.

[58] Ullery L, Gibbs J, Ames G, Senecal F, Slattery J. Busulfan clearance in renal failure and hemodialysis. Bone Marrow Transplant 2000;25:201–3.

[59] Ben Venue Laboratories Inc. BiCNU (carmustine) kit. Bedford, OH: Ben Venue Laboratories; 2011.

[60] Weiss RB, Issell BF. The nitrosoureas: Carmustine (bcnu) and lomustine (ccnu). Cancer Treat Rev 1982;9:313–30.

[61] National Center for Biotechnology Information. Carmustine – compound summary. PubChem Compound. Bethesda MD, National Library of Medicine. Downloaded form http://pubchem.ncbi.nlm.nih.gov on July 22, 2013.

[62] Henner WD, Peters WP, Eder JP, Antman K, Schnipper L, Frei 3rd E. Pharmacokinetics and immediate effects of high-dose carmustine in man. Cancer Treat Rep 1986;70:877–80.

[63] Lin H-S, Weinkam RJ. Metabolism of 1,3-bis(2-chloroethyl)-1-nitrosourea by rat hepatic microsomes. J Med Chem 1981;24:761–3.

[64] Rosenberg B, Vancamp L, Krigas T. Inhibition of cell division in Escherichia coli by electrolysis products from a platinum electrode. Nature 1965;205:698–9.

[65] Rosenberg B, Van Camp L, Grimley EB, Thomson AJ. The inhibition of growth or cell division in Escherichia coli by different ionic species of platinum(IV) complexes. J Biol Chem 1967;242:1347–52.

[66] Rosenberg B, VanCamp L, Trosko JE, Mansour VH. Platinum compounds: a new class of potent antitumour agents. Nature 1969;222:385–6.

[67] Brivet F, Pavlovitch JM, Gouyette A, Cerrina ML, Tchernia G, Dormont J. Inefficiency of early prophylactic hemodialysis in cis-platinum overdose. Cancer Chemother Pharmacol 1986;18:183–4.

[68] Chu G, Mantin R, Shen YM, Baskett G, Sussman H. Massive cisplatin overdose by accidental substitution for carboplatin. Toxicity and management. Cancer 1993;72:3707–14.

[69] Teva Parenteral Medicines Inc. Cisplatin injection package insert. Irvine, CA: Teva Parenteral Medicines Inc; 2007.

[70] Hirai K, Ishiko O, Sumi T, Kanaoka Y, Ogita S. Kinetics of plasma platinum in a hemodialysis patient receiving repeated doses of cisplatin. Oncol Rep 2000;7:1243–5.

[71] Marnitz S, Kettritz R, Kahl A, Lehenbauer-Dehm S, Forster L, Budach V, et al. Simultaneous chemoradiation with cisplatin in a patient with recurrent

cervical cancer undergoing hemodialysis: analysis of cisplatin concentrations in serum and dialysate and therapy-related acute toxicity. Strahlenther Onkol 2011;187:831–4.

[72] Tomita M, Kurata H, Aoki Y, Tanaka K, Kazama JJ. Pharmacokinetics of paclitaxel and cisplatin in a hemodialysis patient with recurrent ovarian cancer. Anticancer Drugs 2001;12:485–7.

[73] Zahra MA, Taylor A, Mould G, Coles C, Crawford R, Tan LT. Concurrent weekly cisplatin chemotherapy and radiotherapy in a haemodialysis patient with locally advanced cervix cancer. Clin Oncol (R Coll Radiol) 2008;20:6–11.

[74] Watanabe R, Takiguchi Y, Moriya T, Oda S, Kurosu K, Tanabe N, et al. Feasibility of combination chemotherapy with cisplatin and etoposide for haemodialysis patients with lung cancer. Br J Cancer 2003;88:25–30.

[75] Bristol-Myers Squibb Company. Paraplatin (carboplatin) injection, solution package insert. Princeton, NJ: Bristol-Myers Squibb Company; 2007.

[76] Calvert AH, Newell DR, Gumbrell LA, O'Reilly S, Burnell M, Boxall FE, et al. Carboplatin dosage: prospective evaluation of a simple formula based on renal function. J Clin Oncol 1989;7:1748–56.

[77] Shord SS, Bressler LR, Radhakrishnan L, Chen N, Villano JL. Evaluation of the modified diet in renal disease equation for calculation of carboplatin dose. Ann Pharmacother 2009;43:235–41.

[78] Lindauer A, Eickhoff C, Kloft C, Jaehde U. Population pharmacokinetics of high-dose carboplatin in children and adults. Ther Drug Monit 2010;32: 159–68.

[79] Oguri T, Shimokata T, Inada M, Ito I, Ando Y, Sasaki Y, et al. Pharmacokinetic analysis of carboplatin in patients with cancer who are undergoing hemodialysis. Cancer Chemother Pharmacol 2010;66:813–7.

[80] de Lemos ML, Hamata L, Conklin J. Comment: evaluation of the modified diet in renal disease equation for calculation of carboplatin dose. Ann Pharmacother 2009;43:1914–5. author reply 1915.

[81] LLC s-aU. Eloxatin® (oxaliplatin) powder, for solution for intravenous use. Bridgewater, NJ: sanofi-aventis US LLC; 2011.

[82] Horimatsu T, Miyamoto S, Morita S, Mashimo Y, Ezoe Y, Muto M, et al. Pharmacokinetics of oxaliplatin in a hemodialytic patient treated with modified FOLFOX-6 plus bevacizumab therapy. Cancer Chemother Pharmacol 2011;68:263–6.

[83] Honecker FU, Brummendorf TH, Klein O, Bokemeyer C. Safe use of oxaliplatin in a patient with metastatic breast cancer and combined renal and hepatic failure. Onkologie 2006;29:273–5.

[84] Gewirtz D. A critical evaluation of the mechanisms of action proposed for the antitumor effects of the anthracycline antibiotics adriamycin and daunorubicin. Biochem Pharmacol 1999;57:727–41.

[85] Rubin EH, Hait WN. Holland-Frei Cancer Medicine. In: Kufe DW, Pollock RE, Weichselbaum RR, Bast RC, Gansler TS, Holland JF, et al., editors. 6th ed. Hamilton: ON. BC Decker; 2003.

[86] Lundbeck Inc. Cosmegen (dactinomycin) product information. Deerfield, IL: Lundbeck, Inc; 2009.

[87] Tattersall MH, Sodergren JE, Sengupta SK, Trites DH, Modest EJ, Frei 3rd E. Pharmacokinetics of actinomycin D in patients with malignant melanoma. Clin Pharmacol Ther 1975;17:701–8.

[88] den Hartig J, McVie JG, van Oort WJ, Pinedo HM. Pharmacokinetics of mitomycin C in humans. Cancer Res 1983;43:5017–21.

[89] Verweij J, den Hartigh J, Stuurman M, de Vries J, Pinedo HM. Relationship between clinical parameters and pharmacokinetics of mitomycin C. J Cancer Res Clin Oncol 1987;113:91–4.

[90] Teva Parenteral Medicines Inc. Irvine, CA: Teva Parenteral Medicines Inc; 2007.

[91] Crooke ST, Luft F, Broughton A, Strong J, Casson K, Einhorn L. Bleomycin serum pharmacokinetics as determined by a radioimmunoassay and a microbiologic assay in a patient with compromised renal function. Cancer 1977;39:1430–4.

[92] Pfizer Labs. Doxorubicin hydrochloride for injection. New York, NY: Pfizer Labs; 2011.

[93] Goto M, Yoshida H, Honda A, Kumazawa T, Ohbayashi T, Inagaki J, et al. Delayed disposition of adriamycin and its active metabolite in haemodialysis patients. Eur J Clin Pharmacol 1993;44:301–2.

[94] Yoshida H, Goto M, Honda A, Nabeshima T, Kumazawa T, Inagaki J, et al. Pharmacokinetics of doxorubicin and its active metabolite in patients with normal renal function and in patients on hemodialysis. Cancer Chemother Pharmacol 1994;33:450–4.

[95] Ben Venue Laboratories Inc. Daunorubicin prescribing information. Bedford, OH: Bedford Laboratories; 1999.

[96] Pharmacia & Upjohn Company. Idamycin PFS prescribing information. New York, NY: Pharmacia & Upjohn Company; 2006.

[97] Crivellari D, Lombardi D, Spazzapan S, Veronesi A, Toffoli G, Crivellari D, et al. New oral drugs in older patients: a review of idarubicin in elderly patients. Crit Rev Oncol Hematol 2004;49:153–63.

[98] Pfizer Injectables. Camptosar (irinotecan hydrochloride injection) prescribing information. New York, NY: Pfizer Inc; 2010.

[99] Czock D, Rasche FM, Boesler B, Shipkova M, Keller F. Irinotecan in cancer patients with end-stage renal failure. Ann Pharmacother 2009;43:363—9.

[100] Fujita K, Sunakawa Y, Miwa K, Akiyama Y, Sugiyama M, Kawara K, et al. Delayed elimination of SN-38 in cancer patients with severe renal failure. Drug Metab Dispos 2011;39:161—4.

[101] Huang SH, Chao Y, Wu YY, Luo JC, Kao CH, Yen SH, et al. Concurrence of UGT1A polymorphism and end-stage renal disease leads to severe toxicities of irinotecan in a patient with metastatic colon cancer. Tumori 2011;97:243—7.

[102] GlaxoSmithKline. Hycamtin (topotecan hydrochloride) prescribing information. Research Triangle Park, NC: GlaxoSmithKline; 2010.

[103] Herrington JD, Figueroa JA, Kirstein MN, Zamboni WC, Stewart CF. Effect of hemodialysis on topotecan disposition in a patient with severe renal dysfunction. Cancer Chemother Pharmacol 2001;47: 89—93.

[104] Iacono LC, Adams D, Homans AC, Guillot A, McCune JS, Stewart CF. Topotecan disposition in an anephric child. J Pediatr Hematol Oncol 2004;26: 596—600.

[105] O'Reilly S, Rowinsky EK, Slichenmyer W, Donehower RC, Forastiere AA, Ettinger DS, et al. Phase I and pharmacologic study of topotecan in patients with impaired renal function. J Clin Oncol 1996;14:3062—73.

[106] Bristol-Myers Squibb Company. Vumon (tenoposide injection) prescribing information. Princeton, NJ: Bristol-Myers Squibb Company; 2011.

[107] Allen LM, Creaven PJ. Comparison of the human pharmacokinetics of VM-26 and VP-16, two antineoplastic epipodophyllotoxin glucopyranoside derivatives. Eur J Cancer 1975;11:697—707.

[108] Company Pharmacia & Upjohn. Toposar brand of etoposide injection, USP prescribing information. Kalamazoo, MI: Pharmacia & Upjohn Company; 1998.

[109] Takezawa K, Okamoto I, Fukuoka M, Nakagawa K. Pharmacokinetic analysis of carboplatin and etoposide in a small cell lung cancer patient undergoing hemodialysis. J Thorac Oncol 2008;3:1073—5.

[110] Inoue A, Saijo Y, Kikuchi T, Gomi K, Suzuki T, Maemondo M, et al. Pharmacokinetic analysis of combination chemotherapy with carboplatin and etoposide in small-cell lung cancer patients undergoing hemodialysis. Ann Oncol 2004;15:51—4.

[111] Stewart CF. Use of etoposide in patients with organ dysfunction: pharmacokinetic and pharmacodynamic considerations. Cancer Chemother Pharmacol 1994;34(Suppl):S76—83.

[112] Novartis Pharmaceuticals Corporation. Prescribing information Gleevec (imatinib mesylate) tablets for oral use, East Hanover. New Jersey: Novartis Pharmaceuticals Corporation; 2012.

[113] Pappas P, Karavasilis V, Briasoulis E, Pavlidis N, Marselos M. Pharmacokinetics of imatinib mesylate in end stage renal disease. A case study. Cancer Chemother Pharmacol 2005;56:358—60.

[114] AstraZeneca AB. Macclesfield, Cheshire, UK, AstraZeneca UK Limited, Gefitinib Prescribing Information. July 22, 2013. Available at: http://www.iressa.com/_mshost5259502/content/6906430/Gefitinib-product-informationasdad.

[115] Shinagawa N, Yamazaki K, Asahina H, Agata J, Itoh T, Nishimura M. Gefitinib administration in a patient with lung cancer undergoing hemodialysis. Lung Cancer 2007;58:422—4.

[116] Pfizer Inc. Sutent prescribing information. New York, NY: Pfizer Labs; 2011.

[117] Izzedine H, Etienne-Grimaldi MC, Renee N, Vignot S, Milano G. Pharmacokinetics of sunitinib in hemodialysis. Ann Oncol 2009;20:190—2.

[118] Park CY, Park CY. Successful sunitinib treatment of metastatic renal cell carcinoma in a patient with end stage renal disease on hemodialysis. Anticancer Drugs 2009;20:848—9.

[119] Thiery-Vuillemin A, Montange D, Kalbacher E, Maurina T, Nguyen T, Royer B, et al. Impact of sunitinib pharmacokinetic monitoring in a patient with metastatic renal cell carcinoma undergoing hemodialysis. Ann Oncol 2011;22:2152—4.

[120] Bayer HealthCare Pharmaceuticals Inc. Nexavar prescribing information. Wayne, NJ,: Bayer HealthCare Pharmaceuticals Inc; 2011.

[121] Castagneto B, Stevani I, Giorcelli L, Montefiore F, Bigatti GL, Pisacco P, et al. Sustained response following sorafenib therapy in an older adult patient with advanced renal cancer on hemodialysis: a case report. Med Oncol 2011;28:1384—8.

[122] Ferraris E, Di Cesare P, Lasagna A, Paglino C, Imarisio I, Porta C. Use of sorafenib in two metastatic renal cell cancer patients with end-stage renal impairment undergoing replacement hemodialysis. Tumori 2009;95:542—4.

[123] Hilger RA, Richly H, Grubert M, Kredtke S, Thyssen D, Eberhardt W, et al. Pharmacokinetics of sorafenib in patients with renal impairment undergoing hemodialysis. Int J Clin Pharmacol Ther 2009;47:61—4.

[124] Kennoki T, Kondo T, Kimata N, Murakami J, Ishimori I, Nakazawa H, et al. Clinical results and pharmacokinetics of sorafenib in chronic hemodialysis patients with metastatic renal cell

carcinoma in a single center. Jpn J Clin Oncol 2011;41:647—55.

[125] Bristol-Myers Squibb. Sprycel (dasatinib) prescribing information. Princeton, NJ: Bristol-Myers Squibb; 2011.

[126] Novartis Pharmaceuticals Corporation. Tasigna (nilotinib) prescribing information. East Hanover, NJ: Novartis Pharmaceuticals Corporation; 2011.

[127] Fishbein WN, Carbone PP. Hydroxyurea: mechanism of action. Science 1963;142:1069—70.

[128] Rodriguez GI, Kuhn JG, Weiss GR, Hilsenbeck SG, Eckardt JR, Thurman A, et al. A bioavailability and pharmacokinetic study of oral and intravenous hydroxyurea. Blood 1998;91:1533—41.

[129] Kotla V, Goel S, Nischal S, Heuck C, Vivek K, Das B, et al. Mechanism of action of lenalidomide in hematological malignancies. J Hematol Oncol 2009;2:36.

[130] Cvek B, Dvorak Z. The ubiquitin-proteasome system (UPS) and the mechanism of action of bortezomib. Curr Pharm Des 2011;17:1483—99.

[131] Nikrad M, Johnson T, Puthalalath H, Coultas L, Adams J, Kraft AS. The proteasome inhibitor bortezomib sensitizes cells to killing by death receptor ligand trail via BH3-only proteins BIK and BIM. Mol Cancer Ther 2005;4:443—9.

[132] Hospira Inc. Methotrexate injection, USP. Lake Forest, IL: Hospira Inc; 2008.

[133] Garlich FM, Goldfarb DS. Have advances in extracorporeal removal techniques changed the indications for their use in poisonings? Adv Chronic Kidney Dis 2011;18:172—9.

[134] Bristol-Myers Squibb Company. Droxia (hydroxyurea) capsule. Princeton, NJ: Bristol-Myers Squibb Company; 2012.

[135] Dogruel M, Gibbs JE, Thomas SA. Hydroxyurea transport across the blood—brain and blood—cerebrospinal fluid barriers of the guinea-pig. J Neurochem 2003;87:76—84.

[136] Merck & Co. Inc. Elspar (asparaginase). West Point, PA: Merck & Co. Inc; 2000.

[137] Celgene Corporation. Thalomid® (thalidomide) capsules for oral use. Summit, NJ: Celgene, Inc; 2012.

[138] Eriksson T, Hoglund P, Turesson I, Waage A, Don BR, Vu J, et al. Pharmacokinetics of thalidomide in patients with impaired renal function and while on and off dialysis. J Pharm Pharmacol 2003;55: 1701—6.

[139] Ando Y, Fuse E, Figg WD. Thalidomide metabolism by the CYP2C subfamily. Clin Cancer Res 2002;8: 1964—73.

[140] Celgene Corporation. Revlamid (lenalidomide) prescribing information. Summit, NJ: Celgene Corporation; 2011.

[141] Chen N, Lau H, Kong L, Kumar G, Zeldis JB, Knight R, et al. Pharmacokinetics of lenalidomide in subjects with various degrees of renal impairment and in subjects on hemodialysis. J Clin Pharmacol 2007;47:1466—75.

[142] Millenium Pharmaceuticals Inc. Velcade (bortezomib) for injection. Cambridge, MA: Millennium Pharmaceuticals Inc; 2012.

[143] Morabito F, Gentile M, Ciolli S, Petrucci MT, Galimberti S, Mele G, et al. Safety and efficacy of bortezomib-based regimens for multiple myeloma patients with renal impairment: a retrospective study of Italian Myeloma Network GIMEMA. Eur J Haematol 2010;84:223—8.

Cancer in Renal Transplant Patients

Aleksandra M. De Golovine, Horacio E. Adrogue
The University of Texas Medical School at Houston, Houston, TX, USA
Memorial Hermann Hospital, Texas Medical Center, Houston TX, USA

In the current era of immunosuppression, renal transplantation is considered the gold standard for renal replacement therapy. In addition to excellent 1-year (95%) and 5-year (80%) graft survival, the mortality advantage over those remaining on dialysis makes it the therapy of choice. This success is due to the use of better immunosuppressant regimens that have prevented graft loss; however, it has resulted in the increased risk of infection and malignancy. In fact, the three most common causes of death of patients with a functioning kidney graft are cardiovascular, infectious and malignancy related.

The increased risk of malignancy is thought to be multi-factorial. The issues include: (1) increased risk of genitourinary and thyroid malignancies related to chronic kidney disease; (2) immunosuppression that suppresses the immune system's tumor surveillance, promotes the development of pro-oncogenic viruses and intrinsically causes the development of malignancies, and (3) the spread of donor-derived malignancies via grafts.

INTRODUCTION

Renal transplantation today is possible because of the powerful, specific immunosuppressive agents available. These same agents are responsible for the most common chronic complications post-transplantation. These include infection and malignancy. The rate of malignancy is greatly increased in the transplant population as a whole as compared to the general population. It is especially increased in the grafts that require the most immunosuppression. Hematopoietic stem cell transplants require the most, followed by intestinal, lung, heart, pancreas, kidney and finally liver. Immunosuppressives are thought to increase the incidence of cancer by decreasing the immune system's ability to detect cancer cells and pro-oncogenic viruses and destroy them, and because some of the immunosuppressive agents directly cause the proliferation of certain cancer cells.

The most common cancers in kidney transplant patients are non-melanoma skin cancers

(NMSC) of which squamous cell are seen the most often and may have an association with the human papillomavirus (HPV). Post-transplant lymphoproliferative disorder (PTLD) is another common malignancy in renal transplant which ranges in its presentation from a mononucleosis-like syndrome to a fulminant non-Hodgkin lymphoma. It is thought to be related to Epstein–Barr virus (EBV). Finally, genitourinary cancers, also very common malignancies in renal transplant recipients, occur just as frequently as in the end stage renal disease population and are thought to be secondary to the effects of the causes of chronic kidney disease like NSAID nephropathy and inherited cystic disease, and chronic kidney disease itself manifested by decreased urine output and acquired cystic disease.

Donor-derived malignancies are uncommon and have become rarer with better donor selection. However, with the increasing number of patients on the waiting list and the shortage of donors, living and cadaveric, there is a bigger push to use more high-risk kidneys and with this comes the added risk of transmitting malignancy.

There are no established guidelines on how to screen transplant patients for malignancies except that the same cancer screening applied to the general population should be applied to transplant patients. Areas of interest in cancer screening of post-kidney transplant patients include surveillance of native and transplant kidneys with ultrasounds to screen for renal cell carcinomas and EBV and HPV vaccines in unexposed patients pre-transplantation.

There are also no established guidelines on what to do with immunosuppression once a patient is diagnosed with a malignancy. The mammalian target of rapamycin (mTOR) inhibitors are known to have anti-oncogenic and immunosuppressive qualities and seem to be useful in some malignancies. Their role in post-kidney transplant malignancies has not been firmly established.

In this chapter, the above concepts will be explored and the most practical approaches will be offered to help the clinician screen for malignancy and manage immunosuppression in a post-kidney transplant recipient who is always at an increased risk for malignancy.

INCIDENCE

Malignancy is now the third leading cause of death in transplant recipients [1]. Between 5 and 10 years post-transplantation 14% of deaths are secondary to malignancy with the rate increasing to 26% after 10 years [1]. The overall rates of *de novo* malignancies in kidney transplant recipients without a history of cancer are two- to three-fold increased over the rate of cancer in the general population. The incidence of lymphoma, NMSCs and Kaposi sarcoma are 20 times higher than the general population with kidney cancer being 15 times higher [1]. There is a five-fold increase in the occurrence of melanoma, leukemia, hepatobiliary, cervical and vulvovaginal cancers, a three-fold increase in testicular and bladder cancers, and a two-fold increase in the incidence of common tumors like colon, lung, stomach, esophagus, pancreas and ovary as compared to the general population [2]. Table 16.1 shows the standardized incidence rates for various types of cancer, virus association and risk after kidney transplant. Data from the Australia and New Zealand Dialysis and Transplant Registry, ANZDTR, which includes 15,183 people who received a transplant from 1963 to 2004, showed that the risk of *de novo* cancers was inversely related to age, with younger recipients exhibiting the greatest risk compared with the general population [1]. The 2008 ANZDTR report showed that post-transplant malignancy was the leading cause of death in kidney transplant recipients, accounting for 32% of all deaths [3].

TABLE 16.1 Standardized Incidence Rates of Malignancies in Post Kidney Transplant Patients and Their Virus Associations

Malignancy > 10 per 100,000 population		Virus association
High Risk (SIR>5)	Kaposi Sarcoma	HHV-8
	Vagina	HPV
	Lymphoproliferative Disease	EBV
	Lip	HPV
	Thyroid	—
	Penis	HPV
Moderate Risk (SIR 1–5)	Small Intestine	—
	Oropharynx	HPV
	Esophagus	EBV/HPV
	Bladder	HPV
	Leukemia	HTLV-1
No Increase Risk (SIR<1)	Breast	—
	Prostate	—
	Rectum	HPV

Abbreviations: HHV-8, Human herpes virus-8, Human papilloma virus; EBV, Epstein-Barr virus; HTLV, human T lymphotropic virus; SIR, standardized incidence rate.

The average time to presentation of cancer in renal transplant recipients varies, but can be approximated to 3 years after transplantation [2]. Cancers tend to occur earlier and grow and metastasize at a faster rate than in the general population and so survival is worse. The average 5-year survival for all cancers in the Australia and New Zealand transplant population is less than 10% [4].

NMSCs are the most common cancer type after transplantation with >90% being basal cell and squamous cell carcinomas. Unlike in the general population where basal cell carcinomas are the most common NMSCs, squamous cell carcinomas are the most common in transplant recipients, with the squamous cell/basal cell carcinoma ratio being around 5:1. This represents an almost perfect reversal from the expected 1:4 ratio in the general population [4]. The incidence of squamous cell carcinoma of the eye is 20 times greater than in the general population. The risk of basal cell carcinomas is 10 times greater than the general population [2]. It is for this reason that in addition to informed consent about this risk, we recommend pre-transplant screening of high-risk patients. A yearly visit to the dermatologist is also expected of all our transplant recipients.

PTLD is another dreaded but common malignancy in transplant recipients. A study that analyzed the United States Renal Data System (USRDS) data from 66,159 adult Medicare-covered kidney transplant recipients found that PTLD developed in 1169 patients or 1.8% over an average follow-up duration of 10 years [2]. In pediatric renal transplant recipients, the incidence is increased to 5% at 10 years post-transplantation when compared to our adult patients. Data from the USRDS also show that the incidence of PTLD is highest for people in the first year post-transplant and decreases thereafter [4].

There is an increased risk of recurrence of malignancy post-renal transplantation. A retrospective review that looked at the recurrence of 1297 pre-existing cancers in renal transplant recipients done by Israel Penn and colleagues in 1997 showed an overall cancer recurrence rate of 21% in kidney transplant recipients with a history of cancer. Fifty-four percent occurred in the first 2 years post-transplant, 33% between 2 and 5 years, and 13% for recipients greater than 5 years post-transplant. The highest risk of recurrence was for symptomatic renal cell carcinoma, sarcoma, melanoma, bladder cancer and multiple myeloma. Breast, prostate and colorectal cancers had a smaller risk, but this may be stage related for prostate cancer with stage I and II having a much lower risk than stage III [4]. This study forms the basis for our current recommendation of waiting 2–5 years post-malignancy cure before proceeding with transplantation.

Chronic kidney disease itself has been postulated to be a risk factor for malignancy in the post-kidney transplant population. The increased risk of cancer in the dialysis population was studied by combining the data from the USRDS, the European Dialysis and Transplant Association (EDTA) and ANZDTR. This included 831,804 patients who were followed up for a mean of 2.5 years. There was an increased risk of cervical, bladder, thyroid and renal cell carcinoma and there was no significant increase in the risk of breast, colorectal and prostate cancers when compared to the general population. The risk seemed higher in patients younger than 35 years [5]. A 2009 study using the ANZDTR showed that the risk of certain malignancies, namely that of the thyroid, kidney and urinary tract, seen in dialysis patients does not increase in transplant patients, unlike immune deficiency-related cancers or cancers with a viral etiology like PTLD and Kaposi sarcoma whose risk is greatly increased [6]. The risk of dialysis-related cancers was increased four-fold in dialysis and transplant patients. The risk of immune deficiency-related cancers was 1.5 times increased in dialysis patients and 5 times increased in transplant patients [6].

A very rare but feared complication in transplant is the accidental transmission of malignancy through a donor organ. The risk of a donor having an undetected malignancy is around 1.3% and the risk of transmitting a malignancy from donor to recipient is 0.2% [7].

CAUSES

Known Cancer Risks

Similar to the general population, there is an increased risk of malignancy in transplant recipients who use tobacco products and drink alcohol above the recommended amount. There is a definite increase in NMSCs in those persons

who have had a lot of exposure to UV radiation pre-transplantation and post-transplantation, especially sunburns.

Chronic Kidney Disease/End Stage Renal Disease

The increased risk of cancer in chronic kidney disease is thought secondary to the systemic effects of advanced renal failure and dialysis. Renal failure is thought to contribute to impairment in immunity and, even though there is no evidence of increased malignancy secondary to dialysis itself, theoretically, pre-dialysis carcinogenic exposures can be prolonged with dialysis because of decreased clearance. Other risks are impaired anti-oxidant defenses, vitamin D deficiency, the use of erythropoiesis stimulating agents and cytotoxic therapies used to treat certain primary renal diseases [5]. The cancers associated with chronic kidney disease are renal cell carcinomas, urinary tract cancers and thyroid cancers [6]. The increased risk of renal cell carcinoma is thought secondary to inherited and acquired cystic disease of the kidney that is present in around 40% of graft recipients when they are transplanted and appears in around 16% after transplantation [5,6]. Acquired renal cysts are associated with a 1.6 to 7% incidence of renal cell carcinoma. The rate of urinary tract cancers is thought to be increased because of analgesic nephropathy as a cause of the chronic kidney disease, especially cancers of the renal pelvis and ureters, and perhaps the reduction in urinary flow. The increase in thyroid cancer may be secondary to the reduced production of the selenocysteine-containing enzyme, glutathione peroxidase because of damage to proximal tubular epithelium which is the main source of the enzyme, or from uremia-related selenium deficiency. Glutathione peroxidase is a free radical scavenger in the thyroid gland and its deficiency could potentially lead to an increase in cancer. Detection bias may also be present because of imaging of parathyroids secondary to hyper-parathyroidism in chronic kidney disease patients [6].

State of Immunosuppression

Because of the use of immunosuppressives to ensure graft survival, the immune system is impaired in renal transplant patients. This results in impaired immunosurveillance of neoplastic cells, DNA damage and disruption of DNA repair mechanisms and upregulation of cytokines that can increase tumor growth [2].

There is an increased risk of the development of malignancy with more intense and longer duration of immunosuppressives [2]. The use of lymphocyte depleting agents like OKT3, ATG and thymoglobulin are associated with an increased risk of PTLD and carcinoma of the cervix, vulva and vagina as compared to the use of anti-IL-2 receptor antibodies [2–8]. There are still little data about whether alemtuzumab increases the risk of malignancy compared to other induction agents. A large multicenter prospective randomized trial that compared alemtuzumab versus thymoglobulin and basiliximab as induction therapies in renal transplantation showed a worse safety profile in the alemtuzumab group with a higher incidence of malignancies compared with the conventional therapy group [10].

Calcineurin inhibitors are associated with an increased cancer risk [4]. Table 16.2 describes the effects of calcineurin inhibitors on pro-oncogenic mechanisms. Tacrolimus and cyclosporine have been shown to promote tumor progression via inducing transforming growth factor beta overexpression in the host [2–4]. Transforming growth factor beta promotes tumor cell invasion and metastasis [1]. Other studies have shown that cyclosporine used in mouse models enhances tumor growth by promoting angiogenesis and increasing expression of vascular endothelial growth factor, VEGF. Cyclosporine also upregulates the expression of IL-6 which promotes

TABLE 16.2 The Pro-oncogenic and Immunosuppressive Effects of Calcineurin Inhibitors

	Mechanism	Effect
Calcineurin inhibitors	Increases TGF-beta$_1$	Decreases IL-2 stimulated T-cell proliferation Promotes tumor invasion and metastatic growth
	Increases VEGF	Increases angiogenesis and potential tumor growth
	Increases IL-6	Increases B-cell growth, activation and immortalization, potentially increasing risk of PTLD
	Decreases DNA repair capability	Increases tumor genesis
	Decreases IL-2	Decreases T-cell proliferation

Abbreviations: TGF-beta$_1$, transforming growth factor-beta$_1$; IL-2, interleukin-2; VEGF, vascular endothelial growth factor; IL-6, interleukin-6.

B-cell activation and growth and potentially can contribute to the development of PTLD [1–9]. The European and the US Multicenter Trial reports comparing maintenance immunosuppression with tacrolimus versus cyclosporine showed no significant difference in cancer incidence [8].

The antimetabolite azathioprine has been shown to increase the incidence of UV radiation-induced skin cancers in mice [1]. Mycophenolate mofetil (MMF) and the prodrug mycophenolic acid (MPA) have conflicting data about the pro- vs. anti-oncogenic properties of the drugs [1]. The drug was initially developed as a neoplastic agent [9]. The US Randomized and Tricontinental Multicenter study comparing MMF and azathioprine in cadaveric renal recipients showed no difference in the incidence of malignancy between the two drugs. An independent report using data from the SRTR database on 17,145 patients with pre-existing diabetes mellitus showed a significantly higher incidence of malignancy in azathioprine-treated patients than in MMF-treated patients [8].

There are no studies available in the transplant population that address if corticosteroids increase the risk of malignancy. There are some reports of an association of NMSCs with corticosteroid therapy in nontransplant patients and an association of an increased incidence of non-Hodgkin lymphoma [8]. There is also an association of an increased incidence of Kaposi sarcoma with chronic steroid use [9].

The newest immunosuppressive, belatacept, a co-stimulation blocker, showed an increase in the incidence of PTLD compared to cyclosporine in a phase II study. The extension of the trial that followed the patients for 5 years showed no difference in malignancies between the two drugs [11].

The mTOR inhibitors, sirolimus and everolimus, have shown anti-oncogenic as well as immunosuppressive properties. Table 16.3 shows the anti-oncogenic and immunosuppressive properties of mTOR inhibitors. Signaling of mTOR is deregulated in cancer. The binding of ligands to membrane receptors, IL-2 receptors and growth factor receptors activates mTOR signaling. Phosphatidylinositol-3′kinase, PI3K, and Akt are proto-oncogenes and phosphorylate mTOR. Genetic alterations result in excess stimulation of the Akt−mTOR pathway and are common in malignancies. PTEN, a protein that downregulates the P13K−Akt pathway, is inhibited by deletions or mutations in a lot of cancers, activating the Akt−mTOR pathway and downstream pathways involving p70S6 kinase, 4E-binding protein 1 and c-myc that cause proliferation of various cell types [12]. Sirolimus, an mTOR inhibitor, inhibits these pro-oncogenic pathways. Sirolimus upregulates E-cadherin, which increases cell adhesiveness and may reduce cancer metastasis [9]. Sirolimus also reduces cyclin D1 and increases p27 kip 1 which inhibits G1 to S transition and can slow

TABLE 16.3 The Anti-oncogenic and Immunosuppressive Properties of mTOR Inhibitors

	Mechanism	Effect
mTOR inhibitors	Decreases mTOR signaling blocking the effects of IL-2 and VEGF, decreases p70S6 kinase	Decreases cell proliferation of lymphocytes, endothelial cells and tumor cells, decreases angiogenesis
	Increases E-cadherin	Increases cell adhesion and decreases the metastatic potential of cancers
	Increases inhibitors of cyclin D1 molecules that control the cell cycle	Decreases cell proliferation, including tumor cells
	Decreases IL-10 and blocks the activity of STAT1 and STAT3	Decreases the chance of EBV-associated B-cell lymphoma in mice

Abbreviations: mTOR inhibitors, mammalian target of rapamycin inhibitors; IL-2, interleukin-2; VEGF, vascular endothelial growth factor; IL-10, interleukin-10; STAT 1, signal transducers and activators of transcription 1; STAT 3, signal transducers and activators of transcription 3; EBV, Epstein−Barr virus.

tumor growth [1]. Sirolimus has been shown to decrease tumor neovascularization in mice through antiangiogenic activity via impaired VEGF production and decreased responsiveness of endothelial cells to VEGF [12]. Sirolimus has also been shown to decrease IL-10 secretion in mice which prevents STAT1 and STAT3 activation associated with EBV-associated B-cell lymphomas [9]. Because of these potent anti-oncogenic and simultaneous immunosuppressive effects, the mTOR inhibitors may be the solution to the problem of increased malignancy in the setting of immunosuppression. Conversion from calcineurin inhibitors to mTOR inhibitors has been shown to lead to the regression of Kaposi sarcoma in renal transplant recipients and is part of the standard of care for this setting [13]. The Akt−mTOR pathway is thought to be aberrant in Kaposi sarcoma [1]. The CONVERT trial that followed 830 kidney transplant recipients for 2 years randomly assigned to stay on calcineurin inhibitors or change to sirolimus found that sirolimus conversion among patients with a baseline GFR more than 40 mL/min was associated with great patient and graft survival. There was no difference in rejection rate, but there was an increase in urinary protein excretion and lower incidence of malignancy, especially skin cancers, compared with calcineurin inhibitor continuation [14].

Pro-oncogenic Viruses

Exposure to immunosuppression disrupts the antiviral activity of the immune system resulting in *de novo* viral infections and reactivation of previously controlled viral infections. These infections can then lead to malignancies. The major cancer causing viruses are human papillomavirus (HPV), associated with squamous cell carcinoma of the oral cavity, genital tract and skin; Epstein–Barr virus (EBV), associated with PTLD; human herpes virus 8 (HHV-8), associated with Kaposi sarcoma (KS), primary effusion lymphoma and Castleman's disease and hepatitis B (HBV) and C viruses (HCV), which are associated with hepatocellular carcinoma [3,15,16].

HPV

HPV is a papillomavirus, a DNA virus, with worldwide distribution. There are many genotypes and some are associated with oropharyngeal, esophageal and anogenital cancers. There is a link between NMSC and HPV infection in the transplant population as well that may explain why skin cancer is so common and why squamous cell cancer (SCC) is much more common than basal cell cancer in transplant recipients [17,18]. HPV-induced warts or verruca vulgaris occur in up to 90% of transplant recipients and individual incidence increases with increased graft survival. These warts can progress to dysplastic lesions and invasive SCC in immunosuppressed patients. HPV DNA has been detected in 70–90% of cutaneous SCC in transplant recipients, much higher than in non-immunosuppressed persons [19,20]. One study found a predominance of HPV types 5 and 8 in SCC specimens from transplant recipients [19]. On the other hand, HPV DNA has been found in equal amounts of around 35–40%, in basal cell carcinomas from transplanted and non-immunosuppressed persons [19]. The mechanisms by which HPV could play a role in skin cancer development may be the prevention of UV-induced apoptosis and similar immunosuppressive activities that minimize the local immune responses to persistent HPV infections and the elimination of neoplastic cells [19].

EBV

EBV is a gamma herpesvirus, a DNA virus, with worldwide distribution. About 95% of adults have serologic evidence of previous EBV infection. The primary infection is usually subclinical in childhood but in adolescence or adulthood manifests as mononucleosis and then the virus becomes dormant for the lifetime of the host in most cases. The virus is associated with Hodgkin and non-Hodgkin lymphomas, nasopharyngeal carcinoma, gastric carcinoma and leiomyosarcoma and with most cases of PTLD [2,21,22]. PTLD is almost always EBV related. EBV infection can lead to cell transformation and in the setting of chronic immunosuppression can lead to tumor growth. In EBV-associated PTLD which tends to be B-cell large, non-Hodgkin lymphoma, EBV infects the B-cells and induces a B-cell proliferation and later transforms and immortalizes them. In non-immunocompromised hosts, EBV-specific cytotoxic T-lymphocytes (CTLs) kill infected B-lymphocytes expressing more active infection thereby selecting for more dormant infected B-cells. In the immunocompromised organ transplant recipient the more infected cells are not destroyed and eventually may lead to PTLD [23].

Transplant recipients most at risk for developing PTLD are those that are EBV negative and receive an EBV-positive organ, usually children and those that have received a high cumulative dose and type of immunosuppression, especially tacrolimus and lymphocyte depleting agents [23]. In both cases, the increased risk of acquiring or reactivating EBV is the main reason for the increased risk.

The use of monitoring EBV viral load post-transplant has been investigated and there are no clear evidence-based recommendations on how to proceed. Plasma EBV levels are probably more accurate than whole blood levels [21,22]. There is no set cut-off level to begin a change in therapy, but in general a rising EBV viral load may necessitate a reduction of immuno-suppression versus treatment with antivirals, rituximab or EBV-specific CTLs [22,23]. The use of EBV viral load and the quantification of recipient EBV-specific CTLs may be more helpful in determining who is more at risk for developing PTLD.

EBV vaccination is considered in EBV seronegative recipients, but so far no vaccine has been able to produce long-lasting antibodies [23].

CMV

CMV is a gamma herpesvirus that has a worldwide distribution as well. CMV infection occurs in 20–60% of all transplant recipients and is the most common viral infection after kidney transplantation [17,18]. CMV infection is associated with immune deregulation of helper/suppressor T-cells and this can cause rejection, other opportunistic infection and the development of PTLD [18].

HHV-8

HHV-8 is a gamma herpesvirus and it is mostly seen in people of Arab, Jewish, African, Turkish, Greek or Italian descent. Only 0–5% of adults are positive for HHV-8 antibodies and about 12% of transplant recipients develop

HHV-8 antibodies post-transplant in the United States [18]. Transplant recipients either acquire primary infection with HHV-8 or reactivate it. Primary infection in transplant recipients can present with fever, splenomegaly, rash, lymphoid hyperplasia and pancytopenia [15]. The virus can infect B-cells, endothelial cells, macrophages and epithelial cells and then go into a latent phase. HHV-8 has several oncogenes. It can modulate the host immune system by directing inflammatory cell recruitment away from a T-helper 1 type to a T-helper 2 type, thus evading the cytotoxic immune response [2]. The virus can also impair host antigen presentation and T-cell activation and lead to tumor development by prevention of apoptosis [2]. It also induces secretion of IL-6 which promotes B-cell proliferation and other angiogenic cytokines that stimulate VEGF expression [15]. Kaposi sarcoma is the most common cancer associated with HHV-8, but the virus is also associated with primary effusion lymphoma and Castleman's disease, a non-neoplastic condition.

Currently, there is no standard serological test for HHV-8 for clinical use. HHV-8 DNA quantification using plasma and peripheral blood mononuclear cells has been used to diagnose active HHV-8 infection. HHV-8 PCR can be used for surveillance of HHV-8 infection in high-risk individuals, including those who are HHV-8 negative and receive HHV-8-positive organs and HHV-8-positive recipients who are receiving high-dose immunosuppression [15]. Studies have shown no difference in survival between HHV-8-positive recipients, and those who are mismatched or have positive donors. The role of antiviral treatment of HHV-8 is not yet determined. Ganciclovir, foscarnet and cidofovir have activity against HHV-8 *in vitro*, but *in vivo* data are limited [15].

HTLV-1 and HTLV-2

Human T-lymphotrophic viruses 1 and 2 are RNA retroviruses that are more common in people from the Caribbean, Africa and Japan.

HTLV-1 causes a myelopathy/tropical spastic paraparesis and is associated with T-cell leukemia and lymphoma. Donors who are HTLV-1 positive should not be used. HTLV-2 is serologically similar to HTLV-1 but no disease has yet been associated with it [18].

HBV and HCV

Hepatitis B virus, a DNA virus, and hepatitis C virus, a RNA virus, both increase the risk of hepatocellular carcinoma in those infected. It is not uncommon for kidney transplant recipients to be infected with these viruses since both are easily transmitted in the blood. A retrospective registry analysis of 225,000 patients found that the standardized incidence ratio for hepatocellular carcinoma was 6.5 per 100,000 person years among kidney, heart and lung recipients and 25 per 100,000 person years among liver recipients. The incidence of hepatocellular carcinoma among non-liver recipients was independently associated with hepatitis B surface antigenemia, HCV infection and diabetes [24]. Hepatitis C infection is associated with an increased risk of PTLD in organ transplant recipients [23].

Donor Transmission

Transmission of malignancies through donor organs is fortunately much less common than during the early years of transplant when the risk of these transplantations was not yet known. Most recently, transmission of undiagnosed cancer to recipients has been reported to be around 1–3% [4].

Unknown transmission of cancer from organs of donors with malignancy may occur. This can happen when the cause of death is intracranial hemorrhage from an assumed brain aneurysm or arteriovenous malformation. These hemorrhages may actually be secondary to brain metastasis [25]. To avoid accidental transmission of malignancies from donors to recipients, careful attention must be paid to the history of the donor, including prior history of cancer and menstrual irregularities after a pregnancy or abortion, and a beta HCG level on all women of child-bearing age to evaluate for choriocarcinoma [25].

In general, donors who have malignancies should not be used. Exceptions are low-grade NMSCs, carcinoma in situ of the cervix and primary low-grade brain tumors with low incidence of spread outside of the CNS and not treated with radiotherapy, chemotherapy, ventriculoperitoneal and ventriculoatrial shunts or extensive craniotomies because these can all cause tumor spread [4,25].

The ideal situation is when autopsies are performed on all cadaveric donors to truly evaluate for malignancies. This is difficult to do since consent is not always obtained for autopsy and it takes a while for the results to come back, especially of the brain which has to be fixed in a preservative for a week [25]. The task of obtaining the results is the responsibility of the recipient's transplant team, which is an added burden on the transplant center.

All living donors should be screened for malignancy based on age and history with appropriate cancer screening recommendations.

DIAGNOSIS AND TREATMENT

Premalignant Skin Lesions and NMSC

Warts or premalignant lesions are usually treated with cryotherapy, electrosurgery, laser vaporization, or with salicylic acid, podophyllin, podophyllotoxin and trichloroacetic acid. Imiquimod, a cream FDA approved for the treatment of anogenital warts, is also an option. It stimulates natural killer cell activity, augments T-cell activity and induces cytokines all of which directly stimulate the immune system to destroy the lesions [20].

NMSCs are usually diagnosed by biopsy and treated with excision. Metastatic NMSCs, which are mostly squamous cell carcinomas, are treated with wide excision as well as chemotherapy and radiotherapy if appropriate. In extreme cases, immunosuppression can be decreased or readjusted. As mentioned before, mTOR inhibitors have been shown to decrease the incidence of NMSCs, but NMSCs still develop in patients on mTOR inhibitors.

PTLD

Recipients with PTLD present anywhere between 1 week and more than a decade after transplant; median 6 months post-transplant. About 86% of the tumors are B-cell predominant, 81% are EBV positive and 64% are monoclonal. The spectrum of disease involves early lesions with reactive plasmacytic hyperplasia, polymorphic PTLD with polyclonal or monoclonal expansion of atypical lymphoid cells and monomorphic PTLD with lymphoma histopathology [23]. The monomorphic histopathology is most commonly diffuse large B-cell lymphoma, but can be Burkitt/Burkitt-like lymphoma, myeloma or rarely T-cell lymphoma or, even more rare, Hodgkin lymphoma [23]. The majority of kidney transplant recipients have extra-allograft involvement that includes lymph nodes, spleen, intestines, liver, lung and the central nervous system. Symptoms usually are lymphoma related B-cell symptoms that include fever, night sweats, weight loss, kidney transplant dysfunction and mass lesions [26]. Diagnosis involves checking EBV PCR, tissue diagnosis and using an FDG-PET/CT scan or CT scan with oral and intravenous contrast to identify nonvisible lesions. Special studies with immunophenotyping by flow cytometry or immunohistochemistry and molecular studies like fluorescent *in situ* hybridization for the EBV genome are used on the tissue that is obtained to help further diagnose PTLD [26].

Treatment first involves reduction of immunosuppression which always carries the risk of allograft rejection. General guidelines involve cutting the calcineurin dose by 50% and stopping the antimetabolite [22]. The predictors of lack of response include serum LDH greater than 2.5 times the upper limit of normal, organ dysfunction and multiple sites of disease [26]. EBV-positive tumors may respond to antiviral therapy, but there has not been any clear evidence for this. If disease is localized, complete surgical excision or radiation is effective and recommended. Patients who fail to respond to decreased immunosuppression and surgical excision are candidates for chemotherapy. Rituximab, an anti-CD20 monoclonal antibody, is tried first in CD20-positive lymphomas. The CHOP regimen, cyclophosphamide, doxorubicin, vincristine and prednisolone alone or in combination with rituximab are used if there is not an adequate response to rituximab alone or if the lymphoma is CD20 negative [24,26]. Cytokine therapy has also been tried in an attempt to establish a competent immune system. Other therapies have included interferon alpha and intravenous immunoglobulin G infusion but their efficacy is difficult to assess since the organ recipients that have received these regimens were also on antivirals and have had their immunosuppression reduced [24]. Another therapy that has been attempted with some success in patients with EBV-positive PTLD is T-cell immunotherapy using EBV-positive cytotoxic T-lymphocytes [24].

Prognosis is variable because of the different grades of PTLD, but those with poor performance status, age >60, more than one site of disease, PTLD of T-cell origin, monoclonality and nondetection of EBV and need for chemotherapy do worse [22].

Kaposi Sarcoma

Transplant-associated Kaposi sarcoma usually presents as angiomatous, red, blue or purple lesions mostly affecting the legs. The next most common sites are the trunk and hard palate. Lesions are also visceral and can appear on mucosal surfaces, lungs, gastrointestinal tract and lymphoid tissue in about 10% of transplant recipients [2]. Lesions may cause hemoptysis, intestinal bleeding and lymphedema from large obstructing lymph nodes. Diagnosis is by biopsy and once diagnosed, recipients need to have an oral exam, upper and lower endoscopies and CT scan of the chest, abdomen and pelvis to evaluate for visceral disease. HHV-8 can be identified in affected tissue by *in situ* hybridization or immunohistochemistry.

Treatment involves reduction of immunosuppression, especially replacing calcineurin inhibitors with mTOR inhibitors which can cause tumor regression through their antiproliferative properties, mainly their antiangiogenic activity by the impairment of VEGF production [15]. Despite these positive results, poor response to mTOR inhibitors has been documented and there are some reports of recipients developing KS while on mTOR inhibitors. Surgical resection and radiotherapy is attempted in isolated lesions and chemotherapy is tried with visceral lesions. The most common chemotherapy is CHOP, but doxorubicin, bleomycin and vincristine have been successfully used and paclitaxel has also shown to be effective in visceral and skin involvement [15].

Prognosis is good for cutaneous involvement, but poorer for visceral disease, especially vital organ involvement.

Despite the theoretical benefit of decreasing immunosuppressives, there are no evidence-based established guidelines on what do with immunosuppression when a transplant recipient has a malignancy. A logical approach is assessing the type of malignancy and its prognosis. A malignancy with a poor prognosis does not necessitate any change in immunosuppression since the outcome is poor no matter what. Malignancies with a better prognosis necessitate a decrease in immunosuppression with the goal of cure. Kidney transplant recipients have the advantage over other organ recipients of having access to life-saving dialysis if their allografts fail and this must also be factored into the decision of decreasing or even stopping immunosuppression in a renal transplant recipient.

The potential antineoplastic effects of mTOR inhibitors have definite positive results in Kaposi sarcoma and these patients should be started on the drug in place of calcineurin inhibitors, but there are still not enough data to start mTOR inhibitors in kidney recipients with other malignancies, including NMSC and PTLD.

PREVENTION

Screening for cancer prior to solid organ transplant is a standard part of the transplant evaluation process. Unfortunately, there is no universally agreed-upon process on how best to accomplish this task. The American Cancer Society recently published the 2012 cancer screening guidelines and we feel that these are appropriate general standards to use in the kidney transplant population [27]. The guidelines are shown in Table 16.4.

Breast Cancer

Breast self-exams should start at age 20 and any abnormal masses should be reported to a health professional. Since breast cancer is the second most common cause of cancer death and the most common cancer type in US women, the importance of early screening cannot be overstated. Annual mammography starting at age 40 is the official recommendation of the America Cancer Society (ACS) and we support this view.

Women who have a proven or suspected *BRCA* mutation will need a more aggressive and individualized screening and should be referred to an expert in that field.

Lung Cancer

The recommendation to screen for lung cancer comes from the National Lung Screening

TABLE 16.4 Screening Guidelines for the Most Common Cancers

Cancer screened	Patient screened	Test recommended
Breast	All women 40 years and older	Mammogram once per year
Lung (2)	All current or past smokers (≥30 pack-years)	Low-dose helical chest CT (once per year for 3 years)
Cervical	All women within 3 years of first intercourse or at 21 years	Papanicolaou test once per year *prior* to transplant and twice during the first year *post-transplant*
Adenomatous polyps and colorectal cancer	All average-risk adults 50 years and older Start at an earlier age if risk factors are present	gFOBT/FIT or sDNA or FSIG or CSPY or DCBE or CT colonography (see text for details)
Prostate	All men over 50 who "have at least a 10-year life expectancy" and have been provided informed consent of risks of screening Start at earlier age if risk factors present	PSA with or without DRE
Endometrial cancer	All women, at menopause or sooner based on gynecology recommendation (high-risk patients)	Endometrial biopsy
Ovarian cancer	Consider in women with mutations on BRCA1 or BRCA2 or 2 or more first degree relatives with ovarian cancer	Serial CA 125 and TVU
MGUS/Multiple myeloma	Men and women 50 years or older	SPEP with IF and serum free light chain analysis

Abbreviations: gFOBT/FIT, guaiac fecal occult blood test/fecal immunochemical testing; sDNA, stool for exfoliated cell DNA; FSIG, flexible sigmoidoscopy; CSPY, colonoscopy; DCBE, double contrast barium enema; TVU, transvaginal ultrasound.

Trial Research Team which screened over 53,000 patients [28].

In this randomized trial, they found that in those with a heavy smoking history, doing three yearly low-dose computed tomography (CT) scans significantly reduced mortality from lung cancer by 20% versus doing three chest radiographs over a 7-year follow-up. This was done in a non-transplant population so we feel it is reasonable to screen kidney transplant candidates who are planned to be maintained on lifelong immunosuppression. Also of interest in this study was that the rate of death from any cause was significantly lower in the CT group by 6.7%. The risk of false-positive exams must be weighed against the possible benefit of early detection in high-risk patients. There is still controversy over the appropriateness of screening for lung cancer. However, for the select group at risk after a transplant, we feel it is reasonable to consider screening.

Cervical Cancer

All women should have regular follow-up with a gynecologist once per year before and after a transplant. The US Public Health Service and Infectious Disease Society of America recommend that all immunocompromised patients should be tested twice during the first year after diagnosis of the immune-deficient condition. Any patient found to have HPV or cervical intraepithelial neoplasia will need close follow-up by a gynecologist expert in management of such patients. The use of HPV vaccination is recommended by the ACS for females 11–12 years and 13–18 for those that missed in the younger group. There are insufficient data to recommend for or against vaccination in 19–26-year-olds. While in theory it does make sense to vaccinate the kidney transplant candidates, this recommendation is not supported by any data.

Colorectal Cancer

There is an increased risk of colorectal cancer (CRC) in transplant patients and thus standard screening is encouraged. Guaiac fecal occult blood testing (gFOGT), fecal immunochemical testing (FIT) and testing stool for exfoliated cell DNA (sDNA) are non-invasive initial screening for colorectal cancer. While these are used for non-transplant evaluation patients, we proceed to colonoscopy (CSPY) instead of the above non-invasive testing. Since colorectal cancer may be missed with flexible sigmoidoscopy (FSIG) and double-contrast barium enema (DCBE) the use of CSPY is preferred. If available, CT colonography (virtual CSPY) may be used but cannot be recommended over the standard CSPY. These recommendations are based on the fact that these patients are knowingly immunosuppressed and it must be ensured they are free of disease prior to transplantation. In addition to the screening CSPY, those patients known to be at higher risk for CRC will get more frequent follow-up with CSPY every 2–3 years as indicated by risk. Those high-risk patients include those with: (1) familial adenomatous polyposis or hereditary nonpolyposis colon cancer; (2) adenomatous polyps; (3) prior colorectal cancer; (4) family history of CRC or adenomas in first degree relatives; and (5) a long history of inflammatory bowel disease.

Prostate Cancer

This is a very controversial area in the general population and somewhat so in the transplant population. Recent publications have changed the way many centers approach this topic. In the non-transplant population, all men over 50 who have at least a 10-year life expectancy and have been provided informed consent of risks of screening should be offered screening. Since there are false-positive rates with PSA and this may lead to unnecessary biopsies and anxiety, general screening is now done with caution. In a recent evidence update for the US Preventive Services Task Force in the non-transplant population, it was concluded that the potential benefits remain unclear for PSA testing and that psychological harm may occur [29].

Endometrial Cancer

Standard-risk women at time of menopause may start screening. There are insufficient data to recommend average-risk women prior to menopause to start screening while asymptomatic. This average-risk population includes women with hypertension, obesity, diabetes, or nulliparity. The risk and benefit of screening should be discussed and the patient asked to report spotting and unexpected bleeding. While the recommendations for screening are mainly based on expert opinion, high-risk women should strongly consider early screening starting at 35 years. High-risk factors include a known personal history of HNPCC (hereditary nonpolyposis colorectal cancer) and family history of HNPCC. An expert in the field should perform a patient-specific risk stratification prior to solid organ transplantation.

Ovarian Cancer

While this is an uncommon malignancy, it is the one associated with the highest mortality of more than 50% at 5 years. Still, the data will only support routine screening in high-risk patients including those with two or more first degree relatives with ovarian cancer or personal diagnosis of mutations in BRCA1/ BRCA2, HNPCC or breast—ovarian cancer syndrome. The key to screening may be serial CA 125 determinations and trans vaginal ultrasound (TVU). A recent US randomized, controlled trial of over 78,000 average-risk women aged 55–74 years screened with CA 125 and TVU for 4 years did not show a difference in ovarian cancer deaths. With a maximum follow-up of 13 years, there were 3.1 ovarian cancer deaths per 10,000 women-years in the screening group versus 2.6 deaths per 10,000 women-years in the control group (RR was 1.18 with 95% confidence interval which crossed 1 (0.82–1.71)). The conclusion was that screening this group was not helpful in reducing deaths [30]. An expert in the field should perform a patient-specific risk stratification prior to solid organ transplantation.

MGUS/Multiple Myeloma

Monoclonal gammopathy of undetermined significance (MGUS) is defined as the presence of a serum monoclonal protein in a small but elevated concentration (≤ 3 g/dl). Criteria also include a bone marrow biopsy with less than 10% plasma cells; no lytic lesions; small amount or absent urinary light chains; lack of anemia, chronic kidney disease and hypercalcemia related to the paraproteinemia [31]. In the general population over 50 years old, the incidence is 3.2% and a recent study in the end stage renal disease (ESRD) population found 9.2% of those screened had MGUS. The study screened 1215 patients and found 675 patients were 50 and older. Thirty-one (9.2%) of the 336 for which a serum protein electrophoresis (SPEP) with immunofixation (IF) was found had MGUS. This may imply that even this high percentage may be an underestimate. During the study period, nine of the patients with pre-transplant MGUS received a kidney transplant and these were compared to 25 well-matched patients with MGUS who remained on dialysis. With a median follow-up of 18.7 months, the transplanted patients with MGUS had a 78% mortality compared to 20% of those with MGUS who remained on dialysis ($p = .00008$). The mortality in transplanted patients without MGUS was 7.8%. Infectious and non-myeloma cancer deaths were the cause of most of the deaths. Kidney transplant did not seem to confer a survival benefit for this population but a larger study is needed before MGUS could be considered a contraindication for kidney transplant [32]. Another very large study reported on 42 patients (23 patients with pre-transplant MGUS and 19 after transplant) out of a population of 3518 kidney transplant recipients. At 8.5 years median follow-up (range 0.3–37), four (17.4%) of the pre-transplant MGUS patients developed a hematological malignancy and two (10.5%) of the post-transplant MGUS patients developed EBV-negative T-cell lymphoproliferative disorders [33]. Not all centers agree that MGUS should be screened for prior to transplantation and this remains a controversial area.

CONCLUSION

Renal transplant is still the best choice of renal replacement therapy for most patients with end stage renal disease and is known to have the best mortality benefit out of all available therapies. The current immunosuppression regimens are responsible for much of that success. Unfortunately, just like most drugs, they have adverse side-effects that must be taken into account. One of the most dangerous side-effects of immunosuppressives and immunosuppression is the increased risk of malignancy. Knowing this, and the fact that there is an increased risk of malignancy related to chronic kidney disease itself, the goal of future research in malignancy prevention in transplant patients should be further investigation of immunosuppressive agents like mTOR inhibitors that have antineoplastic activity and effective immunosuppressive activity, investigation of malignancy prevention posttransplantation by improved, evidence-guided screening protocols in chronic kidney disease patients and improved, standardized guidelines for screening for malignancy in donors.

References

[1] Kapoor A. Malignancy in kidney transplant recipients. Drugs 2008;68(Suppl. 1):11−9.

[2] Rama I, Grinyo J. Malignancy after renal transplantation: the role of immunosuppression. Nat Rev Nephrol 2010;6:511−9.

[3] Alberu J. Clinical insights for cancer outcomes in renal transplant patients. Transplant Proc 2010;42: S36−40.

[4] Wong G, Chapman J. Cancers after renal transplantation. Transplant Rev 2008;22:141−9.

[5] Nayak-Rao S. Cancer screening in end-stage renal disease. Saudi J Kidney Dis Transpl 2009;20(5):737−40.

[6] Stewart JH, et al. The pattern of excess cancer in dialysis and transplantation. Nephrol Dial Transplant 2009;24:3225−31.

[7] Cohen D, Vella J. Transplantation NephSAP. J Am Soc Nephrol 2011;10(6):593−6.

[8] Kauffman M, et al. Post-transplant de novo malignancies in renal transplant recipients: the past and present. Journal compilation with European Society for Organ Transplantation 2006;19:607−20.

[9] Guba M, et al. Pro- and anti-cancer effects of immunosuppressive agents used in organ transplantation. Transplantation 2004;77(12):1777−82.

[10] Gallon L, Chhabra D, Skaro A. T-cell-depleting agents in kidney transplantation: is there a place for alemtuzumab? Am J Kidney Dis 2011;59(1):15−8.

[11] Vincenti F, et al. Five-year safety and efficacy of belatacept in renal transplantation. J Am Soc Nephrol 2010;21:1587−96.

[12] Dantal J, Soulillou J-P. Immunosuppressive drugs and the risk of cancer after organ transplantation. N Engl J Med 2005;352:1371−3.

[13] Campistol JM, et al. Use of proliferation signal inhibitors in the management of post-transplant malignancies − clinical guidance. Nephrol Dial Transplant 2007;22(Suppl. 1):i36−41.

[14] Schena FP, et al. Conversion from calcineurin inhibitors to sirolimus maintenance therapy in renal allograft recipients: 24-month efficacy and safety results from the CONVERT trial. Transplantation 2009;87:233−42.

[15] Savani BN, Goodman S, Barrett J. Can routine posttransplant HPV vaccination prevent commonly occurring epithelial cancers after allogeneic stem cell transplantation? Clin Cancer Res 2009;15: 2219−21.

[16] Prendergast MB, Mannon R. Malignancies before and after transplantation. Kidney Transplant 2010: 311−26.

[17] Wilkinson A, Kasiske B. Long-term post-transplantation management and complications. Handbook Kidney Transpl 2010:232−42.

[18] Stockfleth E, et al. Human papillomaviruses in transplant-associated skin cancers. Dermatol Surg 2004;30:604−9.

[19] Tan H-H, Goh C-L. Viral infections affecting the skin in organ transplant recipients. Am J Clin Dermatol 2006;7(1):13−29.

[20] Loren AW, et al. Post-transplant lymphoproliferative disorder: a review. Bone Marrow Transplant 2003;31:145−55.

[21] Gulley ML, Tang W. Using Epstein−Barr viral load assays to diagnose, monitor, and prevent posttransplant lymphoproliferative disorder. Clin Microbiol Rev 2010;23(2):350−66.

[22] Jacobson CA, Lacasce AS. Lymphoma: risk and response after solid organ transplant. Oncology 2010;24(10):936.

[23] Ariza-Heredia EJ, Razonable RR. Human herpes virus 8 in solid organ transplantation. Transplantation 2011;92:837−44.

[24] Vella JP, Cohen DJ. Malignancy after kidney transplantation. NephSAP 2009;8(6):480−3.

[25] Penn I. Spontaneous and transplanted malignancy. Organ Transplant 2003:520−7.

[26] Vella JP, Cohen DJ. Posttransplant complications. NephSAP 2011;10(6):593−6.

[27] Smith RA, et al. Cancer screening in the United States, 2012. CA Cancer J Clin 2012;62(2):129−42.

[28] The National Lung Screening Trial Research Team. Reduced lung-cancer mortality with low-dose computed tomographic screening. NEJM 2011;365: 395−409.

[29] Lin K, et al. Benefits and harms of prostate-specific antigen screening for prostate cancer: an evidence update for the U.S. Preventive Services Task Force. Ann Intern Med 2008;149:192−9.

[30] Buys SS, et al. Effect of screening on ovarian cancer: the Prostate, Lung, Colorectal and Ovarian (PLCO) Cancer Screening Randomized Controlled Trial. JAMA 2011;305:2295−303.

[31] International Myeloma Working Group. Criteria for the classification of monoclonal gammopathies, multiple myeloma and related disorders: a report of the International Myeloma Working Group. Br J Haematol 2003;121:749.

[32] Soltero L, et al. Initial survival data of kidney transplant patients with pre-transplant monoclonal gammopathy. Clin Transplant 2011. epub Nov 2. PMID: 22044717.

[33] Naina HV, et al. Long-term follow-up of patients with monoclonal gammopathy of undetermined significance after kidney transplantation. Am J Nephrol 2012;35(4):365–71.

Index

Note: Page numbers with "*f*" denote figures; "*t*" tables; and "*b*" boxes.

Color Plates

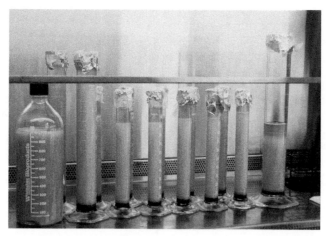

FIGURE 4.1 **Leukemia cells removed by leukapheresis.** The graduated cylinders contain leukemic cells removed by leukapheresis from a patient with T-cell acute lymphoblastic leukemia and hyperleukocytosis (white blood cell count 365,000 per cubic millimeter). Each cylinder contains straw-colored clear plasma at the top, a thick layer of white leukemic cells in the middle, and a thin layer of red cells at the bottom. *Reprinted from Howard et al. [92] with the permission of the publisher.*

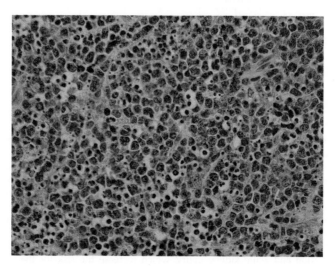

FIGURE 4.2 **Burkitt lymphoma of the appendix.** The highly cellular nature of Burkitt lymphoma is evident (hematoxylin and eosin). *Reprinted from Howard et al. [92] with the permission of the publisher.*

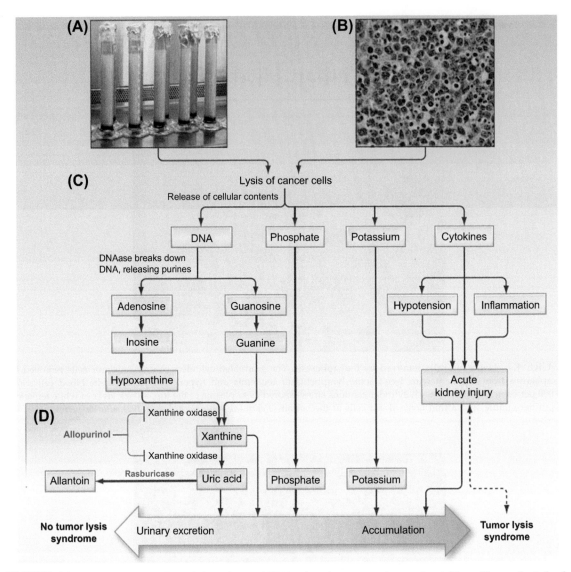

FIGURE 4.3 Lysis of tumor cells and the release of DNA, phosphate, potassium and cytokines. The graduated cylinders shown in Panel A contain leukemic cells removed by leukapheresis from a patient with T-cell acute lymphoblastic leukemia and hyperleukocytosis (white cell count, 365,000 per cubic millimeter). Each cylinder contains straw-colored clear plasma at the top, a thick layer of white leukemic cells in the middle and a thin layer of red cells at the bottom. The highly cellular nature of Burkitt lymphoma is evident in Panel B (Burkitt lymphoma of the appendix, hematoxylin and eosin). Lysis of cancer cells (Panel C) releases DNA, phosphate, potassium and cytokines. DNA released from the lysed cells is metabolized into adenosine and guanosine, both of which are converted into xanthine. Xanthine is then oxidized by xanthine oxidase, leading to the production of uric acid, which is excreted by the kidneys. When the accumulation of phosphate, potassium, xanthine, or uric acid is more rapid than excretion, the tumor lysis syndrome develops. Cytokines cause hypotension, inflammation and acute kidney injury, which increase the risk for the tumor lysis syndrome. The bidirectional dashed line between acute kidney injury and tumor lysis syndrome indicates that acute kidney injury increases the risk of the tumor lysis syndrome by reducing the ability of the kidneys to excrete uric acid, xanthine, phosphate and potassium. By the same token, development of the tumor lysis syndrome can cause acute kidney injury by renal precipitation of uric acid, xanthine and calcium phosphate crystals and by crystal independent mechanisms. Allopurinol inhibits xanthine oxidase (Panel D) and prevents the conversion of hypoxanthine and xanthine into uric acid but does not remove existing uric acid. In contrast, rasburicase removes uric acid by enzymatically degrading it into allantoin, a highly soluble product that has no known adverse effects on health. *Reprinted from Howard et al. [92] with the permission of the publisher.*

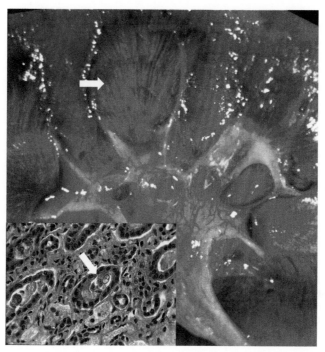

FIGURE 4.5   Renal findings in a child with fatal tumor lysis syndrome. The kidney shown was examined at the autopsy of a 4-year-old boy who had high-grade non-Hodgkin lymphoma and died of acute tumor lysis syndrome. Linear yellow streaks of precipitated uric acid in the renal medulla are shown (arrow); a single tubule containing a uric acid crystal (arrow) is shown in the panel. *Reprinted from Howard et al. [18] with the permission of the publisher.*

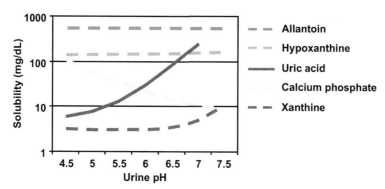

FIGURE 4.7   Solubility of metabolites important in tumor lysis syndrome over a range of physiologic urine pH values. Uric acid solubility is highly pH dependent. As urine pH rises from 5 to 7, the solubility increases 25-fold, from 8 to 200 mg/dL. This increased uric acid solubility and consequent decreased risk of crystal formation and acute kidney injury is the reason urine alkalinization was standard for patients at risk for tumor lysis syndrome prior to the advent of rasburicase. In contrast to uric acid, calcium phosphate becomes less soluble and more likely to crystallize as urine pH increases. Xanthine has low solubility and hypoxanthine relatively high solubility, regardless of urine pH. Note that the scale is logarithmic. *Reprinted from Howard et al. [18] with the permission of the publisher.*

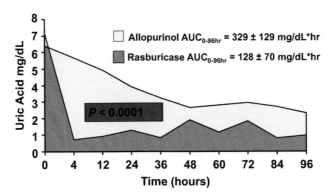

FIGURE 4.10 Uric acid levels during the first four days of treatment in patients at risk for tumor lysis syndrome randomized to receive rasburicase versus allopurinol. In patients at risk for tumor lysis syndrome, rasburicase was associated with a rapid decrease in uric acid and a corresponding lower area-under-the-concentration-time curve for uric acid, as measured over the first 4 days of therapy (128 ± 70 versus 329 ± 129 mg/dL*hr, $p < 0.0001$). *Adapted from Goldman et al. [66].*

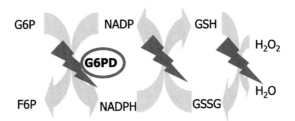

FIGURE 4.11 Role of glucose-6-phosphate dehydrogenase deficiency during oxidative stress. Reduced glutathione (GSH) is necessary to reduce hydrogen peroxide (H_2O_2) to water and remove the oxidative stress, forming oxidized glutathione (GSSG) in the process. However, for each molecule of hydrogen peroxide reduced, one molecule of GSH is needed. Oxidized glutathione is reduced by NADPH, which is oxidized to NADP, and requires glucose-6-phosphate dehydrogenase to reduce it back to its active form. Deficiency of G6PD inhibits reduction of NADP to NADPH, thereby inhibiting the reduction of GSSG back to GSH, and thus leaving hydrogen peroxide and other oxygen radicals free to damage red blood cell membranes and hemoglobin. G6P, glucose-6-phosphate; F6P, fructose-6-phosphate; G6PD, glucose-6-phosphate dehydrogenase; NADP, nicotinamide adenine dinucleotide phosphate; NADPH, reduced NADP; GSH, reduced glutathione; GSSG, oxidized glutathione; H_2O_2, hydrogen peroxide.

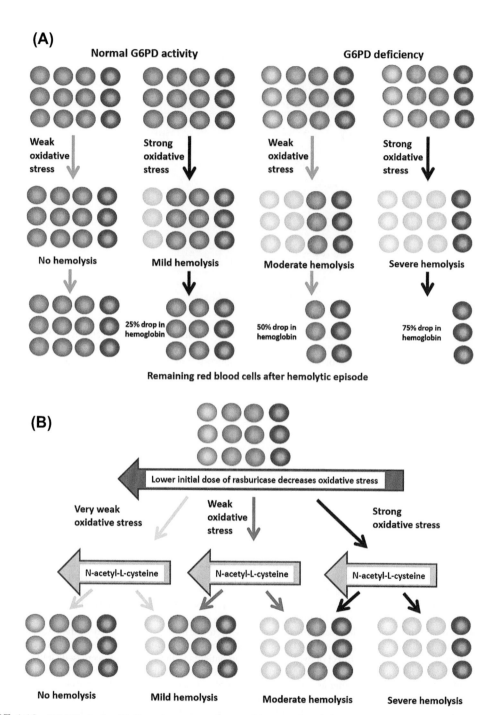

FIGURE 4.12 (A) Effect of oxidative stress on patients with normal and decreased glucose-6-phosphate dehydroge-nase activity. (B) Potential mitigating strategies for patients with glucose-6-phosphate dehydrogenase activity who require rasburicase. Red blood cells circulate for 120 days, but gradually lose their glucose-6-phosphate dehydrogenase

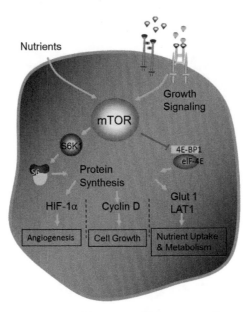

FIGURE 8.2   mTOR activation supports cancer cell growth. mTOR = mammalian target of rapamycin; S6K1 = ribosomal protein S6 kinase beta-1; 4E-BP1 = eukaryotic translation initiation factor 4E-binding protein 1; elF-4E = eukaryotic initiation factor 4E; HIF-1α = hypoxia-inducible factor 1 alpha; Glut 1 = glucose transporter 1; LAT1 = large neutral amino acid transporter.

(G6PD) activity. In this figure, cells with the highest G6PD activity are shown in red and those with decreased activity in green. At any given age, circulating red blood cells have less G6PD activity in people with mutations in this enzyme, but the youngest cells of a G6PD deficient person may have more activity than the oldest cells of a normal person. In patients with tumor lysis syndrome, the higher the uric acid, the more hydrogen peroxide produced and the greater the oxidative stress when rasburicase is administered. A decrease of uric acid from 9.0 to 2.2 mg/dL, as occurred in the patient reported by Elinoff et al. [50], is associated with a production of 2 mmol of hydrogen peroxide, a quantity sufficient to hemolyze two-thirds of the patient's erythrocytes. (A) Effect of oxidative stress on patients with normal and decreased G6PD activity. Note that red blood cells that remain after a hemolytic episode are those that contain the highest G6PD activity; thus, measurement of G6PD activity immediately after an episode is not advisable, since it would yield falsely elevated activity levels. (B) Potential mitigating strategies for patients with G6PD deficiency who require rasburicase. Use of an initial small "test dose" of rasburicase (e.g. 1.5 mg) results in a smaller oxidative stress and potentially less hemolysis than use of the regular dose. N-acetyl-L-cysteine may partially protect red blood cells from oxidative damage and decrease the amount of hemolysis at any given degree of oxidative stress. *Reprinted from Howard et al. [101] with the permission of the publisher.*

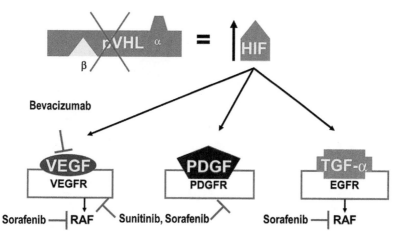

FIGURE 8.3 Targets of therapeutic agents − IFN alpha? pVHL = Von Hippel−Lindau tumor suppressor; HIF = hypoxia-inducible factors; VEGF = vascular endothelial growth factor; VEGFR = vascular endothelial growth factor receptor; PDGF = platelet-derived growth factor; PDGFR = platelet-derived growth factor receptor; TGF-α = transforming growth factor alpha; EGFR = epidermal growth factor receptor; RAF = a serine/threonine-specific protein kinase.

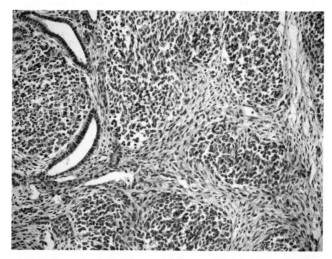

FIGURE 9.3 Triphasic favorable histology Wilms tumor consisting of blastemal, epithelial and stromal components.

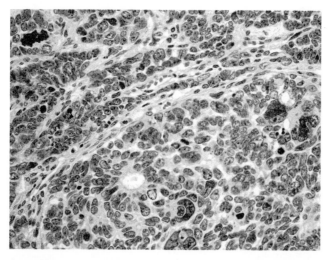

FIGURE 9.4 Anaplastic Wilms tumor with large nuclei, hyperchromasia and multipolar mitotic figures.

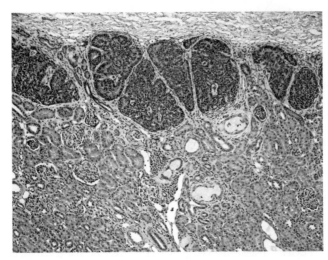

FIGURE 9.5   Perilobar nephrogenic rests in patient with Beckwidth–Weideman syndrome. Undifferentiated cells make up the small multiple nephrogenic rests just beneath renal capsule with sharp demarcation from cortex.

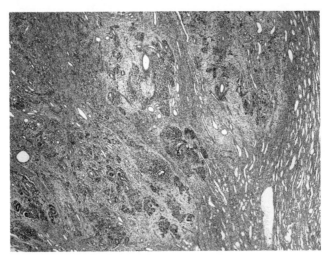

FIGURE 9.6   Intralobar nephrogenic rests with irregular margins with nephrons intermingled within the rest with prominent stroma.

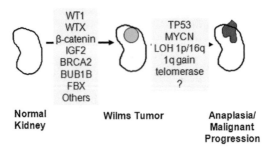

FIGURE 9.8   Model of Wilms tumor development.

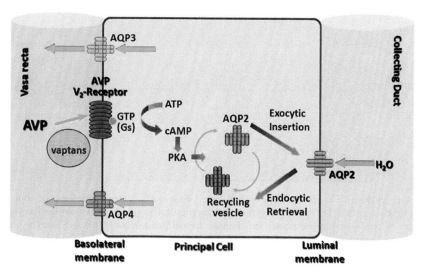

FIGURE 11.1 **The principal cell of the kidney collecting duct.** The V2 vasopressin receptor (V2-receptor) located in the basolateral cell surface binds to AVP present in the interstitial fluid, and activates the heterotrimeric protein G. Activated protein G increases the activity of the membrane-bound enzyme adenylyl cyclase (AC) causing an increase in the intracellular levels of cAMP. This in turn stimulates the activity of the cAMP-dependent protein kinase A (PKA), triggering a phosphorylation cascade that promotes the insertion of aquaporin 2 (AQP2) into the apical membrane of the cell. AVP-regulated AQP2 increases the water permeability of the apical membrane and allows the reabsorption of water from the hypotonic processed filtrate into the surrounding hypertonic interstitium. The water can exit the cell through the aquaporin 3 and aquaporin 4 water channels, constitutively present in the basolateral surface of the cells. Vaptans are synthetic vasopressin receptor antagonists. By interfering with AVP–V2R interaction they prevent aquaporin-mediated water reabsorption. *Modified from Mayinger and Hensen [9].*

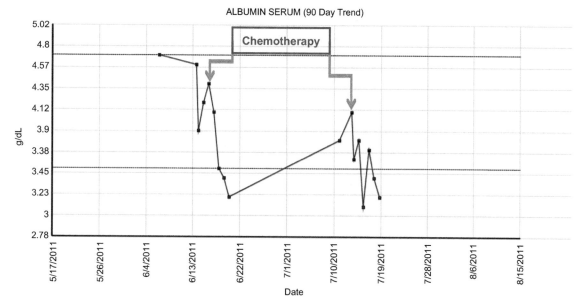

FIGURE 11.2 **Acute depressive effect of chemotherapy on serum albumin levels.**

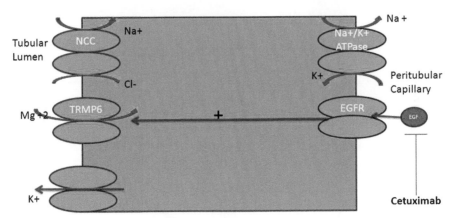

FIGURE 11.3 **EGFR pathway.** The epidermal growth factor (EGF) was discovered as the first hormone to regulate active magnesium reabsorption through TRPM6. Reabsorption of magnesium is primarily driven by the luminal membrane potential established by the voltage-gated potassium channel. Cetuximab targets EGFR and leads to decreased TRMP6-mediated magnesium reabsorption.

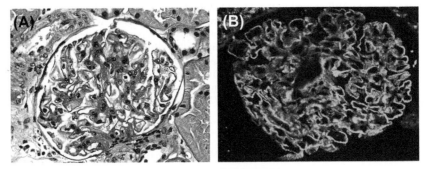

FIGURE 14.1 **Paraneoplastic membranous glomerulonephritis.** (A) A 69-year-old woman with breast cancer developed nephrotic syndrome. The glomerulus shows global, moderate thickening of the capillary walls. PAS ×400. (B) Immunofluorescence demonstrates global, granular, polyclonal IgG and C3 along the capillary walls. FITC IgG ×400.

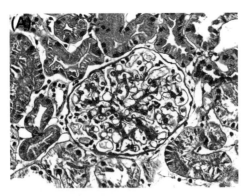

FIGURE 14.2 **Paraneoplastic minimal change disease.** (A) A 63-year-old man with renal cell carcinoma. Glomerulus showing preserved capillary architecture without significant changes. PAS ×600.

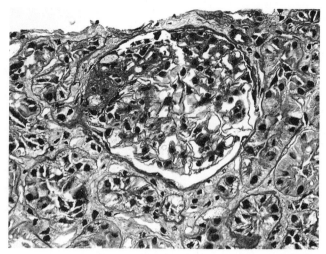

FIGURE 14.3 **Paraneoplastic focal segmental glomerulosclerosis.** A 40-year-old man presented with nephrotic syndrome and subsequently diagnosed with thymoma. The figure shows a normal appearing glomerulus showing segmental collapse and sclerosis containing a trapped foam cell at the periphery with adhesion to the Bowman capsule.

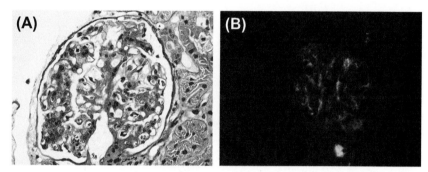

FIGURE 14.4 **Paraneoplastic IgA nephropathy.** A 72-year-old man presented with hematuria and flank pain, diagnosed with renal cell carcinoma, followed by total nephrectomy. The non-neoplastic portion of kidney examined. (A) Glomerulus shows global, mild mesangial hypercellularity and increased matrix. PAS ×400. (B) Immunofluorescence microscopy localized IgA deposits, mainly in the mesangial areas. FITC IgA ×300.

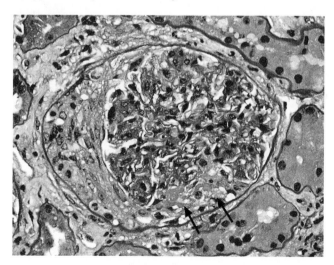

FIGURE 14.5 **Paraneoplastic crescentic glomerulonephritis.** A 59-year-old woman diagnosed with squamous cell carcinoma of the lung has hematuria, mild proteinuria and renal insufficiency. Serology for ANCA was negative. The figure shows the glomerulus showing a cellular crescent in the Bowman space partly compressing the underlying glomerulus. An area of fibrinoid material due to necrosis is visible (arrows). PAS ×400.

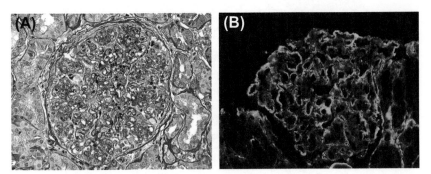

FIGURE 14.6 Paraneoplastic membranoproliferative glomerulonephritis. An elderly man with hematuria and nephrotic syndrome recently treated for lung cancer. (A) Glomerulus is enlarged and hypercellular with a lobulated configuration, infiltrated by mononuclear cells and cell proliferation as well as peripheral capillary wall thickening with double contours. PAS ×400. (B) Immunofluorescence microscopy reveals segmental, granular, capillary wall and mesangial deposits of polyclonal IgG, C3 and lesser IgM with an irregular distribution. FITC IgG ×400.

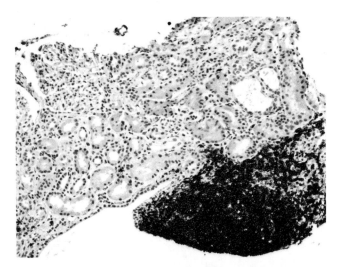

FIGURE 14.8 Paraneoplastic minimal change disease and infiltrating small B-cell lymphoma in the kidney. The figure shows a large lymphoid aggregate in the renal cortex, with positive CD20 and lambda light chain. Adjacent glomeruli appear normal. Immunoperoxidase CD20 ×200.

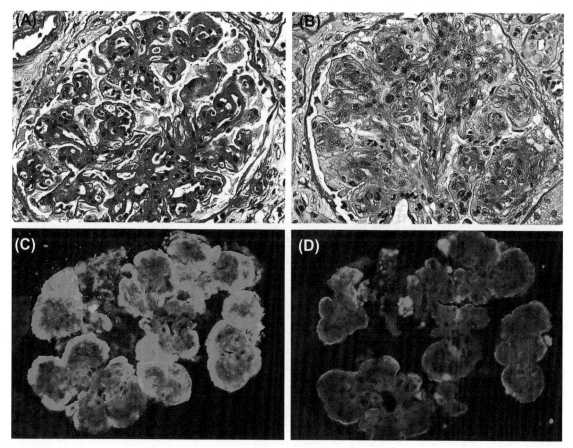

FIGURE 14.9 Paraneoplastic membranoproliferative glomerulonephritis and chronic B-cell lymphocytic leukemia (CLL). (A) Glomerulus showing enlargement, increased mesangial cellularity and global thickening of the peripheral capillary walls with frequent double contours and focal cellular interposition. (B) Glomerulus from another case of CLL demonstrates hypercellularity and nodular mesangial sclerosing changes leading to narrowing of the capillary lumina with thickening of the capillary walls. PAS ×400. (C) Immunofluorescence microscopy shows mainly monoclonal IgG and kappa light chain deposits along the capillary walls and focally in the mesangial areas. FITC kappa LC ×400. (D) Immunofluorescence microscopy using FITC lambda light chain is mostly negative in a similar distribution. ×400.

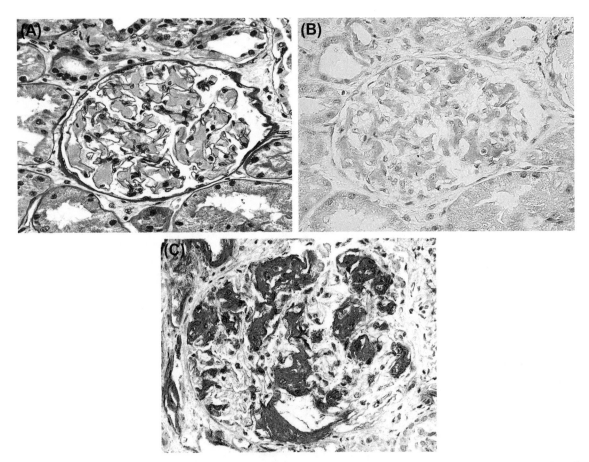

FIGURE 14.11 **Paraneoplastic amyloidosis.** An 18-year-old girl presented with lymphadenopathy in the neck and axilla of 2 years' duration diagnosed as Hodgkin disease and now has nephrotic syndrome. See Chapter 14 for details. (A) Glomerular infiltration of pale staining amorphous material, replacing mainly the mesangial areas, without significant proliferative change. PAS ×400. (B) Special staining for amyloid (Congo red) is strongly positive in the mesangial areas with amorphous deposits. ×400. (C) Amyloid A protein is localized in the glomerulus and small arterial vessels with amyloid deposits. Immunoperoxidase stain ×400.

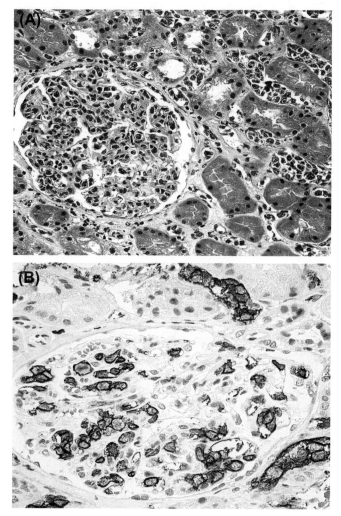

FIGURE 14.12 **Angiotropic B-cell lymphoma/leukemia in the kidney with acute renal failure.** (A) Glomerular and peritubular capillaries occluded and distended by malignant lymphoid cells. PAS ×400. (B) Malignant lymphoid cells are positive for monoclonal B-cell markers including CD20 (seen here). × Immunoperoxidase stain ×400.

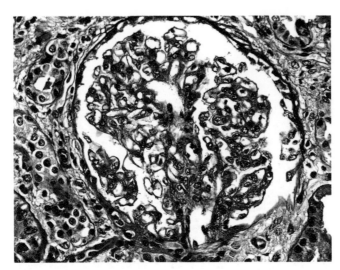

FIGURE 14.13 Myeloproliferative disorder and mesangial disease presenting as nephrotic range proteinuria. Glomerulus showing mild mesangial hypercellularity, without immune deposits, but significant epithelial injury by electron microscopy. PAS ×400.

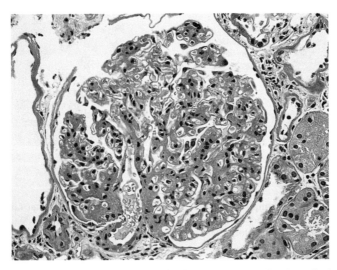

FIGURE 14.14 Myeloproliferative disorder and glomerular disease with proteinuria and microhematuria. Glomerulus showing diffuse mesangial sclerosis, focal compromise in capillary lumina and peripheral capillary wall thickening with focal double contours (without immune deposits), suggestive of chronic endothelial injury or thrombotic microangiopathy. PAS ×400.

Printed and bound by CPI Group (UK) Ltd, Croydon, CR0 4YY

08/05/2025

01864987-0001